To My Beloved Brother,
Teague
Who's health
is veddy veddy
important
t'me

XOX
Jay

Dr. Timothy Johnson's

OnCall Guide to Men's Health

Dr. Timothy Johnson's OnCall Guide to Men's Health

Dr. Timothy Johnson

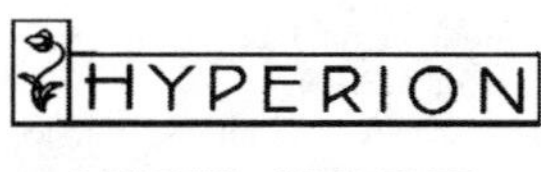

NEW YORK

This book is not intended to substitute for an individual's medical treatment. It is not the equivalent of, nor is it intended as a replacement for, any professionally supervised medical treatment. All matters regarding your health require medical supervision. The author and the publisher disclaim any liability arising directly or indirectly from the use of this book.

A ROUNDTABLE PRESS BOOK

For Roundtable Press, Inc.
Directors: Julie Merberg and Marsha Melnick
Writing and Research: Ginny Graves
Additional Writing and Research: Curt Pesmen
Design: Charles Kreloff
Illustrations: Judy Francis
Production Editors: John Glenn and Sara Newberry
Fitness Consultant: Karen Andes
Psychological Consultant: Barbara Freedgood-Lopato

ISBN: 0-7868-8669-2
Hyperion books are available for special promotions and premiums. For details contact Hyperion Special Markets, 77 West 66th Street, 11th floor, New York, New York. 10023, or call 212-456-0100

FIRST EDITION
10 9 8 7 6 5 4 3 2 1

CREDITS: Glycemic Index and Glycemic Load Values for Major Carbohydrate Sources (Relative to White Bread) on page 7 reprinted with the permission of Simon & Schuster from *Eat, Drink, and be Healthy* by Walter C. Willett, M.D., Dr. P.H. Copyright (c) 2002 by the President and Fellows of Harvard College
Glycemic index taken from:
Jenkins, D.J.A., et al. "Glycemic Index of Foods: A Physiological Basis for Carbohydrate Exchange." American Journal of Clinical Nutrition, 34 (1981): 363–66.
Wolever, T.M.S. "Glycaemic Index of 102 Complex Carbohydrate Foods in Patients with Diabetes." Nutrition Research, 14 (1994): 651–69.
Jenkins, D.J.A. Provisional data. (October 1995).
Brand Miller, J., et al. "The Glycemic Index of Foods Containing Sugars: Comparison of Foods with Naturally Occurring Vs. Added Sugars." British Journal of Nutrition, 73 (1995): 613–23.
Jenkins, D.J.A., et al. "The Glycaemic Response to Carbohydrate Foods." Lancet (1984): 388–91.
Brand Miller, J., et al. "Rice: A High or Low Glycemic Food?" American Journal of Clinical Nutrition, 56 (1992): 1034–36.
Brand Miller, J., et al. "In Search of More Low Glycemic Index Foods." Proceeding of the Nutritional Society of Australia, 19 (1995): 177.

For Nancy, Nana, Nolden, Beth, Cooper, Kiplee,
—and Mozart, Spot and Fraidy

I have been encouraged and helped by many friends in the process of writing this book. However, I would like to thank three people in particular. Bob Miller, the Publisher at Hyperion, was the first to enthusiastically suggest how helpful my particular way of discussing health information might be to men like himself - too busy to read something encyclopedic but wanting to know the bottom line. Peternelle van Arsdale, Executive Editor at Hyperion, has been a cheerful interface between the world of health information, about which I know a lot, and the world of publishing, about which I know almost nothing. And finally, a very special word of thanks to Julie Merberg of Roundtable Press, who has made all the distracting details of this effort seem like effortless pleasure. She has always been joyful, on the phone, via e-mail, and especially in person.

Contents

Part Two: Common Health Problems

Part Three: Minding The Mind

Part Four: Fit For Life

Preface

Right up front I want to let you know what this book is—and is not. As the title emphasizes, this book is a *guide* to men's health, meaning it is not an encyclopedia that says at least a little something about every possible health problem a man might face. Quite frankly, there are several such encyclopedias already available, and the internet is basically a constantly changing encyclopedia of health information—some of it very good, some of it very bad, a lot of stuff in between. But as most of you know, such sources can often be overwhelming and/or confusing—that is, too much or too little information on a subject without any sorting out of what is really important or any advice about what to really pay attention to. This book attempts to be different in several ways, all of them designed to fulfill the mission to be a true guide.

First, I have carefully selected what I think are the relatively few essential topics I believe every man should know at least something about—and I have left out everything else. (I literally spent more time deciding what to leave out than what to include.) And one of the prime factors in selecting certain topics for extra emphasis, like nutrition and exercise, was that they involved information that men could put into practice in their lives without outside help or assistance. Furthermore, the topics that are included are not treated with the depth of a true reference source that one might turn to for extensive and exhaustive information on a given topic. Therefore, I would hope this is a book that any man would read through in its entirety—not all at once, of course—because it will give him at least a basic knowledge base for making good health choices about the most common problems we men should think about.

Second, within each topic I have emphasized prevention (when there is solid information) and screening or early diagnosis. That's why, for example, I spend a lot of time on colon and prostate cancer—where there are important tests all men should know about—and no time on pancreatic cancer, for which there are no effective screening tests available. Screening means looking for disease before there are any warning symptoms to call it to your attention; early diagnosis means paying attention to such symptoms as early as possible. In most cases, finding a disease early means a much better chance of successful treatment or cure. So I really emphasize these areas whenever possible. That also means I usually spend less time on treatment details which are likely to change rapidly as new information becomes available—and which, quite frankly, are going to be more in the joint hands of you and your doctor as you discuss treatment options. But you are the one ultimately most responsible for preventing illness and maintaining your good health by arranging for appropriate screening tests and being alert to warning symptoms—so those are the areas I emphasize.

Finally, why a special guide for men? Well, as most of you know, we men are often not very good about taking care of ourselves when we are well, or seeking medical attention when we are sick. Study after study has shown that men are more reluctant to face up to worrisome symptoms or go to the doctor for checkups. And that is probably one big reason why men's life expectancy, which in the early 1900s was virtually the same for both sexes, now lags behind women's. So I am speaking specifically to men about problems that can make a big difference in our lives and trying to do so in a way that is not frightening or alarmist but honest and direct.

The outline for the book is fairly logical—starting with basic information about nutrition and exercise that all men should know about—and then moving to more detailed information about the most common health problems that we should all worry about. The next part focuses on the many physical and emotional problems that center around our sexual and reproductive systems. And the final part looks at some important issues of mental and social health, especially from a man's point of view when appropriate.

This book came about because many of the people I work with at ABC News have urged me to put into print form what I so often do in private conversation—which is to give advice about good health practices and choices. As you might expect, I get a lot of letters and calls and requests for hallway consultations about health matters. And I always try to give honest answers, the same answer I would give to family and friends when they call for advice. So you will find throughout the book that I often get to a bottom line and tell you my opinion because I think that is what you expect from me as a guide. I also do not hesitate to tell you about my own personal health choices when appropriate. Indeed, I regard this effort as an opportunity to put down on paper the most important health information I have accumulated during my now 30 years as a medical journalist.

I had a lot of help in putting this book together. However, I must take full responsibility for the content of this book. As a guide, it should get you on the right track. But ultimately you must take primary responsibility, along with your health care advisors, for making the best decisions for yourself. Good luck.

PART ONE:

Taking Care of Yourself

There is one sense in which beginning this book with discussions of nutrition and exercise is an obvious choice: No other activities aside from sleep and work consume so much of our attention and time. Most of us spend a lot of time and energy thinking about and preparing for our traditional "three meals a day," not to mention all the snacks in between. But what about exercise, you might ask—given that for many of us, we are doing well if we spend even a half hour a few times a week in formal exercise? I would argue that when you think of exercise in a less formal way, most of us engage in a lot of activity each day—including walking about our office and to and from our transportation, climbing at least a few stairs, hopefully playing some games or engaging in some sports at least on weekends. And given the latest data which suggests that all activity—not just formal exercise—can be important to our health, I believe this topic is also worth talking about right up front.

Secondly, nutrition and fitness are two areas over which we have significant control. Whereas many other aspects of our health are a function of genetics or random luck, we can make choices about the food we put into our bodies, and the way we work, build, and maintain them. In order to make informed decisions that will have a tremendous impact on our overall health, it's crucial that we're well-informed about diet and exercise.

There is one other reason why I have chosen to discuss nutrition and exercise in the first two chapters: There have been some fairly dramatic changes in our thinking about both subjects in the last several years. Therefore, you might find it both surprising and interesting to learn about some of the new information on these subjects at the very beginning of this journey through the world of health information pertinent to our daily lives.

CHAPTER 1

Nutrition: A Very Basic Primer

I am beginning this book with a topic that part of me would like to avoid altogether, because it is so complicated and even controversial. So I have decided that I will face it right up front, to also acknowledge that it is one of the most important and basic aspects of our lives.

For most of us men, one important question could be put this way: *Shall I eat thoughtfully or shall I eat impulsively, according to my desire and instinct of the moment?* I will be the first to admit that the latter pathway is the easiest. Unfortunately, it is not the healthiest.

So the question now becomes: *How can I eat in a way that is reasonably healthy and pleasurable as well?* I have come to believe that it is important to consider both—our health and our pleasure—when we eat. If we think only about our health, eating will become a burden.

But even if you do your research and follow the "rules," you've probably noticed that the conventional wisdom on healthy eating shifts from month to month, from study to study. For years, we've heard that ample fiber was a dietary must, but today we're hearing that it's not all that important. Red wine, eggs, and oat bran have been in and out of fashion. Much of the reason behind inconsistencies in study results lies in differences in their methodologies. Studies that are the most reliable—randomized, controlled, "double-blind" studies—are the most difficult and expensive studies to perform. It's not easy to recruit enough people to participate in such rigid studies long enough to produce meaningful statistical results.

Other types of investigations—particularly those in which researchers must discern subtle differences between subjects' eating habits, or studies which rely on people to remember what they ate weeks, months, or years earlier—can easily yield contradictory results. The resulting flood of inconsistent nutritional messages does not make it any easier for you to make healthy choices. So I'm going to try to help you do that by:

- First, looking at the three basic sources of calories in our diets: proteins, fats, and carbohydrates.
- Then, looking at some of the controversial nutrition topics like fiber, alcohol, vitamins, and supplements.
- And finally, looking at the issues surrounding ideal weight and how to best lose excess weight.

My hope is that by the end of this section, you will have a clearer idea of how to eat in a manner that is both healthy and pleasurable.

We are going to begin by looking at the three major sources of calories in our diet—carbohydrates, fats, and proteins. You will probably be surprised to learn how much nutritional experts have changed their thinking about these foods in recent years—particularly carbs and fats—and you may be shocked to find out how often the traditional food pyramid is out-of-date.

The Modern Story on Carbohydrates

Even though fats get most of our attention because of their highly publicized relationship to heart disease, the simple fact is that carbohydrates provide 50 to 60 percent of the calories in most American diets. And increasingly, nutritionists have come to appreciate that bad carbohydrates may play just as negative a role in our lives as bad fats do. So what makes a good or bad carbohydrate? The usual answer is that simple carbohydrates are bad and complex carbohydrates are good. Unfortunately, as we have learned in recent years, the answer is not that simple; in fact, it is downright complex!

First, some definitions. Simple carbohydrates refer to sugars like glucose (the form of sugar found in our blood), sucrose (table sugar), fructose (found in fruits and vegetables), and lactose (milk sugar). Complex carbohydrates are basically long chains of simple sugars linked together. (The main complex carbohydrate in our food is starch, which is a long chain of glucose sugars.) When we consume complex carbohydrates, they are digested into simple sugars, which are then absorbed from our intestine into our bloodstream. And that's where the story gets interesting—and much more complicated.

Glucose, the sugar in our bloodstream, is an important fuel for many of our body's tissues, especially our brain cells. Therefore, the levels of glucose in our blood are carefully maintained within a fairly narrow range. One very important substance in keeping our blood sugar levels under control is insulin, a hormone made by special cells in the pancreas. When our blood sugar levels get too high, the pancreas releases more insulin to move the excess glucose into storage, especially in liver and muscle cells. Conversely, when blood sugar levels fall too low, insulin production quickly drops, and the liver starts to release some of its stored glucose. *(See page 196 for information on diabetes and insulin resistance.)*

I take the time to very briefly describe this blood sugar–insulin control system at this point because many nutritionists now believe that carbohydrate foods that are quickly digested and therefore lead to sudden spikes in blood glucose levels—and consequent sudden spikes in insulin levels—might contribute to a vicious cycle of increased hunger and food intake. The idea is that when our blood sugar goes up quickly, insulin levels also go up quickly; this quick rise in insulin leads to a quick drop in blood sugar levels, which then leads to a sense of hunger and a desire for more food. In contrast, carbohydrates that are more slowly digested will cause less of a glucose-insulin "up and down" roller coaster effect and that might result in less hunger and less food intake. And for people who are already overweight, eating quickly digested carbohydrates may be especially dangerous. For example, in the famous Nurses' Health Study, overweight women with a diet high in easily digested carbohydrates were at much higher risk of having a heart attack.

By now you get the main idea: Nutritionists think that it is better to keep blood sugar levels more steady and stable, and that means trying to eat carbohydrates that are more slowly digested into the simple sugars that get into our blood. And until recently, the rule was that simpler carbohydrates in our diet were more likely to be quickly digested than more complex carbohydrates.

The glycemic index and load

Actually, that "rule" is still often true. But when nutritional scientists started testing various carbohydrates in real human beings to see how quickly they were digested into simple sugars, they were surprised at how often the "rule" was not followed. For example, they found that the carbohydrate in ice cream was not converted into blood sugars as quickly as you would expect, and that cornflakes were converted much more quickly than expected. To be fair, many carbohydrates did behave as expected, but there were enough surprises to warrant a new way of "judging" carbohydrates other than the quick labels "simple" or "complex."

That new way is known as the glycemic index. Using white bread as the standard for fast digestion into sugars—and giving it an arbitrary value of 100—equal amounts (50 grams) of various other carbohydrates were compared to white bread in terms of how much your blood sugar rises in the first two hours after consumption. They were then assigned corresponding numbers above or below 100. The higher the glycemic index number, the faster that food is digested into blood sugar. If you look at the chart opposite showing various foods, you can see that an apple is predictably pretty "slow" (with a glycemic index of 55) whereas mashed potatoes are very "fast" (with an index of 104). (Even jam is converted to blood sugar more slowly than mashed potatoes are.)

However, the glycemic index is not enough to tell you the full story. What you really want to know is how much actual blood sugar you will get from a typical portion of that food—the so-called glycemic load. That number is the glycemic index (digestion speed) times the actual grams of carbohydrate in a typical serving. The difference between the index and the load is well illustrated by carrots. Even though carrots have a high index (meaning they are digested quickly), a usual portion of carrots contains a relatively small amount of carbohydrate—so the actual load from that portion is quite small. (That's why it is so unfair to knock carrots, as some of the popular low-carb diets now do.)

Whole versus refined grains

The bottom line—so far—is that when you are comparing two carbohydrate-rich foods in terms of their impact on your blood sugar and insulin system, it is good to know about their glycemic index and load. However, there are some other considerations in choosing carbohydrates—especially their nutrient and fiber content. For example, fruits and vegetables often have high glycemic index values, but they have other strengths, including many vitamins, minerals, and fiber *(see page 8 for more on fiber)*. When it comes to grains, in particular, these other nutrients become important.

Glycemic Index and Glycemic Load Values for Major Carbohydrate Sources

(relative to white bread)

Foods	Serving Size	Glycemic Index (%)	Carbohydrate (grams)	Glycemic Load*
Potatoes, mashed	1 cup	104	37	38
Bread, white	1 slice	100	12	12
Bread, dark	1 slice	102	12	12
Orange juice	6 ounces	75	20	15
Banana	1 medium	88	27	23
Rice, white	1 cup	102	45	45
Pizza	2 slices	86	78	67
Pasta	1 cup	71	40	28
English muffin	1 muffin	86	26	23
Fruit punch	12 ounces	95	44	42
Coke	12 ounces	90	39	35
Apple	1 medium	55	21	12
Milk, skim	1 cup	46	12	54
Pancake	2 six-inch	119	56	66
Sugar, table	1 tsp.	84	4	34
Jam	1 tbsp.	91	14	13
Cranberry juice	1/2 cup	105	18	19
Potatoes, French-fried	4 ounces	95	35	33
Candy	1 ounce	99	27	27
Ice cream	1/2 cup	42	16	7
Carrots, cooked	1/2 cup	131	8	11
Carrots, raw	1/2 cup	131	4	5
Baked beans	1 cup	60	27	16
Breakfast Cereals				
Shredded Wheat	2 biscuits	95	38	36
Raisin Bran	1 cup	88	47	41
Cornflakes	1 cup	114	24	27
Grape-Nuts	1/2 cup	96	23	22
Cheerios	1 cup	106	22	17
All-Bran	1/2 cup	72	24	17
Total	1 cup	109	32	35
Wheaties	1 cup	109	24	26
Bran Flakes	1 cup	74	31	23
Special K	1 cup	74	20	15
Oatmeal	1 cup	82	25	21

*Glycemic load calculated by multiplying grams of carbohydrate by glycemic index of bread (100% = 1.0)

By now you have undoubtedly heard about the importance of distinguishing between "whole" (or intact) and so-called "refined" grains. The word "refined" is quite misleading in this case. It refers to the process of milling whole grain seeds to remove impurities but also to reduce them to a fine flour. Such flour may be easier for baking, cooking, and storing but is much less valuable from a nutritional point of view. Therefore, "reduced" might be a more accurate word than "refined," at least when it comes to nutritional value. During the various stages of the typical milling process, all kinds of valuable vitamins and minerals are lost. No wonder more recent nutritional research has emphasized the value of intact or whole grain foods and products in terms of:

- Reducing the risk for developing Type 2 diabetes.
- Reducing the risk for heart disease.
- Reducing the risk for constipation and diverticulitis, two common intestinal problems.

So the bottom line is not only choosing carbohydrates with lower glycemic numbers but also selecting whole grains whenever possible. For example, whole grain cereals are far preferable for breakfast than the many sugary cereals. Brown rice is whole—white rice is not. Whole grain breads are best for sandwiches. And learning to cook with whole wheat flour is a big plus. Think whole and healthy. They go together.

Another major source of "healthy carbohydrates" is the category of foods known as "fruits and vegetables." There are two major reasons to regard these foods as healthy: They contain all kinds of vitamins and minerals in amounts and combinations that we can't possibly reproduce with pills; and they contain large amounts of the stuff we typically refer to as "fiber."

Fiber, Your Friend

Dietary fiber comes from plant-based foods (fruits, vegetables, and whole grains) and is not actually digestible. *Insoluble* fiber bulks up stools to promote easier passage of solid waste products, and *soluble* fiber slows down absorption of food. High-fiber diets include regular servings of bran, oats, beans, whole wheat bread, fruits, and vegetables.

Insoluble fiber

Composed of cellulose and hemicellulose, insoluble fiber is found mostly in the bran portion of grains, wheat bran being one of the best sources. Insoluble fiber can help prevent digestive problems, from constipation to diverticulitis. If you strive to get the recommended 25 to 30 grams of dietary fiber into your meals and snacks each day, you will get enough insoluble fiber in the process.

Soluble fiber

Pectin, mucilage, gum (not the kind you chew), and other types of soluble fiber are most abundant in fruits, vegetables, and grains. The soluble fiber of oat bran, in particular, has earned praise from health experts for helping slow digestion so you feel full longer, making you less likely to overeat.

Surprisingly Good Fiber Sources

The following foods are relatively high in fiber (7 grams or more); some may surprise you.

FOOD SOURCE	SERVING SIZE	FIBER (grams)
Prunes, dried, stewed	1 cup	16.37
Split peas, boiled	1 cup	16.27
Lentils, boiled	1/2 cup	15.64
Beans, black, boiled	1/2 cup	14.96
Wheat flour, whole grain	1 cup	14.64
Dates, natural, dried	1 cup	13.35
Lima beans, boiled	1 cup	13.16
Avocado	1 medium	12.00
Buckwheat flour, whole groat	1 cup	12.00
Black-eyed peas, boiled	1 cup	11.18
Chickpeas, canned	1 cup	10.56
Cornmeal, enriched, yellow	1 cup	10.21
Pears, Asian, raw	1 pear	9.90
Raspberries	1 cup	8.00
Blackberries	1 cup	7.60

Fiber takes up space in the stomach. It will fill you up during meals but does not translate into calories as it passes through the system. An easy way to add fiber is to eat the skins of fruits and vegetables whenever possible. (Just remember to wash them first, because the skins can harbor illness-causing bacteria.) When you increase the fiber in your diet, you should also increase your daily consumption of water—another way to prevent constipation.

Some highly publicized recent studies have questioned previous claims by researchers that dietary fiber can prevent colon and other cancers. Two major studies published in The New England Journal of Medicine found no evidence that diets rich in high-fiber foods, including fruits and vegetables, lower the risk of colon cancer or the recurrence of polyps (which can turn into cancer). Nonetheless, most experts, including the researchers who performed the two studies, still contend that there is a strong link between fiber-rich foods and reducing the risk for heart disease and diabetes. Research also has shown that fiber helps move food through your colon more rapidly, washing away potentially toxic substances. A high-fiber diet is believed to help prevent diverticulitis, a gastrointestinal disorder. It may also reduce cholesterol levels, lower blood glucose levels in people with diabetes, and help with weight loss because fiber gives you a feeling of fullness.

Both the National Cancer Institute and the American Dietetic Association recommend 20 to 35 grams of fiber each day. Most Americans get half that or less. However, if you don't consume much dietary fiber, don't jump to 30 grams too quickly. Your digestive tract might rebel, causing gas and cramping. Instead, add about five grams of dietary fiber each week, until you reach the appropriate level.

Here are some easy ways to increase your dietary fiber:

Consume *at least* five servings of fruits and vegetables a day. Researchers say 8 to 10 servings are optimal, but don't be frightened off by these numbers. An apple or orange counts as 1 serving. Cooked or raw vegetables in an amount the size of a baseball represents 2 servings. A cup of greens is 1 serving, so a large salad with veggies could easily get you 3 to 4 servings in a single meal. For a head start, make it a point to have a piece of fruit with breakfast.

Add fiber to meals and even snacks. Switch to whole grain breads. Always ask for extra lettuce and tomatoes on your sandwich (rather than double meat). Strange as it might sound, dessert is an opportunity for more fiber. Add fruit or granola to your frozen yogurt or low-fat ice cream. Ask for fresh berries with your biscotti at Italian restaurants. Take this challenge: See if you can add something nutritious to every meal, including your snacks and dessert. You'll be amazed at how much your diet will improve!

Bacteria Alert

In today's world, no discussion of food and health is complete without a mention of the growing problem of food-borne illnesses. Last year 75 million Americans became sick from bacteria in food, with illnesses ranging from upset stomachs and diarrhea to fatal infections. More than 300,000 of them were hospitalized, and more than 5,000 died.

You'd like to think that scientists are right on top of this, identifying the bacteria responsible and devising antibiotics to treat them. Think again. Basically, the bacteria are evolving faster than our antibiotics can keep up with them. You'll find them in just about any food: listeria in cheese and meat; salmonella in raw eggs, meat, and unpasteurized juice and milk; E. coli in beef, milk, and salad bar items; cyclospora on imported berries; Norwalk-like viruses in oysters.

The single most common source of infection these days seems to be grocery store produce, over half of which comes from foreign countries. A lot of that produce was grown in Mexico and South America, and it arrives carrying exotic strains of E. coli and other bacteria people here are not accustomed to. Obviously, thorough washing of foods makes a lot of sense.

High-protein diets have led to more meat consumption. Steaks generally aren't a problem because the bacteria reside on the outside, and even meat that is still pink on the inside is safe if the outside is well browned. But ground beef is another story. The bacteria in ground beef is mixed throughout, so unless the meat is thoroughly cooked all the way through, the bacteria can still survive. Poultry consumption is up, and chicken is almost always cooked well enough, but people often cut up raw chickens on kitchen cutting boards, which then come in contact with tomatoes being sliced for salads—a sure way to transmit any illness-causing bacteria the chicken might contain. If you use a cutting board for meat or poultry, don't use it for other foods no matter how thoroughly you wash it.

Salad buffets are one of the biggest sources of food-borne bacteria. Who knows how long the chicken salad with the mayo dressing has been sitting out there?

Other tips: Don't let foods sit outside the refrigerator. Avoid unpasteurized juices. And consider your vulnerability. The same bacteria that can cause a little vomiting in a healthy middle-aged man can be fatal to an older man, an infant, or someone undergoing chemotherapy.

Consider stirring fiber supplement powder into water or juice. If you prefer to try this route, start slow to avoid diarrhea or gas.

And, finally, don't be fooled by the label "multigrain." That is no guarantee of fiber. Check the nutrition box instead for actual fiber content.

The Modern Story on Fats

Even though we have been taught to think that fats are bad and that we should cut down on the percent of fats in our diet, the current nutritional message is considerably more complicated: Most nutritionists now say we should cut down on bad fats but actually increase good fats in our diet. So the obvious question becomes how to tell the difference.

Saturated or Unsaturated?

Unfortunately, there is no way to avoid a very simple (I promise!) chemistry lesson first. All fats consist of chains of carbon atoms connected to hydrogen atoms. For our purposes, the differences between fats lies in the number of hydrogen atoms they have.

Bad fats

Saturated fats. These fats carry as many hydrogen atoms as they can—they are "saturated" with hydrogen atoms. This makes them solid at room temperature. Such fats are typically found in meat and animal fat, dairy products, and a few vegetable oils (coconut and palm). These are the fats that raise the levels of bad cholesterol and increase our risk for heart disease. *(For more information on heart disease, see page 124.)*

Trans fatty acids (TFA). These are actually made by taking good polyunsaturated fats and heating them in the presence of hydrogen atoms to make them partially saturated (or as they are sometimes called, partially hydrogenated). Now why would anyone want to take good fats and make them into not-so-good fats? Because they are easier to store, ship, and use in cooking. That's why they are so common in processed foods and snacks. The problem is that they are bad for us and they increase the risk for heart disease. Some experts think they may be even more dangerous than saturated fats.

Trans Fatty Acids in Selected Foods

FOOD	TRANS FATTY ACIDS (grams per one serving)
Vegetable shortening	1.4–4.2
Margarine (stick)	1.8–3.5
Margarine (tub, regular)	0.4–1.6
Salad dressings (regular)	0.06–1.1
Vegetable oils	0.01–0.06
Pound cake	4.3
Doughnuts	0.3–3.8
Microwave popcorn (regular)	2.2
Chocolate chip cookies	1.2–2.7
Vanilla wafers	1.3
French fries (fast food)	0.7–3.6
Snack crackers	1.8–2.5
Snack chips	0–1.2
Chocolate candies	0.04–2.8
White bread	0.06–0.7
Ready-to-eat breakfast cereals	0.05–0.5

Adapted from U.S. Department of Agriculture (USDA) food composition data, 1995

Good fats

Monounsaturated fats. These are fats that have two less hydrogen atoms than fully saturated fats. However, this seemingly small difference makes a big difference in how they act in our body; they actually lower bad cholesterol and raise good cholesterol.

Polyunsaturated fats. These have even fewer hydrogen atoms than monounsaturated fats, and they also lower bad and raise good cholesterol. Both monounsaturated and polyunsaturated fats are liquid at room temperature. *(For a full discussion of cholesterol, see page 129.)*

Omega-3 fats. These members of the polyunsaturated fat family seem to provide special protection for the heart, especially in preventing abnormal heart rhythms that are responsible for many sudden deaths *(see page 150)*. Unfortunately, they are not widely available in a typical American diet. The single best source are so-called "fatty fish" like salmon, mackerel, sardines, and herring; I admit that most of us are not going to eat much of those last three, but I do believe, based on my own experience, that you can learn to truly enjoy well-prepared salmon. There are also "fish oil" supplements widely available in drug and health stores; in some studies these pills have been shown to be helpful in preventing heart disease.

Sources of good fats

Unsaturated fats come from plant oils, nuts, seeds, and fish. Avocados, olives, olive oil, nuts, seeds, tuna, salmon, and sardines are excellent sources. Whether monounsaturated or polyunsaturated, these fats are good to include in the diet, especially when they replace saturated fats. Some plant oils are predominantly monounsaturated, such as olive, canola, avocado, and sesame. Other plant oils that are basically polyunsaturated are sunflower, corn, and safflower. Good fats, especially when they are used in place of bad fats, can improve your health and enhance your meals.

One of the best parts about good fats is that including them in your diet may help you control your weight. Nutritionists often suggest that dieters add certain fats, such as an olive oil–based salad dressing or nuts sprinkled over vegetables, to help satisfy their appetite and make meals taste better. If you are making an effort to cut down on calories and lose pounds but still feel hungry most of the time, try including some olive oil, nuts, seeds, and avocados in your meals. Using olive oil in your cooking is a sound nutritional idea.

Sources of bad fats

Saturated fats are easy enough to detect. They are found primarily in animal fats, dairy products, and some tropical oils, such as coconut and palm. Ice cream, butter, whole milk, and full-fat cheese contain saturated fats. Trans fatty acids are typically described on food labels as "partially hydrogenated oils" or "vegetable shortening." These are fats that are naturally found in a liquid form but have been manufactured into solids. They make peanut butter and margarine easier to spread and add shelf life to crackers, cookies, and other packaged baked goods. Hydrogenated oils also are usually used to make french fries and other deep fried foods. Trans fats can behave like saturated fats in the body, often elevating blood cholesterol, but on nutrition labels they are not labeled separately (as of this writing) because of opposition from the food industry.

What about eggs? Because a single egg contains about 200 milligrams of cholesterol (which is about two-thirds of the total recommended cholesterol per day), eggs have long been on the list of "forbidden foods." And I am not about to tell you that you should stop worrying about eggs or, more precisely, about egg yolks, which is where all the cholesterol is. But I will point out two things. First, for many people, the amount of actual cholesterol in the diet—as compared to saturated or trans fatty acids—doesn't seem to make much difference in cholesterol levels. In other words, for most people, fats are a much more important dietary source of increased blood cholesterol than is dietary cholesterol itself. And second, back to eggs, they do contain some other good nutrients, such as protein, folic acid, and some other B vitamins. So I am willing to say, based on some actual study data, that up to one egg per day on average does not seem to be dangerous to your heart, though even that amount may be risky for people with diabetes.

Butter versus margarine. Today, this is a tough question to answer unless you are willing to read the labels. By definition, butter contains a lot of saturated fat that is bad for you. The problem is that some margarines—usually the older stick solid type—contain a lot of trans fats that can make them worse than butter. There are some new margarines that are low in saturated and trans fats that might be safer than butter. But here is the real truth: Olive oil is much better than either and very tasty for bread-dipping.

The bottom line on fats

In a nutshell, not all fats are bad—which is a very different message than we were getting ten years ago. So in thinking about the fats in your diet, it is much more important to think about the kinds of fats you are eating rather than simply the total amount. In fact, we are now in a position to say something that would have sounded like heresy 10 years ago: Cutting down on saturated and trans fats and increasing monounsaturated and polyunsaturated fats is actually good for you as long as you are paying attention to total calories.

The Modern Story on Protein

Most American men have no problem getting enough protein in their diets. Trouble is, there are many different sources of protein, and you might not be consuming the best foods to meet your body's protein needs. Protein helps you see, digest, regulate hormones, fight infection, and repair muscle. Protein is also used for fuel if carbohydrates are depleted. Think of your daily servings of protein as the building blocks of your body. You need to use the right kind of blocks to get the body you want.

Another quick chemistry lesson: Proteins are basically long chains of amino acids. Your body naturally manufactures 11 of the 20 amino acids you need; the other 9, which you have to get from food, are called the essential amino acids. When you hear that a food is a "perfect" or "complete" protein source, it means the item offers an optimal balance of essential amino acids. The newest research shows that egg whites, soy beans, legumes, and fish are all complete proteins for the human body—in other words, great dietary sources of protein.

Dairy products are another source of highly developed protein, but some people can't digest the lactose sugar in them. And they usually contain a lot of saturated fats. Red meat is a powerful protein, but it can include too much saturated fat in the bargain. As a result, it's best to choose lean red meats (look for cuts featuring either "loin" or "round"). Chicken and turkey (without the skin) can be better options, but beware that ground poultry can be quite fatty (check with your meat counter expert for the percentage of fat your favorite types contain). Plants often do not contain complete proteins, so if you're a true vegetarian, it's important to eat a wide variety of vegetables and include legumes on a daily basis; I would recommend that such a person get special nutritional counseling.

How much protein do you need?

You should aim to get 15 to 20 percent of your daily calories from protein. A more precise measuring stick comes from this guideline: Divide your weight in pounds by 2.2 and then take that number and multiply by 0.8 to get the grams of protein you need daily for normal lifestyle activities. For example, a 200-pound man scores 73 grams. If you are moderately active, the multiplication factor is 1.0 (rather than 0.8). Men in serious training (cardiovascular and/or strength) can increase the multiplier to 1.4. Few men, no matter what their athletic status, require more daily protein than this upper end. Don't forget that whole foods are usually best. If you rely in part on protein powder (instead of protein foods that contain a variety of vitamins

Dietary Protein Sources

FOOD SOURCE	SERVING SIZE	PROTEIN (grams)
Tuna salad	1 cup	32.88
Cottage cheese, 1% milkfat	1 cup	28.00
Pork loin, lean, pan-fried	3 oz	27.35
Chicken breast, roasted	1/2 breast	26.68
Sirloin, broiled	3 oz	25.81
Turkey, light meat, roasted	3 oz	25.12
Ham, lean, roasted	3 oz	25.00
Halibut, broiled	3 oz	22.69
Soybeans, green, boiled	1 cup	22.23
Couscous, dry	1 cup	22.07
Ground beef, extra-lean, broiled	3 oz	21.59
Beans, white, canned	1 cup	19.02
Lentils, boiled	1 cup	17.86
Wheat flour, whole grain	1 cup	16.44
Lima beans, boiled	1 cup	14.66
Yogurt, plain, low fat	8 oz	11.92
Milk, 1% milkfat	1 cup	8.03
Tofu, soft	1 piece	7.86
Egg noodles, cooked, enriched	1 cup	7.60
Soy milk	1 cup	6.74
Peanuts, dry-roasted	1 oz	6.71
Spaghetti, cooked, enriched	1 cup	6.68
Wild rice, cooked	1 cup	6.54
Egg, whole, hard-boiled	1 large	6.29

Adapted from: U.S. Department of Agriculture, Agricultural Research Service. 2001. USDA Nutrient Database for Standard Reference, Release 14. Nutrient Data Laboratory Home Page, http://www.nal.usda.gov/fnic/foodcomp

Protein and Muscle: The Myths and the Truths

Truth may be stranger than fiction on occasion, but blurring the facts about protein has helped sell plenty of books and diet products in recent years. Here's what's true about the protein diet craze and how it relates to your muscles:

◆ When you engage in aerobic activity such as running or cycling, your body derives 4 to 10 percent of energy from proteins. During short-burst exercise (weight lifting, softball, sprinting), your body converts mostly carbohydrates into energy and burns no fat and only minuscule amounts of protein.

◆ So why are all these weight lifters consuming protein powders? Studies show that protein needs rise when you add new muscle to the body, especially in the two to three hours after a weight-lifting workout. Getting the extra protein from foods is the recommended route, but it's reasonable for busy people to occasionally replace meals with protein drinks.

◆ Protein powders can serve as handy meal replacements—especially as a mid-morning, mid-afternoon, or post-workout mini-meal. But the convenience comes at a price. A typical serving (powder mixed with juice/milk/water or canned) can be fairly expensive, and the liquid used may be high in fats or calories.

◆ Protein drinks have long been a favorite of bodybuilders who believe extra protein builds muscles faster than eating carbohydrates, though scientific studies show this accelerated effect is less pronounced in seasoned bodybuilders and more pronounced in individuals who are in the beginning phases of weight training programs. Another popular theory is that the powders will help your muscles recover more quickly after heavy-lifting workouts. While that is true to a certain extent, research shows that a relatively small amount will do the job. The danger of protein drinks is in thinking that if some additional protein is good, more is even better.

◆ Be careful about overloading on protein. Your muscles can only process so much; even the most intense athlete requires only about 25 to 50 percent more than a sedentary man. In fact, excess protein in your diet can put an extra nitrogen load on your kidneys. Moreover, too much protein may wash calcium out of your bones, possibly putting you at risk of bone weakness.

and minerals), you may come up short in terms of the zinc and iron you need.

Having a reasonable amount of protein on your plate at every meal has an added benefit: It will make your fuel base last longer and discourage between-meal stops at the refrigerator. This is because proteins (and fats) usually digest more slowly than carbohydrates, and you will actually feel less hungry after eating them. If you like "meat and potatoes" every night, try turkey, beans, or soy foods such as tofu and tempeh instead. For the next six weeks, skip red meat at lunch or dinner and opt for poultry, fish, or soy instead. You can put lean ground turkey in your taco filling or diced tofu in your pasta sauce. Black beans are a good substitute for beef in chili.

Could certain proteins be dangerous? In general, for people without kidney or liver disease, the answer to this question is no. In fact, to the degree that protein foods low in saturated fat replace other saturated fats and simple carbohydrates in the diet, they are a good nutritional bargain. However, there are suggestions in the medical literature that in some people, proteins present in milk or peanuts or soybeans might cause allergic reactions. It is sometimes very hard to prove this effect in a given person, but eliminating suspect foods from the diet may be worth a try. Finally, I should point out that we do not have much good evidence on the long-term safety of large amounts of soy in the diet. Certainly, several servings of soy a week should not be a problem, but large amounts every day—as is the case with some soy enthusiasts—have not been carefully studied for long-term safety.

The Traditional Dietary Guidelines

By now, you are probably sensing that nutritional advice is in a state of flux—that traditional advice is no longer sacred. Nowhere is this more apparent than in a critical examination of the famous Food Guide Pyramid developed by the U.S. Department of Agriculture (the USDA). At this point I want to recommend a superb nutrition book written by Walter Willett, M.D., who is Chairman of the Department of Nutrition at the Harvard School of Public Health and Professor of Medicine at Harvard Medical School. His book, *Eat, Drink, and Be Healthy,* is the best book on nutrition for the general public I have read to date. (Full disclosure: I have a Master's Degree from the Harvard School of Public Health and I have known Walter for many years.) Not only is his book very readable and informative, but it is very brave. Dr. Willett is not afraid to call a spade a spade, and he is not afraid to criticize some sacred cows—including the USDA Food Pyramid. I would urge you to buy this book and read it all for yourself; it will be well worth your time. But at this point I am going to summarize his major criticisms of the USDA Food Pyramid, criticisms you will now better understand after reading this chapter thus far. His major concerns are that:

- The USDA's recommendation to use fats "sparingly" ignores the fact that some fats—namely polyunsaturated and monounsaturated ones—are actually good for you and should be increased in most diets.
- The USDA's suggestion of 6 to 11 servings of bread, cereal, rice, and pasta is too simplistic and ignores the fact that many of these carbohydrates have a high glycemic index that may mean they are not as healthy as other carbohydrates or even unsaturated fats. (Willett also criticizes the USDA for mentioning potatoes in their guidelines as a vegetable when it is really more like a starchy carbohydrate with a very high glycemic index.) To quote directly from Willett's book, "The central message in the USDA Pyramid is that you should feel good about eating carbohydrates, especially if you are eating them in place of fats. But if you eat too much of the wrong kinds of carbohydrates and too little of the good kinds of fats, you can set yourself up for the same problems you may be trying to solve [page 19]."
- The USDA's recommendation of 2 to 3 servings a day of the "meat, poultry, fish, dry beans, eggs, and nuts group" does not seem to recognize that meat should not be an equal with the others because it usually also contains too much saturated fat.
- The USDA's recommendation of 2 to 3 servings of the "milk, yogurt, and cheese group" does not sort out whole milk products from 1 percent or skim milk products—or seemingly recognize that other sources of calcium may be healthier for many people. (See section on calcium below.)

Finally, Willett criticizes the USDA Pyramid for not offering guidance on weight, exercise, alcohol, and vitamins. So I am now going to turn to some of the issues left out of the USDA Pyramid because they are clearly important to our overall health.

The Modern Story on Vitamins and Minerals

Here is my main message right up front: Almost always, it is better to get essential vitamins and minerals from eating food rather than depending on supplements. That's because when it comes to nutrition, it is hard to beat Mother Nature. Nutrition experts stress that even though we have learned a lot, we really still know very little about the kinds and combinations of vitamins and minerals that occur naturally in foods. That's one reason why studies that might show certain kinds of diets to be beneficial in reducing the risk for heart disease or cancer may not show the same result with man-made supplements.

Having said this, it is also important to acknowledge that there are some potential gaps in the produce of Mother Nature's bounty—such as the difficulty in getting enough vitamin D for some people or the deficit in certain B vitamins in people with restricted diets. Therefore along with many others, I have come to the conclusion that it makes sense for almost anyone to take a daily multivitamin that includes the recommended daily intake for various vitamins and minerals. Today, this is expressed as Daily Values (DVs) on supplement bottles. Such amounts are usually safe and provide a kind of backup to our diet. I would recommend buying the cheapest brand possible, usually the store's own brand, that meets the manufacturing standards of the United States Pharmacopeia (USP) as indicated either by a label or the advice of the pharmacist.

Before going to a list of the specific vitamins and minerals that are typically included in a daily supplement, I wish to briefly explain the concept of antioxidation—which is one of the main selling points for many supplements. Antioxidation refers to the neutralizing of so-called free radicals, which are produced by the action of oxygen on our body tissues (called oxidation). An excess of these free radicals can damage all kinds of cells and tissues in the body—and it is this damage that has been linked to a broad range of diseases and even the process of aging. So "anti-oxidants" have been promoted as the answer to almost any problem, in many cases way beyond what good evidence can support.

However, there is suggestive evidence that antioxidants may at least modestly help reduce the risk for heart disease, some cancers, macular degeneration, cataracts, and some aspects of cellular aging. The problem is that most of this evidence comes from population studies of diets—not from good research supporting individual antioxidants. That's why most nutrition experts still advocate eating foods rich in vitamins and minerals—especially fresh fruits and vegetables—rather than taking an assortment of individual supplements. As Dr. Willett puts it in the book I so highly recommend, "No single antioxidant can do the work of the whole crowd. Taking high-dose beta-carotene or vitamin A pills, then, is like listening to a single violin play a Mozart symphony—you get a little something, but not the full, glorious effect. It's also possible that the imbalance that occurs by taking too much of any one antioxidant may be like listening to an orchestra in which one section is playing with damaged, eardrum-shattering instruments [page 155]."

What Every Man Should Know about Dietary Supplements

VITAMIN A: A fat-soluble vitamin that can be stored in your body for indefinite periods, vitamin A can build up and be toxic in large doses. Indeed, there is some evidence that daily intakes of 10,000 or more international units (IU) of vitamin A (retinol) can increase the risk for hip fractures and even birth defects if taken during pregnancy. Consequently, beta-carotene, which helps your body manufacture vitamin A, is often recommended as a full or partial substitute for vitamin A supplementation. Beta-carotene also is an antioxidant, which means it can help neutralize free radicals that otherwise might damage healthy cells, while vitamin A is not. Vitamin A keeps your eyes healthy, and is essential for the growth and health of cells in many tissues including skin, hair, eyes, and bones.

Foods: *For vitamin A*, fortified milk, eggs, cheese, liver, fish oil. *For beta-carotene*, apricots, cantaloupe, carrots, collard greens, fennel, kale, mustard greens, peaches, pumpkin, red pepper, romaine lettuce, spinach, sweet potatoes, Swiss chard, winter squash.

Supplements: 5,000 IU of a combination of beta-carotene and vitamin A.

VITAMIN B: There are actually eight different "B-complex" vitamins: thiamine, riboflavin, niacin, B-6, pantothenic acid, B-12, biotin, and folic acid. The B vitamins are water-soluble, which means your body eliminates what it doesn't use, but in some cases not before a vitamin can do harm. For example, megadoses of niacin can be toxic to your liver. Nutritionists often recommend taking a B-complex supplement, because the vitamins probably work best in combination. Folic acid, B-6, and B-12 also lower levels of blood homocysteine, which may help to reduce the risk for heart disease, and even Alzheimer's disease.

Foods/Supplements: Here are foods rich in the various B vitamins, plus the current recommended daily intake for male adults for each vitamin:

B-1 (thiamine): Pork, legumes, nuts, fortified cereals (1.5 mg, or milligrams).

B-2 (riboflavin): Milk, yogurt, meats, leafy greens, whole grain or fortified cereals, breads (1.7 mg).

NIACIN: Meats, fish, legumes, nuts, whole grain or fortified cereals, breads (20 mg).

PANTOTHENIC ACID: Whole grains, fish, poultry, organ meats, yogurt, legumes (10 mg).

B-6: Chicken, fish, brown rice, whole wheat, eggs (2 mg).

B-12: Meat, fish, poultry, milk, eggs (6 micrograms).

FOLIC ACID (folate): Fortified cereals, dark green leafy vegetables, fruits, legumes, yeast breads, wheat germ (400 micrograms).

BIOTIN: Liver, soy, oatmeal, rice, barley, legumes, cauliflower, whole wheat (300 micrograms).

VITAMIN C: Experts agree that this vitamin is a powerful antioxidant, but they still hotly debate how much is too much in supplement form. Vitamin C helps regulate your metabolism during times of stress or illness, which makes it a popular home remedy when you feel a cold coming on. However, there is little hard evidence that it makes much difference in preventing or treating the common cold.

Foods: Citrus fruits, green vegetables, fortified cereals, brussels sprouts, cantaloupe, cauliflower, kiwi, papaya, peaches, red cabbage, red pepper, strawberries, potatoes.

Supplements: 60 mg.

VITAMIN D: This vitamin promotes the absorption of calcium and phosphorus, which in turn nourishes bones and teeth. It's also a key player in keeping your nervous system and muscles functioning at optimal levels. Your body usually manufactures vitamin D from exposure to sunlight. Some people in Northern climes and people who do not get outside may not make enough of it. *(For more information on vitamin D and calcium absorption, see Osteoporosis on page 245.)*

Foods: Fortified milk, cold-water fatty fish, such as salmon.

Supplements: 400 IU.

VITAMIN E: Some research has suggested vitamin E might protect against heart disease, retinal eye disease, various cancers, and dementia. Vitamin E also may boost your immune system and neutralize the dangers of secondhand smoke. It's a difficult vitamin to get from food, however. Because it is a fat-soluble vitamin, it is potentially dangerous in megadoses. If you take blood-thinning drugs or aspirin for cardiovascular health, consult a physician before taking a vitamin E supplement.

Foods: Wheat germ, vegetable oils, almonds, hazelnuts, sunflower seeds, leafy greens, whole grains, avocados, peanuts.

Supplements: 30 IU is the current recommended daily value but many nutritionists suggest 200 to 400 IU.

VITAMIN K: This nutrient is essential for blood clotting. Fortunately, your body gets most of what it requires from an average diet. However, some surveys show that younger people who do not eat green leafy vegetables may not get enough.

Foods: Kale, Swiss chard, other leafy greens, broccoli, brussels sprouts.

Supplements: You will get enough vitamin K by adding leafy greens to your diet, but many multivitamin tablets contain 25 micrograms.

In the following discussion of minerals, I am not going to recommend specific amounts, because in most cases there is much less data on minerals than there is on vitamins.

CALCIUM: There's been a great deal of media coverage about this mineral's role in keeping women's bones strong. However, men (especially those who are 65 and older) can face similar bone-thinning problems if they're not careful about getting enough calcium. This nutrient also is important for proper heart and muscle contractions and nerve impulses. *(For a more thorough discussion of calcium and recommended amounts, see Osteoporosis on page 245.)*

Foods: Milk, yogurt, cheese, fortified orange juice, canned salmon and sardines, collard greens, arugula, broccoli, almonds.

MAGNESIUM: Involved in hundreds of chemical reactions in the body, magnesium helps metabolize food and transmit messages between cells.

Foods: Nuts, legumes, whole grains, green vegetables, bananas.

POTASSIUM: This nutrient helps the body transmit nerve impulses and is responsible for the contraction of muscles, making it important for athletes. People who take water pills (diuretics) and/or drink lots of coffee (also a diuretic) can develop dangerously low levels of potassium.

Foods: Fruits (especially bananas, oranges), vegetables (especially potatoes), legumes, meats. People with kidney disease should take extra potassium only under a physician's supervision.

COPPER: This underrated mineral may be helpful in preventing cardiovascular disease, promoting fertility, and maintaining healthy skin. Newer research shows it may help protect against osteoporosis and bone loss.

Foods: Shellfish, legumes, whole grains (especially rye and wheat), mushrooms, liver, peas, artichokes, avocados, tomatoes, potatoes, prunes, bananas.

IRON: This mineral helps carry oxygen in your bloodstream and is critical to forming red blood cells. Because of menstruation, younger women are at much greater risk of iron deficiency, while men are more likely to have a surplus. The theory that iron surplus causes heart disease is not generally accepted. Unless directed by your physician, get your iron from food.

Foods: Liver, beef, lamb, clams, oysters, mussels, dark-meat chicken, beans, peas, leafy greens, dried apricots and raisins, fortified cereals, kelp, blackstrap molasses.

SELENIUM: This trace mineral wasn't shown to be essential until 1979, but it has fast become recognized as a potential disease-fighter by researchers. It may work in tandem with vitamin E to help prevent certain cancers, including prostate cancer. A major trial is now under way to see if 200 micrograms of selenium plus 400 IU of vitamin E a day will protect against prostate cancer.

Foods: Brazil nuts, seafood, meats, oats, brown rice.

CHROMIUM: This mineral has become popular as a dietary supplement because of media reports and manufacturer claims about its ability to enhance the burning of fat. Chromium is indeed vital for digesting fats, carbohydrates, and protein, but claims about its use in weight loss remain controversial at best.

Foods: Whole grains, whole-grain breads and cereals, potatoes, prunes, peanut butter, nuts, seafood, brewer's yeast.

ZINC: You may have seen media reports linking zinc to healthier immune systems and fewer colds. Whether it actually has any value in this role remains controversial. But we do know that this mineral fuels enzymes that perform hundreds of cellular tasks, ranging from making DNA to healing wounds. For men, low zinc might contribute to fertility problems or symptoms of an enlarged prostate.

Foods: Beef, pork, liver, dark-meat poultry, eggs, seafood (especially oysters), nuts, beans, wheat germ.

I would especially warn against high cost vitamin programs that are heavily promoted as having a unique formulation that ensures good health. Indeed, before you ever commit to such a program or to megadoses of any vitamin or mineral, I would strongly advise consulting with a registered dietician (RD). Most regular physicians are not always well versed on the details of modern nutrition research, but RDs usually are and can be readily found in most major hospitals and clinics.

On pages 22 through 25 you will find a brief summary list of common vitamins and minerals sold as supplements. In each case I have provided good food sources for the particular nutrient—and the current recommended Daily Values for vitamins. Obviously, people with special needs (such as restricted diets or digestive diseases) may need to take special supplements under the direction of a dietician.

The Modern Story on Essential Liquids

Actually, when it comes right down to it, there is only one essential liquid and that, of course, is water. Nutritionists often say that our bodies need the equivalent of about eight 8-ounce glasses of water for a 2,000 calorie diet—which is probably where the traditional advice for drinking that much water a day comes from. However, that doesn't mean you should be a slave to that formula—getting your eight glasses a day no matter what. Sometimes you will need more because of the heat and/or increased exercise. And often you will get your "water" from other sources—such as a diet rich in fruits and vegetables (which contain a lot of water) or other kinds of beverages that are mostly water. But the reason we tend to emphasize the "eight glasses a day" is to remind ourselves how important water is to our health—and to stress that often we cannot rely on our thirst as a reliable guide to our water needs. We should, of course, drink water when we are thirsty. But under circumstances of intense heat and/or exercise, we should force ourselves to drink water on a regular basis *before* we get thirsty, at which point we may be in danger under those circumstances.

Now, what about other "liquid refreshments" as a source of water? Unfortunately, they all have their drawbacks in comparison. Regular soda is a terrible nutritional bargain because it is so loaded with simple sugar—about 10 teaspoons of sugar in a typical 12-ounce can! (No wonder some critics call regular soda "liquid candy.") Diet soda is obviously better in terms of sugar (and calories), but many brands contain caffeine, which may be problematic for some people. Fruit juices are a better nutritional bargain, but they too are usually loaded with sugar and calories. As described earlier, whole milk products are also loaded with saturated fats, though skim milk is certainly more acceptable. So that leaves two other categories that deserve more detailed attention.

Coffee, Tea, and Caffeine

My own personal opinion (and that of many other nutritionists and physicians) is that caffeine in moderation is fine for most people. There are some among us who are exquisitely sensitive to caffeine as a stimulant, and even small amounts will make such people "jittery" in unacceptable fashion—and wide awake at night! And most regular caffeine consumers (from any source, including colas) will develop a mild "addiction," meaning headaches with sudden withdrawal. But for the rest of us, several average-size cups of coffee or tea a day should pose no problem—and, without added sugar or cream, offer no calories! Past reports suggesting that coffee might cause cancer or heart disease have been disproved; those studies, by and large, failed to rule out the effect of smoking that so often went along with regular coffee drinking.

In fact, more modern research suggests some potential health benefits from regular coffee drinking, such as reduced risk for kidney stones and gallstones. And some studies have even suggested a lower suicide rate among coffee drinkers, possibly from the mild stimulant/antidepressant effect. Teas have the added potential benefit of plant nutrients that might lower the risk of some cancers, particularly stomach cancer. So in moderation—which I will arbitrarily define as three or less average-size cups a day—coffee and tea should pose no health hazard for the vast majority of us and might confer modest health benefits.

The Pros and Cons of Alcohol

This is the section many of you have been waiting for. And I must respond to this question with care, given the enormous destruction, both physical and emotional, caused by alcohol abuse in our society. In fact, my own personal view—and I stress that this is entirely personal and opinionated—is that overall, alcoholic beverages do more harm than good, even accounting for all the social and financial (to the companies that make and distribute them) benefits from truly moderate drinking.

But the fact is that "drinking" is here to stay. So what about the potential health benefits from alcohol? There is no doubt that truly moderate drinking—which I define as one to two average-size alcoholic drinks per day—confer modest protection against heart disease and strokes. And, by the way, the latest research shows such benefit from any kind of alcoholic beverage; there does not appear to be anything truly magic about red wine. The total explanation for this effect is not in, but clearly in most people, alcohol helps raise levels of good cholesterol and reduces the chance of blood clot formation that might block blood flow in critical arteries. (The health benefit equation for women is more complicated because in them, alcohol also seems to slightly raise the risk for breast cancer.) However, even moderate drinking may be dangerous for people prone to alcoholism because of a family history of such problems or in people taking certain medications, including painkillers, antidepressants, or sedatives. Therefore, I typically say the following:

- If you already drink safely in moderation and have no family history of alcoholism or other contraindications (such as liver disease or if you are taking certain medications), by all means continue unless your medical circumstances change.
- If you do not drink, don't start just because of potential health benefits. They are relatively modest, and you can usually gain similar benefits from increased exercise and/or dietary changes.

In summary, while I have respect for the research that shows health benefits from moderate alcohol consumption, I have even more respect for the dangers posed by potential alcohol abuse.

The Modern Story on Weight Control

First, of course, we have to agree on the importance of weight control—and, quite frankly, you will find some disagreement among scientists on this question. Obviously no one thinks true obesity is good for you. But the questions of defining what "overweight" should mean and the strategies for reducing weight are matters of great debate. I will now "weigh in" with my opinions, but I would urge you to read other sources on this one, including Dr. Willett's outstanding book, mentioned earlier *(see page 19)*. His opinion about the danger of excess weight is clear: "But next to whether you smoke, the number that stares up at you from the bathroom scale is the most important measure of your future health. Keeping that number in the healthy range is more important for long-term health than the types and amounts of antioxidants in your food or the exact ratio of fats to carbohydrates [page 35]." And the recent Surgeon General's report on obesity seconds this concern by suggesting that 300,000 deaths a year in this country are "associated" with obesity—and that obesity may someday overtake smoking as the leading cause of death in the U.S. The report goes on to state that obesity is "associated" with heart disease, certain types of cancer, Type 2 diabetes, stroke, arthritis, breathing problems, and psychological disorders such as depression. That's an impressive list by any accounting.

The importance of abdominal fat. Before getting to the cosmic view of weight concerns, I want to address a common question about men in particular—namely the importance of abdominal fat (the so-called beer belly) versus other fat distribution. As you may know, there is a theory that fat around the waist is more dangerous to our health than fat elsewhere. Some proponents of this theory like to use the waist-hip ratio as a marker of this danger and talk about apple (abdominal fat) versus pear (hip fat) shapes. But others say just keeping an eye on the waist is good enough. Men in particular tend to replace muscle with fat in the abdominal area as they age, and just looking down at your waist may be your first clue that you are developing a problem even though your total weight initially remains the same. However, ultimately your total weight is also very important, and it is to this issue that I now turn.

What is "overweight?" I once attended a conference on obesity where experts spent a whole day on the question of how to best measure obesity. At the end of

Body Mass Index Table

	Normal						Overweight					Obese										Extreme Obesity						
BMI	**19**	**20**	**21**	**22**	**23**	**24**	**25**	**26**	**27**	**28**	**29**	**30**	**31**	**32**	**33**	**34**	**35**	**36**	**37**	**38**	**39**	**40**	**41**	**42**	**43**	**44**	**45**	**46**
Height (inches)														**Body Weight (pounds)**														
58	91	96	100	105	110	115	119	124	129	134	138	143	148	153	158	162	167	172	177	181	186	191	196	201	205	210	215	220
59	94	99	104	109	114	119	124	128	133	138	143	148	153	158	163	168	173	178	183	188	193	198	203	208	212	217	222	227
60	97	102	107	112	118	123	128	133	138	143	148	153	158	163	168	174	179	184	189	194	199	204	209	215	220	225	230	235
61	100	106	111	116	122	127	132	137	143	148	153	158	164	169	174	180	185	190	195	201	206	211	217	222	227	232	238	243
62	104	109	115	120	126	131	136	142	147	153	158	164	169	175	180	186	191	196	202	207	213	218	224	229	235	240	246	251
63	107	113	118	124	130	135	141	146	152	158	163	169	175	180	186	191	197	203	208	214	220	225	231	237	242	248	254	259
64	110	116	122	128	134	140	145	151	157	163	169	174	180	186	192	197	204	209	215	221	227	232	238	244	250	256	262	267
65	114	120	126	132	138	144	150	156	162	168	174	180	186	192	198	204	210	216	222	228	234	240	246	252	258	264	270	276
66	118	124	130	136	142	148	155	161	167	173	179	186	192	198	204	210	216	223	229	235	241	247	253	260	266	272	278	284
67	121	127	134	140	146	153	159	166	172	178	185	191	198	204	211	217	223	230	236	242	249	255	261	268	274	280	287	293
68	125	131	138	144	151	158	164	171	177	184	190	197	203	210	216	223	230	236	243	249	256	262	269	276	282	289	295	302
69	128	135	142	149	155	162	169	176	182	189	196	203	209	216	223	230	236	243	250	257	263	270	277	284	291	297	304	311
70	132	139	146	153	160	167	174	181	188	195	202	209	216	222	229	236	243	250	257	264	271	278	285	292	299	306	313	320
71	136	143	150	157	165	172	179	186	193	200	208	215	222	229	236	243	250	257	265	272	279	286	293	301	308	315	322	329
72	140	147	154	162	169	177	184	191	199	206	213	221	228	235	242	250	258	265	272	279	287	294	302	309	316	324	331	338
73	144	151	159	166	174	182	189	197	204	212	219	227	235	242	250	257	265	272	280	288	295	302	310	318	325	333	340	348
74	148	155	163	171	179	186	194	202	210	218	225	233	241	249	256	264	272	280	287	295	303	311	319	326	334	342	350	358
75	152	160	168	176	184	192	200	208	216	224	232	240	248	256	264	272	279	287	295	303	311	319	327	335	343	351	359	367
76	156	164	172	180	189	197	205	213	221	230	238	246	254	263	271	279	287	295	304	312	320	328	336	344	353	361	369	377

the day, an eminent researcher in the field stood up and offered this time honored method of answering this question: Take off all your clothes, stand in front of a mirror, and "if you look fat, you are fat." In fact, that usually works if we are willing to be honest about our appearance. (This may be one of those times when a second opinion could be very helpful.) But many of us want a more precise way of determining our "weight status," and there is a relatively simple one—the so-called Body Mass Index, or BMI for short. This is the new standard and simple method of relating weight to height. I could offer you a formula for calculating it, but the much faster way is to look it up on the chart on page 29.

If you look at the left-hand column to find your height (in total inches) and then move right across that line to find your weight (without clothes), you then simply look at the top of that column to find your BMI. Here is the good or bad news, depending on what your BMI turns out to be: People with BMIs between 25 and 29 are considered to be "overweight," and those with BMIs of 30 and over are considered to be "obese." (The only real exception to this—and it is very rare!—is the extremely muscular person who may be in the 25 to 30 range because of muscle versus fat.)

Do Diets Work?

Now I realize that many of you are in a state of shock right now because you just determined your BMI and were labeled as overweight or even obese. So I urge you to take any bad news not as a death sentence but as motivation to do something about your weight. And that "something" really boils down to two ultimately very simple pieces of advice: Consume fewer calories, and exercise more. Now obviously, while the advice is simple, the execution is not. So I will spend the rest of this chapter talking about diet strategies and the next chapter talking about exercise strategies.

First I will acknowledge that almost any diet will work for the short term if you stick to it because it will inevitably result in fewer calories than your usual consumption. Even those diets that suggest you can "eat all you want" of certain foods tend to work because you will usually quickly get bored with those "certain foods" and actually consume fewer calories than you usually do, even though it might not seem like it. And forget all the talk about different kinds of calories being important; in the long run, a calorie is a calorie, and they all count!

Unfortunately, losing weight short term is seldom the problem. Any fad diet can help you lose weight in the short term, but none of them—no diet, plan, or pill—can guarantee that you will keep it off long term. The number commonly agreed upon by researchers is that only 5 percent of people who try to lose weight succeed in keeping it off at least eight years.

Antiaging Diet

There's really only one medical intervention proven in the laboratory to lengthen life—a very low calorie (yet highly nutritious) diet. Scientists started measuring the antiaging effect in lab rats, eventually working up to rhesus monkeys. The results have been consistent—less food results in a longer life span. We're talking a 30 percent longer life span for animals fed a diet with 30 percent fewer calories than normal. And they not only lived longer, they lived better, exhibiting increased vitality and fewer age-related diseases. Their blood pressure dropped. Their body temperature and metabolism dropped, as if the entire aging process was slowed. In monkeys, cholesterol levels even improved. (These results—on primates—mean a lot more than similar results that were found in mice in the mid-1980s.)

If the figures were to translate to humans, that might mean scaling down to between 1,500 and 2,000 calories a day and living on average past a hundred. Of course, humans don't live in a lab, so there's no guarantee the diet would be maintained or that the results would be the same. In fact, considering that only 5 percent of people who try to lose weight are able to stick with their diets, it seems unlikely there will be many men committing themselves to a 1,500-calories-a-day regimen for life.

A recent USDA study on popular diets looked at what is working for those who lose weight long term. Those stubbornly successful few consistently consume a diet low in calories, about 1,600 a day for the men. They don't try to eliminate fat from their diet, preferring instead to focus on good fats plus lots of fruits and vegetables, but almost no fried food. Virtually all these people are physically active, burning an average 2,500 calories a week through workouts lasting 30 to 45 minutes a day, with at least 40 percent of that in aerobic exercise (see next chapter). These are people who didn't just decide to rely on a diet or a magic pill to change their body shapes. They changed their lives. There is one bit of good news for you—namely that we men generally have an easier time losing weight than women because our metabolic rates are often higher as long as we remain active.

As you age, you should gradually cut back on the amount you eat. Men usually start noticing the extra pounds in their 40s. Another newer research development suggests that male bodies can handle only about 800 calories at any one sitting.

Men and Eating Disorders

Although many people think of eating disorders as the special province of teenage girls, this is simply not true. Not only do children and older women suffer from eating disorders, so do men and boys. In fact, experts have found that 10 percent of all eating disorder sufferers are male, and some consider that to be a low estimate. Unfortunately, as a result of societal pressures and a general lack of awareness, men tend to be a lot more reluctant to seek treatment for eating disorders than women.

The causes of eating disorders are many. Poor self-esteem, anxiety, the media, phobias, physical abuse, competitive sports, and the desire for control have all been implicated as contributing factors. In truth, the underlying causes of disease are different in each individual case, which is partly why eating disorders can be so tricky to diagnose and treat.

There are four types of eating disorders known to affect men.

Anorexia nervosa

Put in the simplest possible terms, anorexia nervosa is a disease of compulsive self-starvation. Terrified of gaining weight and becoming "fat" anorexics limit their caloric intake severely, such that their body weight drops far beyond what is normal and healthy. In addition, many anorexics adopt grueling exercise regimens and patently bizarre eating habits.

The physical consequences of anorexia range from the relatively mild (icy hands and feet, decreased production of sex hormones, dry skin) to the very severe (irregular heartbeat, anemia, osteoporosis, even cardiac arrest). Anorexia can also lead to many distressing but less tangible problems, such as dizziness, fatigue, and mental fuzziness.

Some classic symptoms of anorexia nervosa include:

- The refusal to maintain body weight at or above a minimally normal weight for one's age and height.
- An intense fear of gaining weight or becoming fat, despite being severely underweight.
- Disturbance in the way one's body weight or shape is experienced, undue influence of body weight or shape on self-evaluation, and/or denial of the dangers posed by low weight.

Bulimia nervosa

The most significant feature of bulimia nervosa is the binge/purge cycle. What this means is that a bulimic will habitually consume large quantities of food very quickly, only to "purge" the calories through self-induced vomiting, abuse of laxatives, excessive exercise, or other means. While bulimia can certainly arise from psychological and emotional causes, it is also particularly prevalent among athletes whose weight is strictly controlled, such as wrestlers, jockeys, and gymnasts.

Because sufferers often stay at or near their normal weight, bulimia can be difficult to detect. Nevertheless, habitual binge eating and purging can have serious physical consequences, including irregular heartbeat, tooth decay, electrolyte imbalances, and kidney and liver damage.

Some classic symptoms of bulimia nervosa include:

- Recurrent episodes of binge eating, accompanied by a feeling of not being able to control what or how much one eats.
- Recurrent inappropriate compensatory behavior aimed at preventing weight gain, such as self-induced vomiting; misuse of laxatives, diuretics, enemas, or other purgatives; fasting; sweating; or excessive exercise.
- Undue influence of body weight and/or shape on self-evaluation.

Binge eating disorder (BED)

As the name suggests, binge eating disorder—also known as compulsive overeating—is characterized by frequent episodes of binge eating, but without the compensatory purging behavior common among bulimics. Many who suffer from BED have a history of failed diets, and may in fact be genetically predisposed to weigh more than is considered desirable by mainstream society.

The most direct physical consequence of BED is obesity, which can in turn lead to heart problems, diabetes, and certain types of cancer. Like all eating disorders, BED can also cause various psychological and emotional problems, such as depression, guilt, anxiety, loneliness, and obsessions and compulsions.

Some classic symptoms of BED include:

- Recurrent episodes of binge eating, accompanied by a feeling of not being able to control what or how much one eats.
- During binge episodes, a tendency to: (a) eat much more rapidly than normal; (b)

eat until uncomfortably full; (c) eat large amounts of food when not physically hungry; (d) eat alone, out of embarrassment over how much one is eating; (e) feel guilt, self-loathing, and/or depression as a result.

- The binge eating is not associated with the regular use of inappropriate compensatory behaviors, such as purging, fasting, or excessive exercise.

Muscle dysmorphia

Sometimes called "bigorexia," muscle dysmorphia is often thought of as being the opposite of anorexia nervosa. Instead of obsessing about weight gain, those who suffer from muscle dysmorphia worry that they are puny and underdeveloped. In an attempt to remedy the perceived frailty of their physique, muscle dysmorphics—often athletes or bodybuilders—begin exercising and lifting weights compulsively. They may also use steroids or other muscle-building drugs, a practice with potentially lethal consequences.

Some classic symptoms of muscle dysmorphia include:

- Preoccupation with the idea that one's body is too small and puny, leading to excessive weight-lifting, compulsive exercise, and/or steroid abuse.
- Anxiety, depression, and/or extreme self-consciousness as a result of this preoccupation.
- The refusal to stop working out and using muscle-building drugs, despite the knowledge that to continue could cause health problems.

Consume more than that and the surplus will likely be ticketed to become fat cells. Consequently, many nutritionists now recommend eating five to six small meals each day rather than two or three larger ones. Another idea is to eat most of your food during the day, when your activity levels are highest. That might make it less likely that you will overindulge at dinnertime.

Now, what about some of the diets highly promoted by their authors?

Low-fat diets. These have been the staple of diet programs for decades, ever since fats got such a bad reputation. But overall, there is no good evidence they work for the long haul. Many people simply substitute high-calorie carbohydrates instead; look at the labels on many low-fat foods and snacks and you will be astounded at the number of calories they contain. Furthermore, these kinds of diets usually fail to make any distinction between good and bad fats, as discussed above. And as is true for all diets limiting your food choices, they usually fail to work over the long haul because we get bored with them.

Low-carbohydrate, high-protein and high-fat diets. These are currently among the most popular diets being hawked by authors. And like the low-fat diets, they often work in the short term. But there is no good evidence that they are any better than other diets over the long term. There is also reason for concern about their safety over the long term, given the potential danger of saturated fats for the heart and large amounts of protein for the kidneys.

Diets based on the glycemic concept. As you will recall from reading the section on carbohydrates, there is great interest in the idea that carbohydrates can be distinguished in terms of how quickly they are digested into simple sugars—and therefore their impact on the insulin system. When it comes to weight control, the use of this concept goes something like this: Quickly digested foods cause a sudden spike in blood sugar, which produces a sudden spike in insulin, which leads to a lower blood sugar, which causes renewed hunger. Therefore, the theory goes, a diet built around lower glycemic foods would miminize this self-defeating cycle. Quite frankly, this concept seems to make more sense to me than some other diet theories. But it has not been proven to be superior in rigorous fashion over the long term.

In fact, no special diet has been proven to be predictably successful for most people over the long term. Any diet that works will do so only if it results in lower calorie intake and/or increased exercise on a permanent basis! Indeed, I am willing to flatly state that no diet program will work in the long run unless it is combined with an increase in exercise. And there are two reasons for that statement. One is that exercise obviously can help in "burning" calories—and that's always important. But, second, exercise by definition builds muscle—and muscle tissue is very important to weight control because muscle tissue tends to use more energy than other tissues, even during rest. So to the extent that we increase muscle tissue and replace fat with muscle, we are "building a better furnace" in terms of burning calories.

At this point, I could offer you a standard list of diet tips (eat small portions, avoid desserts, chew thoughtfully, etc.) that would apply to any diet. But I have so come to believe that exercise is really the key to long-term weight loss that I am going to avoid those tips and trust your own judgment to start selecting better foods based on what you have learned so far—and move instead to a discussion of exercise, the subject of the next chapter.

CHAPTER 2

Fitness for Men

The (Modern) Basics: Why and How

For decades, fitness in men was equated with not being fat. If your belly hung over your belt or you could "pinch an inch" you were unfit. Then, in the 1970s, gyms began featuring an amazing array of equipment and workouts. Images of fit people became more varied—from stick-thin marathon runners possessing incredible aerobic capacities to bodybuilders with bulky, rippled physiques and nearly nonexistent body fat. There seemingly was a fitness choice for every man, depending on his preference.

But what image is the most healthful? What regimen is most likely to benefit the weekend warrior who's trying to squeeze fitness into his daily life? That's where science enters the picture. Over the last two decades researchers have been cranking up their treadmills and wading through years of lifetime data trying to answer a few basic questions. First, which type of exercise is correlated with longer life in men? Second, which fitness program helps stave off the chronic and disabling diseases of middle age and beyond, like heart disease, arthritis, diabetes, and cancer?

The Dallas-based Cooper Institute, which coined the word aerobics, meaning "with air," has made major contributions to these discussions. They have concluded that aerobic fitness—the ability of your heart, lungs, and circulatory system to supply fresh, oxygen-rich blood to muscles and organs—is a lot more important than special body shape. And fortunately, the fitness effort the Institute recommends to begin heading off diseases is quite minimal. They say you need to exercise enough to burn the calories expended in a brisk 30-minute walk every day

There is, of course, a very practical connection between body size and aerobic fitness. If you're significantly overweight or actually obese, you are going to find it much more difficult to do an aerobic activity, because there's simply a lot more of you to move. So, if you currently weigh more than your ideal weight, it's a good idea to consider the suggestions made in Chapter 1 to start shedding the pounds while beginning an aerobic workout regimen.

Your aerobic capacity isn't the only ingredient in the recipe for fitness. Another component is strength. Your doctor knows this. That's why you're often greeted with a handshake when you come in for a checkup. By gauging the strength of your grip, your doctor can get a quick, easy read of your approximate muscle tone. Researchers at the Honolulu Heart Project, who followed a group of men for more than 20 years, discovered that those with the greatest grip strength (they used a mechanical grip-strength testing device at regular checkups) had the lowest risk of death regardless of how much they weighed. The men in the top 25 percent for grip strength in middle age had a two-and-a-half to three times better chance of staying free of chronic illnesses and disabilities as they aged. And you don't increase strength solely through aerobic workouts. You have to lift free weights, get to know the resistance-providing training machines at your health club, or do exercises that use your body weight for resistance. Push-ups, pull-ups, and even athletic forms of yoga can make you significantly stronger.

If you're doing aerobic exercise and strength training, you may think you have a well-rounded fitness regimen, but it's still missing one key ingredient: flexibility. As you age, your tendons (which connect your muscles to your bones), ligaments (the tissue that connects bones to bones and prevents joint dislocation), and the sheaths that bind the muscle fibers together (the myofascia) become more rigid. That's one reason you lose mobility and range of motion. It's also why men, as they age, find themselves injuring their Achilles tendons, lower backs, shoulders, hamstrings, and feet. To prevent these common injuries and keep yourself limber, a good full-body stretching program at least two to three times a week is critical. If you're doing an aerobic or strength training workout, make time to stretch for at least 5 to 10 minutes afterwards when your muscles are warm. If you're just stretching, be sure to warm up for 5 minutes doing calisthenics or light aerobics and then stretch. (Although it's tempting to save time by skipping the warm-up, don't. You'll increase your risk of injury if you try to stretch cold muscles.)

The bad news is that men typically have tight muscles. The good news is whether that tightness comes from lack of stretching or because of genetically-determined structure (short connective tissue, for example), regular stretching can promote permanent gains in flexibility.

Real-World Workout

The idea of a one-size-fits-all workout is, in a word, fantasy. Your own level of fitness, strength, and flexibility will determine how you need to start. And your goals will direct your progress. Any certified trainer at a reputable gym can help you put together a sensible program, but here are a few guidelines:

- Any activity using large muscle groups can be aerobic, from walking to skiing. What matters is that you get your heart working harder than it does at rest and that you keep your heart rate elevated for at least 30 minutes, ideally every day. The target for aerobic benefit should be about 70 to 80 percent of the maximum heart rate predicted for your age. You can roughly calculate your maximum heart rate by subtracting your age from 220. Seventy percent of that number will give you a good starting target rate to maintain during an aerobic workout *(see page 52 for more on target heart rate)*. As discussed below, three 10-minute periods of aerobic exercise may be as effective as one 30-minute period.
- Working with weights and machines is not so simple. Using progressively heavier weights with fewer repetitions best develops muscle *strength*. Muscular *endurance*—the ability of your muscles to work for long periods of time before they become fatigued—comes with using lighter weight and doing a greater number of repetitions. Both are important to help you tackle real-life situations. As you age and lose muscle strength, doing more reps with lower weights becomes more sensible for most men, but you need to take your own goals and past fitness history into account before you decide what approach to take. However you do it, using good form is critical. One moment of sloppy lifting or trying to lift too much, too soon, can leave you sidelined for weeks or months.
- At some point along the way you're going to be faced with the question of how many sets, reps, and exercises to do—and you'll hear many sound yet conflicting theories about this. Fortunately, one of the simplest and most efficient ways to train is also the best for a maturing body. Pick 10 exercises that work your

major muscles. (Hint: Start with the legs, then move up to the chest and back before finishing with shoulders, arms, and abs.) Do one set of each for approximately 10 to 12 reps. Lift slowly (take two seconds or more to lift and the same to lower). But then hustle to get to your next exercise. Don't rest between sets. This works your whole body in less than 45 minutes and helps keep your heart rate elevated so you get a mild aerobic benefit as well. In contrast, training your body in parts (that is, legs one day, back and biceps another, etc.), as *bodybuilders* often do, interferes with the critical resting process, which is when your muscles actually get stronger—not while exercising. Overtraining can leave you feeling weak and worn out.

The American College of Sports Medicine recommends "working out" three to five days a week. If you can, manage five sessions a week; three aerobic and two strength workouts each week make a good mix—but listen to your body if you need extra rest or want to substitute a yoga class for a typical workout. The College also says each aerobic workout should last between 30 and 45 minutes. However, data from the National Runner's Health Study shows that more can be better. Specifically, researchers found that men who ran more than 40 miles a week had a significantly lower risk of heart disease than those who ran 10 miles a week. But not everyone is built for running long distance, so don't compromise your skeletal health for aerobic capacity. What good is a healthy heart if years of pounding leave you unable to walk? Consider lower impact alternatives such as swimming, walking, cycling, or rowing.

The trouble is, most of us find it difficult to squeeze in even 10 miles a week (or its aerobic equivalent), let alone 40, and study after study has confirmed the fact that consistency is key. Even the most flawless workout plan won't help you achieve your fitness and health goals if you can't stick with it, and pie-in-the-sky exercise plans are notoriously difficult to stick with.

Studies show that about 30 percent of men quit their fitness programs within 20 weeks. Lowering your expectations and decreasing the intensity of your workouts, at least at the beginning of your program, may help combat the mental and physical fatigue that leads to frustration. It is also very helpful if you can combine your exercise with your interests. The enjoyment factor is especially important as you age, when competitive sports typically play a diminishing role in most men's lives. Even golf will boost your fitness level as long as you walk around the course. (Walking a typical 18-hole course covers some five to six miles.) Carry your own bag and you'll add a bonus "resistance training" element to your outing, providing your back can take it.

Now that you know the general profile of a well-designed fitness program, let's take a closer look at the three major components of fitness: muscle strength, flexibility, and aerobic stamina.

Exercise Equipment

For anyone just starting out at the gym, I know how intimidating the seemingly endless array of equipment can be. But rest assured: Those machines are not nearly as complicated as they look. What follows is an overview of the two major categories of fitness equipment: cardio/aerobic and strength training. It's always a good idea to read the instructional placard and/or ask for a demonstration when using an exercise machine for the first time!

Cardio machines tend to mimic everyday activities, and as a result are almost always very easy to use. (A treadmill, for example, simulates walking, jogging, and running.) Most modern cardio machines are also equipped with computers and software, allowing users to customize their workouts and keep track of calories burned, distance traveled, heart rate, and so on.

One drawback to cardio machines is boredom. Sitting on a stationary bike in a gym for half an hour is just not the same as bicycling through the park. So if you find boredom to be a problem, you might consider taking along a portable CD player or a good book or magazine the next time you work out.

Here are a few of the most popular kinds of cardio equipment:

- Treadmills
- Stationary bikes (upright & recumbent)
- Cross-country ski machines
- Stair climbers
- Rowers (a.k.a. erg machines)
- Elliptical machines

Strength training machines come in two basic forms. With a selectorized machine, you set the resistance level by inserting a pin into one of several holes in a stack of weights. Because they predefine your motion, and because you are isolated from the weight stack by a system of cables and pulleys, selectorized machines are relatively easy to operate and require no spotting.

With a plate-loaded machine, on the other hand, you set the resistance by attaching weighted plates to "horns" on the machine's movement arms. Like selectorized machines, plate-loaded machines predefine your motion, but they are also similar to free weights, in that they can support very heavy loads and you can also adjust the resistance in very small increments.

Here are some common types of strength training machines:

- Back extension
- Pectoral fly
- Hip adduction/abduction
- Lateral pulldown/raise
- Chest press
- Hack squat
- Preacher curl
- Abdominal crunch
- Leg press/curl

Five Major Muscle Groups and How to Train Them

Muscles aren't just for show. Scientifically speaking, lifting free weights or using resistance machines results in increased lean muscle mass, and the more lean muscle mass you develop, the higher your basal metabolic rate (BMR) will be. That means you'll burn more calories even while your body is at rest—all day long. It also means it will be easier to maintain your weight and, therefore, easier to stave off the usual weight gain (and resulting health problems) that occur with age.

Again, I would stress the importance of starting a weight training program under the guidance of a certified trainer. In general, for each specific muscle group, you should try to lift the maximum amount you can with good form, for about 10 reps, so your muscles are fatigued by the end of each set. Once you're able to lift

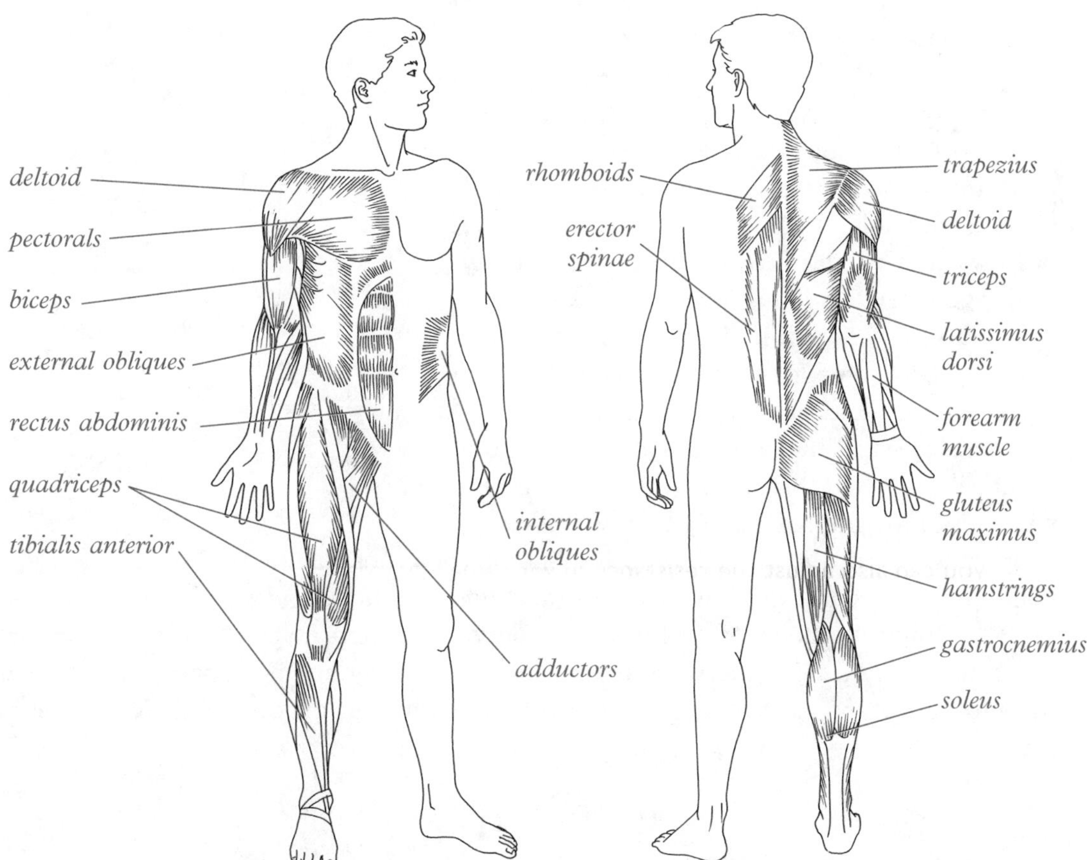

your current weight without straining toward the end of the set, increase the weight or resistance slightly, no more than 10 percent at a time. (Likewise, don't hesitate to lower the weight by 10 percent at the end of a set so that you can complete the exercise with good form. This is called a "drop set." You start a set with heavier weight for a few reps and lighten the weight as you go—a good alternative when you can't lift the heavier weight for the whole set.) Remember to exhale as you lift or resist and inhale while releasing the weight or resistance. The following is a general overview of exercises for five basic muscle groups. Your trainer will help you learn how to do these properly.

1. Primetime Legwork: For knees, ankles, quads, hamstrings, and glutes (gluteus)

The step-back dumbbell lunge

If you're looking for a time-saving, cross training type of move to strengthen the major muscles of the legs (and lower torso), you need not look any farther than the dumbbell lunge. An excellent supplement to leg exercises performed on resistance machines, including leg presses and leg curls, the lunge is easy to do anywhere. The difference with this lunge is you step back instead of forward. The step-forward lunge is a stability-challenge even for young knees that haven't yet worn out. For prime time knees it's even harder. The step back version gives legs a good workout while sparing the delicate knee joints.

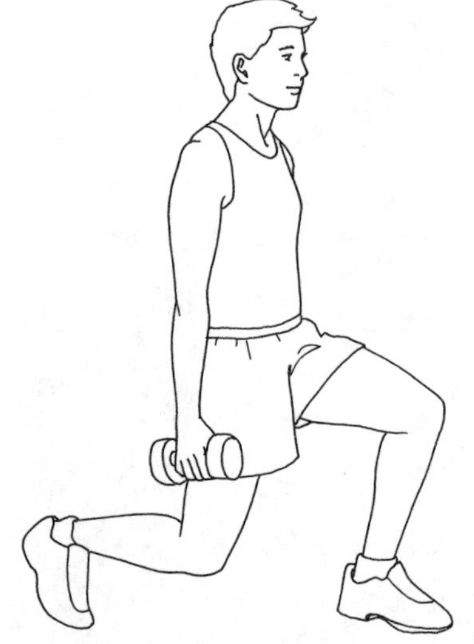

Start by standing with a 10- to 15-pound dumbbell in each hand. Step backward with your right foot, approximately two feet. Keeping your right heel up (step back onto the ball of your foot), allow both your knees to bend until your right thigh is nearly parallel with the floor and your left knee is almost touching the floor. Hold for two seconds, then step forward into the starting position. Try not to let the weights or your torso swing as you lunge. Lunge with the left leg and repeat until you've performed 10 lunges on each side. Work your way up to 15 lunges with each leg.

2. The Lower Torso: For abdominals, obliques, hips, and lower back

The knee rock—side to side

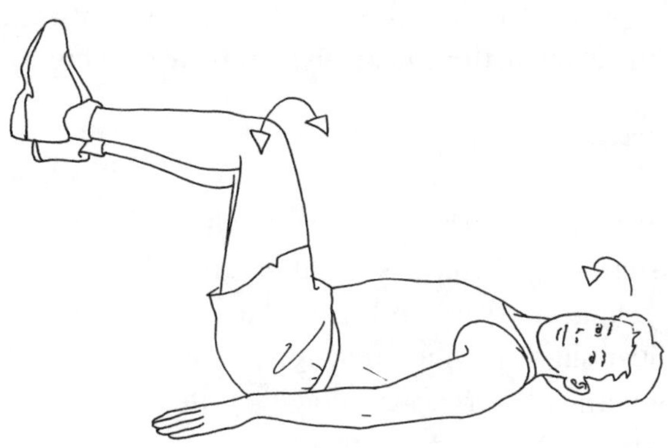

The "knee rock" involves the muscles of your lower torso, from your abs and back muscles through your hip joints, which often become tight and inflexible as you age. Start by lying on the floor, face up with your arms extended to the sides and your pelvis and lower back pressed to the floor. (Slide your hand underneath your lower back to check your press-down "progress.")

Next, bend your legs, bringing your knees to a 90-degree bend, with toes pointing up. Hold for a one count, then gently rock your knees to the right as you turn your shoulders and head to the left. Use the muscles of your hips and spine to initiate the move and allow your legs to follow. Hold for 10 to 30 seconds. Repeat, alternating sides. Work your way up to 10 rocks on each side.

3. The Back: For "lats" (muscles that form the triangular wings of a strong, V-shaped torso), upper back, and rear delts (shoulders)

The dumbbell row

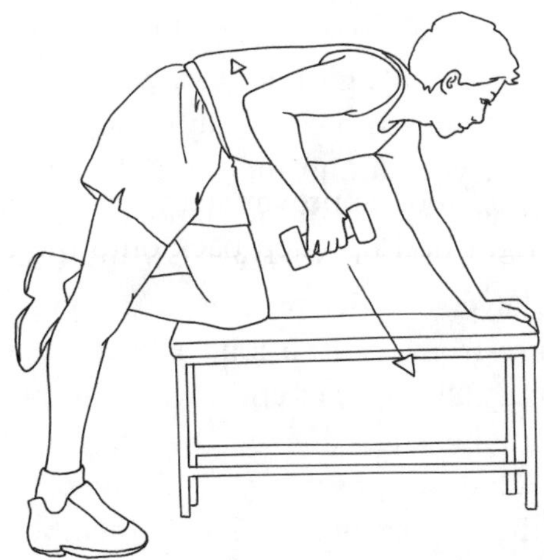

Using a bench and dumbbells, you can easily strengthen some of the most vulnerable real estate on the adult male body—the back muscles involved in twisting and turning motions. Start by resting your left knee and left hand on the bench. Your back should be nearly parallel with the floor, and the lower back should be just slightly arched—and definitely not rounded. Maintaining that "neutral spine" both helps contract your back muscles and protects the vertebrae in your spine. Holding the dumbbell with your right hand, slowly bend and pull your elbow up and back toward your right hip. Your elbow should end up above your back. Be sure to lift the weight with your big back muscles—and not just your shoulders. Think of this more like a bowling motion (an under-hand move) as opposed to a shrug. Squeeze the back muscles at the top of the lift and slowly lower.

The lat pull-down

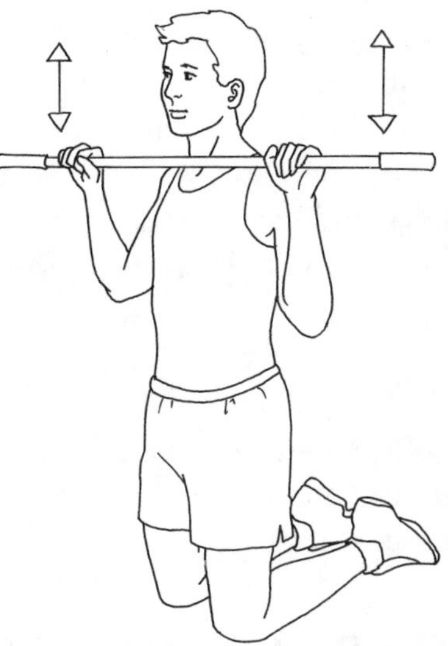

If you're using resistance machines at your gym, the *lat pull-down* is another great back exercise. Using an overhand grip, hands in line with or just slightly wider than your shoulders, pull the overhead bar down slowly, until it grazes your chest. (You can do this whle standing or kneeling.) As the bar touches your chest, arch your upper back slightly while holding in your belly and stabilizing your lower back. The key to doing this properly is to consciously engage the back muscles as you pull the bar. Don't make the mistake of using your arms only. Try 8 to 12 reps with a comfortable weight.

4. The Upper Body: For arms, pecs, and shoulders

The bench press

The "bench press," a health club standard, is a valuable upper body strength builder. It adds girth and strength to the broad pectoral muscles of your chest, the front of your shoulders, and your triceps. (Plus, it's great for confidence building, because you can lift more weight while lying down on a bench than you can while standing.) Although the standard barbell bench press can be a great exercise if you know how to do it properly, it's not the best place to start if you're a beginner or if you have shoulder problems. In gyms there are so many bench press machines to choose from, you no longer have to simply bench press free weights. Also, if you want a full-rounded chest workout, be sure to switch between the flat, incline, and decline benches.

Whatever position you find yourself in, and whatever equipment you use, here are the important things to remember in all bench presses. Sit or lie back so that

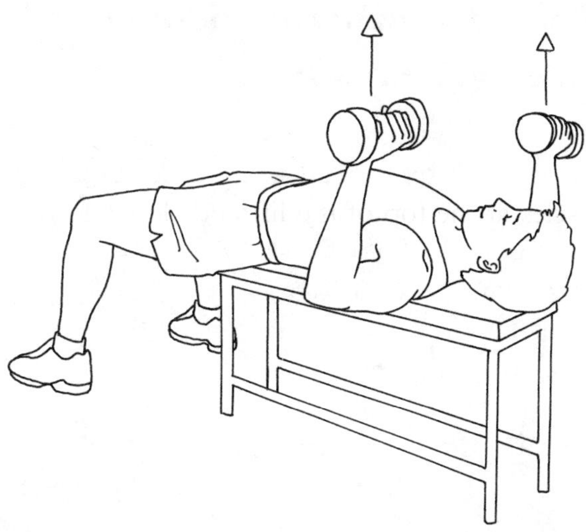

the lower back remains in a small and natural arch. In other words, don't press your lower back flat on the bench. That collapses the chest muscles (i.e., prevents them from contracting properly—defeating the exercise), puts pressure on the discs in your lower back, and tends to throw the work load into the shoulders and not the chest.

Lift the handle, barbell, or dumbbell slowly from chest level (not below because that's hard on shoulder joints) to the point where your elbows are almost (not quite fully) extended. Be careful not to lock the elbows or throw your shoulders forward. Here's the secret of a great bench press: As you lift the weight, also lift your chest! Then lower, just as slowly. A reasonable goal for beginners: 8 to 10 repetitions two to three times a week, starting with nearly half your body weight and working up to 66 percent of your body weight. When you're working with heavy free weights that are difficult for you to lift, always use a "spotter" (partner) to help you with the barbell to prevent injury.

The standing flye

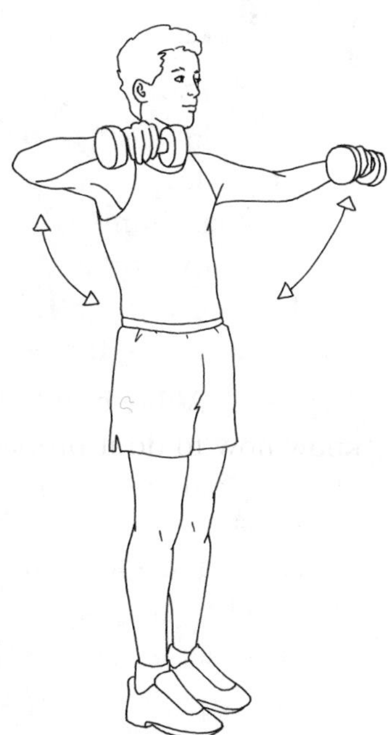

The "standing flye" is great for building shoulder strength. Done improperly, however, or with too heavy a weight, this exercise can damage the very vulnerable rotator cuff—the four small muscles that lift and rotate your arm (you use these when you serve in tennis or volleyball, throw a ball, or swing a golf club). While standing, with arms down and holding light (10-pound) dumbbells, bend your elbows to 45 degrees, and slowly raise the weights to shoulder level (as if you're flapping your wings), but not above—or you'll impinge the delicate shoulder joint and compromise those rotators. Lower slowly as well. Since this is best done with light weight, do as many as 15 reps.

5. The Abdomen: For abdominals

Bicycle legs with twist

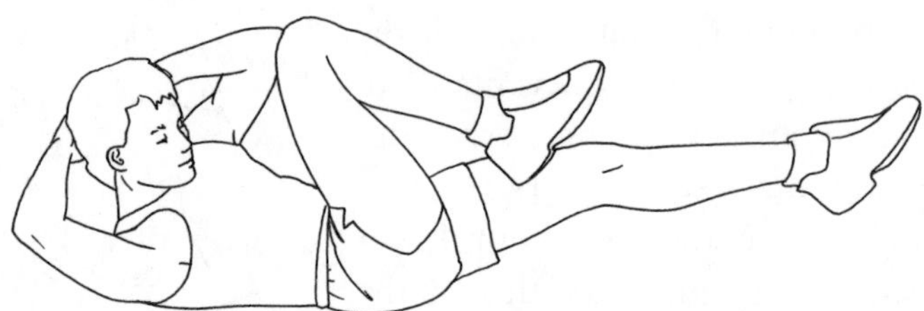

Time to update the old-fashioned sit-up. Studies have shown that the bicycle motion is one of the most effective "ab" exercises because it engages a big percentage of your abdominal muscle fibers. Lie down, place your hands behind your neck with elbows open, bend your knees, and put your feet on the floor. Next, extend one leg in the air. (Hint: The straighter and lower your extended leg, the harder this will be. Work within your range of ability.) Then, keep your other foot on the ground and try to "meet it" in the air with the opposing elbow. (Don't worry about touching at first; close is good enough.) Don't lunge as you curl up. Keep the motion smooth and controlled. Repeat the motion with the other knee and elbow. Work your way up to 15 on each side.

Stretching

In general, men are less flexible than women, a situation that sets us up for a variety of problems when we age—from the old-man shuffle (the result of too-tight hip flexor muscles) to low back pain and other irritating body aches. That's why we stand to gain so much by adding stretching to our routines. (By the way, one of the best flexibility workouts available is yoga.)

Much of our "inflexibility" may be in our "heads," or maybe in our genetic makeup, a relic of the fight or flight response in which we men tend to hold tension in our hips, gluteal muscles, and hamstrings (the big muscles at the backs of our legs) as if poised to spring away at any moment. When our body is in that forward-leaning position, it makes our back work harder than it has to, especially if we're carrying a load or performing exercises (like squats) that place a load on our spine. The result: low back pain and other back problems.

Stretching can help you overcome this inherent tendency, but most people—men especially—tend to skimp on this facet of their workouts. By committing to a flexibility routine, however, you can actually prevent injuries that can sideline you in later years and instead continue to use your body more fully, because you'll maintain greater range of motion in your muscles and joints.

That's why stretching is now routine for all athletes—and should be a routine for all of us. Most mainstream coaches and athletic trainers teach stretches that are derived from yoga poses, whether the athletes realize it or not. Some trainers offer a flexibility assessment, which can help determine which parts of your body need particular attention. Often, they are areas that suffered some previous injury or repeated insult—the torn rotator cuff from a ski trip several years back, the football injury from college, the stiff back from too many hours of staring at a computer screen. The best trainers will help you stretch out by pushing your limbs farther than you could take them yourself, though it's not a good idea to let an untrained person do this for you, because it could result in injury. I personally have found using a stretching machine very helpful in doing systematic and safe stretching; I ordered a machine for under $500 that I saw advertised in a magazine and it has worked well for me.

There are literally hundreds of stretching exercises. The best program will incorporate stretches for all of your main muscle groups. We've listed a number of good options on the next three pages. Whichever you use, here are some things to keep in mind.

Don't stretch when you're cold. Many people hurt themselves by launching into a vigorous stretch without warming up first. A cold muscle doesn't have a lot of give and if you try to force it, you may end up straining a muscle or tearing a ligament instead. (That's why yoga studios are usually kept at 80 degrees Fahrenheit or warmer.) Before you stretch, walk or jog slowly for a few minutes to get your body warm and the blood flowing to your muscles.

Breathe like you mean it. Americans tend to break every activity into its component parts, so they'll stretch but not breathe. But breath control is an integral part of stretching (and yoga) because it helps you work your muscles more effectively. While you're stretching, make sure you continue to breathe deeply throughout the stretch. The resultant calm helps you relax all over and get more from each move.

Take it easy. Flexibility is relative and changes from day to day and hour to hour. You want to stretch muscle, not ligaments, and you have to do so slowly. (Yogis talk about "embracing the bone," by which they mean contracting the muscle, becoming aware of its whole length before trying to elongate it.) Eventually, with regular stretching, your muscles will stay looser and more flexible. But you can overstretch, too, which makes ligaments about as useful as a stretched out elastic band. There are plenty of karate black belts who were once proud of the splits they could do and are now hobbling around like old men.

10 Great Stretches

Here are 10 stretches that will help keep you limber throughout your life. Since I have introduced stretching into my exercise routine, I have noticed much more flexibility in my body for everyday activities such as turning my neck to check oncoming traffic at an intersection. I actually use a stretching machine used by many golfers and advertised in golfing magazines. I find the machine routine, which I do in about 5 minutes after my usual 25 minutes on my cross-country machine, is a very easy and organized way to stretch all my major muscle groups. However, you can accomplish the same goal with simple exercises, such as the following. These stretches focus on the body parts where men hold the most tension—the hips, back and hamstrings. Remember to warm up before you stretch, and be careful not to push your muscles too far.

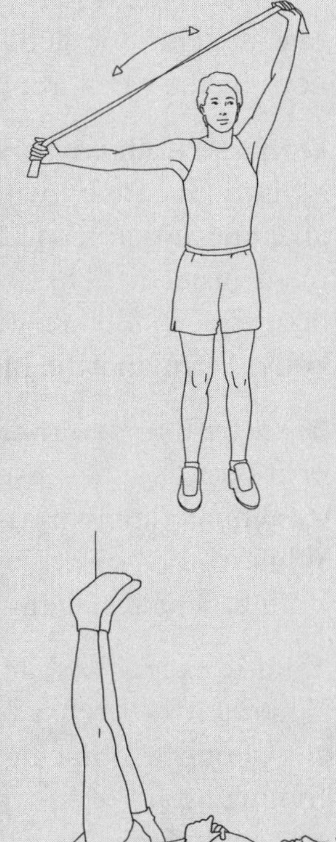

1. Shoulder Stretch. Hold a belt or necktie above your head with your elbows straight and your hands about shoulder-width apart. Keep your wrists straightened and pull gently without gripping so tightly that your knuckles turn white. Hold for at least 10 seconds (that's how long muscles need to stretch with any significance). Hold it for 30 seconds to a minute if you want even more flexibility; improvements tend to diminish after that. Then, widen your grip on the belt and, while maintaining the pull, allow one hand to drop slowly behind you to about waist height. Raise both hands and allow the other hand to drop behind you, to about waist height. Finally, lower both hands behind you and hold the stretch. You should feel your shoulder blades opening.

2. Hamstring and Back Stretch. Lie with your back flat on the floor and your legs up against a wall. You may not be able to straighten your legs completely. Just straighten them until you feel a gentle stretch in your back and hamstrings. This is a more passive stretch than the hamstring stretch with the belt that follows—and a great starter hamstring stretch. To deepen the stretch, lie inside an open doorway, with your leg up on the wall. To increase the stretch, scoot yourself further out the door, toward your feet, as you leave your leg up against the wall. Easy does it, though.

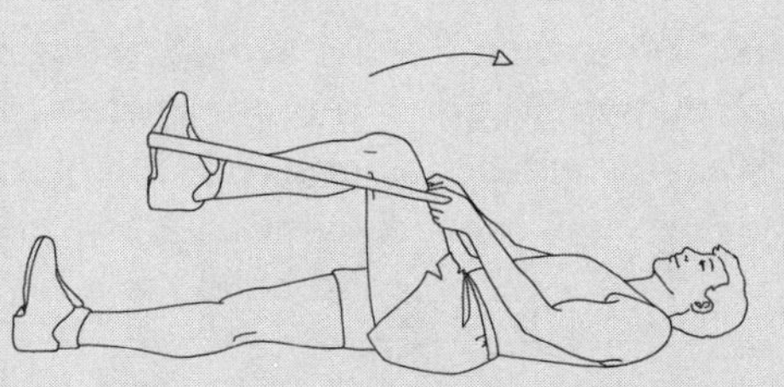

3. Hamstring Stretch with Belt. While lying on your back, keep your right leg straight on the floor and hug your left knee to your chest. Loop a belt around your left foot at the base of your toes. Straighten your left leg and pull on the belt so the foot comes over your chest or head. (If your lower back tightens and arches as you raise your left leg, bend your right knee and rest the right foot on the floor.) This is one of the best hamstring stretches you can do—better than the ones you do while standing. To add an inner thigh stretch, keep pulling on the belt while letting your left leg drift open to the outside. Then switch hands and lower the leg toward the inside to stretch the outer hip. Don't touch the foot to the floor; the point is not to reach all the way to the ground (which would lift the other leg off the ground) but to savor the stretches and increase your ability to balance in your torso.

While stretching, try to breathe into your abdomen so you feel your back expanding and contracting with each breath. You should feel the effects in your hips and back, quads and psoas (in the front of the hip), as well as in your hamstrings. Repeat on the other side.

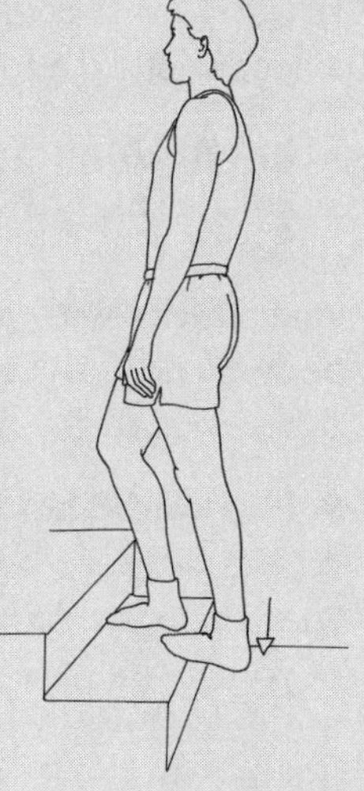

4. Calf Stretch. Facing a step, with your right foot firmly on the step, arrange your left foot so that the front half of the foot is on the edge of the step, with the back half hanging off the edge. Once you're balanced, let the left heel drop so that you feel the stretch in the back of your left leg. Don't bounce—just maintain the stretch for 10 to 30 seconds. Then switch and stretch the right leg.

5. Spine Stretch. Lie flat on your back with your legs straight, toes pointed, and arms stretched overhead, palms together. Gently rock your arms up and down in a short 8- to 12-inch arc. You'll feel your spine stretching between the shoulder blades.

6. Downward Facing Dog. Starting on your hands and knees, raise your butt so that your body forms an upside-down V. Try to straighten your spine so that your lower back is not rounded. If you have tight hamstrings, you probably won't be able to put your heels on the floor right away. To build flexibility at a sensibile pace in this position, bend one knee and straighten the other leg, easing the heel toward the ground. Hold for 10 seconds and alternate. Let the weight of your upper body rest at the base of your fingers, not the palm of your hands. Yogis call this "downward facing dog."

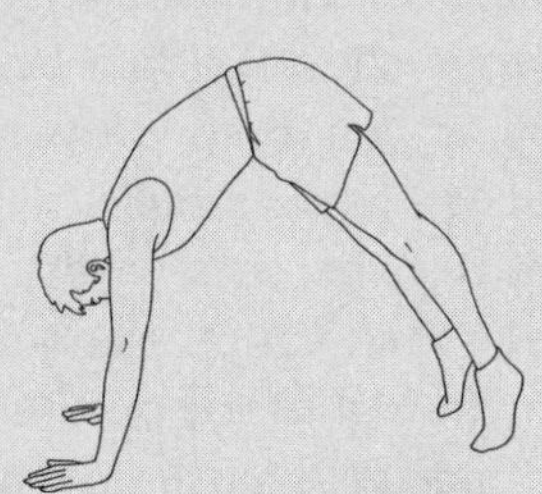

7. Achilles Stretch. Bend one knee and step back with the other leg to get into a lunge position, with your front foot between your hands and your back leg slightly bent or straight and perpendicular to the floor. Relax the back hip. Lower your shoulder toward the ground if you'd like to add a deeper stretch for the groin. Repeat on the other side.

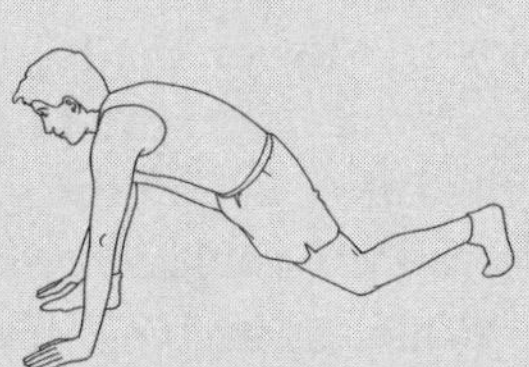

8. Inner Thigh Stretch. Sit up straight on the floor and place the soles of your feet together in front of you. Wrap your hands around your ankles and gently push down on your thighs with your elbows. Avoid tensing your upper body to do this. Let gravity and the weight of your elbows open your thighs.

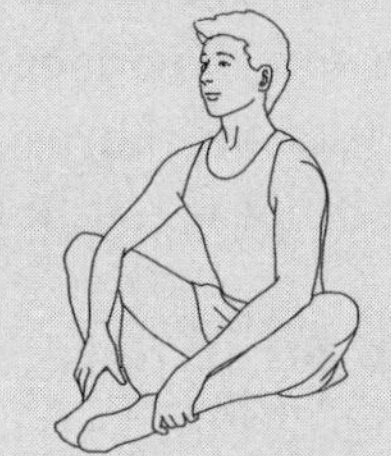

9. Hip and Back Stretch. Sit comfortably cross-legged on the floor with your right leg on top of your left. Lean your upper body forward and walk your arms out in front of you. If you have enough flexibility, place both elbows on the floor. Lean forward until you feel a gentle stretch in the hips and back, then stop. Reverse your legs, placing the left leg on top, and repeat.

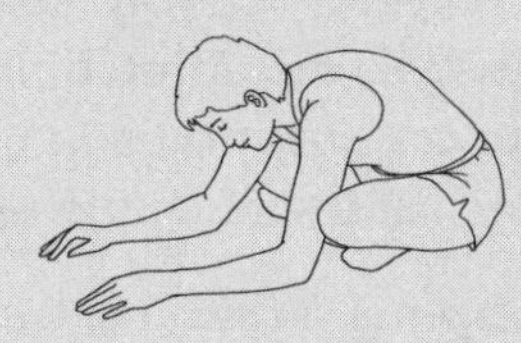

10. Twister Stretch. Sit on the floor with your right leg in front of you and your left leg bent, left foot flat on the floor on the outside of your right knee. Place your left hand behind you and twist at your waist away from your knee. If you can, place your right arm on the outside of your left knee. Repeat on the other side.

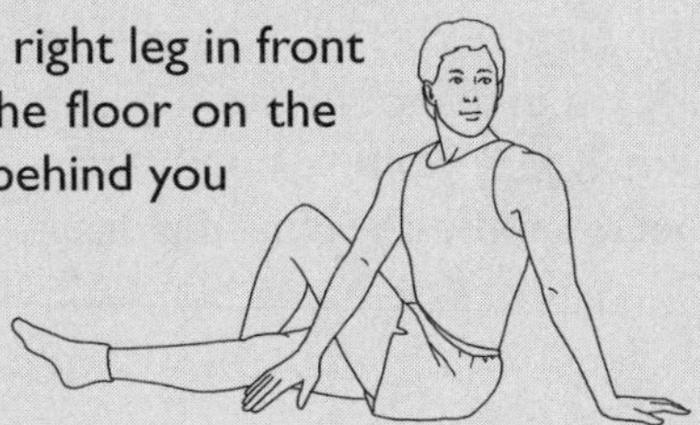

Don't even think about competing. On a recent television sit-com, a pair of male characters talked about attending yoga class together. One pointed a finger at the other, and in an aggressive voice blurted out, "I'll kick your ass in yoga!" It was a comic moment, but like most such moments bore a lot of truth. Men tend to look for the end goal, thinking about reaching the floor with their fingertips rather than about how tight their legs and back are as they reach. Stretching is not a competitive event, and if you try to make it one, chances are you'll injure yourself.

Let yourself relax. Stretching is the yin to the strength-training yang. Instead of pushing yourself into a stretch, allow yourself to relax into it, going only as far as your body can comfortably go. (Don't ever bounce or do ballistic stretches.) Then breathe. You'll be amazed at how rejuvenated you feel when you're done.

Hold each stretch 20 to 30 seconds. By staying in a stretch for that long, you give your muscles time to respond and lengthen. Any shorter time and you may be wasting your time.

Aerobic Conditioning

You undoubtedly know that aerobic exercise is good for your heart. Evidence that this message has reached the masses is everywhere. The streets of cities and towns are often filled with joggers and bikers. Senior citizens dutifully plod through shopping malls before opening hours. Bare-chested doctors rollerblade the beachside trails in Venice Beach and businessmen race up and down the urban mountain trails in Vail at sunset. OK—I've painted an "exuberant" picture, but it's not too far from the truth.

Cardio work, as it's known in health club parlance, isn't just good for your heart. It also helps keep your body weight and body fat in check, probably boosts your immune system, helps your body process blood sugar, and helps lower your blood pressure and cholesterol levels. That's a very impressive list of benefits.

There are countless ways you can get a cardiovascular workout, from health club machines (think: upright and recumbent stationary bikes, treadmills, rowing machines, skiing machines, elliptical trainers, and stair steppers) to aerobic fitness and dance classes. And that doesn't include the wonderful outdoor options, like running, biking, hiking, swimming, and walking. With so many to choose from, you may wonder if there's a "right" aerobic exercise for you. The answer: Whatever you enjoy enough to do safely and regularly is the right workout for you.

The American College of Sports Medicine suggests that you perform 30 to 45 minutes of continuous aerobic exercise three to five days a week, at 60 to 90 percent of your maximum heart rate. Recent studies show that resistance training also confers some cardiovascular benefit, and it's more efficient than aerobic exercise in maintaining lean body mass.

There's good news from more recent research for men who are short on time, too: You don't need to get your aerobic exercise in one long session in order to reap the heart-strengthening benefits. You can further your heart health by taking advantage of aerobic opportunities in everyday life—walking to work, taking the stairs, even working hard in the yard. As mentioned earlier, research has shown that three 10-minute exercise sessions can be as beneficial as one 30-minute session. For many people, brisk walking (3 to 4 miles per hour) for a total of 30 minutes per day is an ideal way to exercise.

The million-dollar question for most busy people is this: How do you stay committed to an exercise program for the long term? That's where enjoyment comes into the equation. Studies have shown that the trait most devoted exercisers share is a love of their chosen activity. For some men this means a health club regimen with a heart monitor and a notebook. For others, it's a meditative run at sunrise or an after-work mountain-bike ride. Others still will find that a brisk lunchtime walk suits their needs best. I have found that first thing in the morning at home on a cross-country machine while watching the news works best for me; once I shower for the day, I seem to lose interest in formal exercise.

Another approach that might keep you motivated and on track is finding an exercise partner. Many cities have swimming programs for adults or running clubs that provide not only company but also structured routines to help you meet your fitness goals. Even a next-door neighbor or someone you pair up with at the gym can serve to boost your commitment, as long as you enjoy their company and share common fitness goals.

Before you launch a full-scale fitness program, ask yourself some questions. Do you like (or loathe) competition? Are you a gadget guy, who likes to know exactly how many calories he's burned or miles he's walked? Do you enjoy the outdoors? What activities did you like best as a child? Are you a joiner or a lone ranger? And, perhaps most importantly, what are your fitness goals? Do you want to lose weight? Improve your cardiovascular health? Have more energy? Buff up? There's almost certainly a program already in place that's tailor-made for someone like you. And if there's not, there are plenty of exercise trainers who are qualified to help you create an individual program. They can also teach you how to make any exercise program as safe and efficient as possible.

I believe it's a good idea to see your doctor for a stress test before starting a new exercise program, especially past age 50. Such a test will tell you how fit you really are and it should also detect any heart irregularities that would preclude vigorous exercise. A stress test report will include the maximum number of METS that you were able to achieve during your test. (METS are the standard way of expressing energy expenditures during various activities.) Many studies now show that the higher your MET number, the better your chances of living longer—giving new meaning to the phrase "survival of the fittest." For example, a recent study showed that men with a MET level of 5 or less on their stress test had twice the risk of dying during the next 6 years as men with MET levels of 8 or more. The good news is that if your MET level is low, you can increase it with regular aerobic exercise. Studies show that such exercise can increase fitness levels by 15 to 30 percent within 3 to 6 months.

Know Your Limits

There's another fitness issue that often crops up for men, and it's this urge that many of us have to push ourselves to our physical limits, to go faster or farther than we went yesterday (or at least faster and farther than the guy down the street). It raises the question: Can you be fit without being so driven? And where should you draw the line? The reality is you can feel good after a 15-minute bike ride or run. It's not necessary to hammer away at it for 45 minutes, especially if your body isn't up to it. Overtraining can actually cause you to lose fitness.

Fitness should be about health, first and foremost. It's easy to lose sight of that when we get caught up in the frenzy of competition. And health clubs may inadvertently feed our need to compare ourselves to other guys by surrounding us with mirrors. It's surprising how tough it is to steer clear of the "I-can-press-more-weight-than-he-can" frenzy when you're regularly a part of that environment. But it's important to try, because there's more than the size of your biceps at stake.

As healthy as exercise is, it carries a risk of injury. High-impact activities like running are hard on your hips and knees. Lifting free weights, which certainly looks more macho than using the resistance machines, also carries a higher price tag if you perform exercises incorrectly or let your form falter as you get tired. The reality is, if you're a driven, type A exercise fanatic, you may be pushing yourself so hard that you aren't able to perform at your peak. Many exercise trainers have men scale back their routines and their weights in order to train properly and therefore get the most from their bodies. Your muscles need rest and recovery time, and your body needs to be treated with respect in order to perform well for you for years to come. The bonus: If you train "smart" instead of just training "hard," it can make you faster, stronger, and healthier.

All that said, injuries do happen, which is why I've included the following section.

Sports-Related Injuries and Concerns

The only real down side to exercise—injury—can typically be prevented with attention to form and a consciousness about your body's abilities and limitations. What follows is a run-down of the most common sports-related injuries, with advice on how to prevent and treat them.

Athlete's Foot

Your body normally plays host to a variety of different fungi, which don't cause any problems. But under certain conditions—like the damp, moist environment inside your shoes and socks—some types thrive. These fungi often set up camp on the outermost layer of skin on your foot, particularly between your toes, causing your skin to produce more cells than usual and making it thick and scaly. The resulting condition is commonly called athlete's foot. About 70 percent of people in the U.S. develop athlete's foot at least once in their lives, and the condition is more than twice as common in men than women, although scientists aren't certain why.

Keeping your feet clean and dry—and drying them thoroughly after showering or swimming—can help prevent a bout with a foot-loving fungus. Choose breathable cotton or wool socks over synthetic ones, which tend to trap heat and moisture next to your skin. If your feet sweat a lot, stick with natural-fiber shoes, like leather, and alternate your footwear on a daily basis to allow each pair to dry thoroughly between wearings. Antifungal or drying powders sprinkled inside your sock and shoe may be helpful if you're particularly prone to the problem. Because the fungi are contagious, wearing rubber thongs in public showers or swimming pools can help prevent the problem as well.

Your doctor will probably diagnose the problem based on your symptoms, which may include:

- Itching and stinging between your toes, particularly the fourth and fifth ones, or on the soles of your feet.
- Blisters on your toes or feet.
- Cracking and peeling or thickened skin.

- Foul odor.
- Thick, discolored toenails that seem to be pulling away from the nail bed.

If your doctor is uncertain of the diagnosis based on a visual exam, he may also want to examine skin scrapings or a fluid sample from your foot under a microscope, which can easily identify the fungus.

If you have a fairly mild case of athlete's foot, your doctor will probably recommend using an over-the-counter or prescription antifungal ointment, such as clotrimazole (Lotrimin) or terbinafine (Lamisil). More severe bouts might require a prescription oral medication, such as itraconazole (Sporanox), fluconazole (Diflucan), or terbinafine, but those drugs are under some scrutiny because they have been linked to rare cases of liver failure.

Bursitis

Bursae are tiny, fluid-filled sacs that provide cushioning and lubrication for the tendons and bones of many joints. When you overuse your joints by playing sports or put pressure on them, such as kneeling for a long time, these sacs can become inflamed and painful, creating a condition known as bursitis. It most commonly affects the joints in your shoulder, elbow, or hip. It is often associated with inflammation of associated tendons *(see Tendonitis on page 62)*. Although there are no good statistics on bursitis, the condition is common, particularly in young, active men.

You may be able to avoid a bout of bursitis by strengthening the muscles all over your body, which helps protect your joints, and taking frequent breaks from repetitive tasks.

Your doctor will most likely be able to diagnose bursitis based on your symptoms, which are primarily pain and inflammation in the affected joint, and a physical exam, which will reveal tender and swollen joints. Bursitis typically goes away within two weeks if you rest the injured joint and use over-the-counter nonsteroidal anti-inflammatories for the pain and inflammation. In rare cases, your doctor may need to remove fluid from the bursa with a needle or give you an injection of corticosteroids to tame the inflammation. Once the pain goes away, your doctor will probably start you on a muscle-strengthening program to avoid a repeat episode.

Jock Itch

The same fungus that infects your feet, causing athlete's foot, can become entrenched in the area under your jock strap or underwear for much the same reason: It's a sweaty, poorly ventilated area. Contrary to its name, jock itch doesn't just strike men or athletes. It affects up to 70 percent of the people in the U.S. at some point in their lives.

In order to avoid a bout of jock itch, you need to keep the area clean and dry. If your underwear becomes sweaty and damp, take it off and change into another pair. Wash workout clothes between wearings, and don't share towels, because you can catch it from someone else. And go for breathable cotton underwear instead of synthetic fibers that trap moisture next to your skin. When you're not exercising, wear boxer shorts, which are well ventilated.

Your doctor will diagnose the problem based on a physical exam and your symptoms, which include a raised, red, itchy rash on your upper thighs, buttocks, genitals, or groin that doesn't go away on its own. Apply over-the-counter antifungal creams, such as clotrimazole or tolnaftate.

Neck Pain

The average head weighs about nine pounds. That's as much as a bowling ball (sorry about that comparison), and your neck is required to carry it around all day! That's why it's easy for necks to get out of whack, especially if you're active, which places extra strain on the muscles and bones in the area. But even desk jockeys suffer from neck pain after long hours of sitting hunched over a computer. Neck pain probably strikes about 45 percent of men at some point in their lives.

Although neck pain may strike despite your best efforts, there are some things you can do to make it less likely. They include:

- Use good posture when you are walking and sitting. Your head should be sitting straight on top of your neck, not jutted forward, which strains the muscles along the back of your neck.
- Make sure your desk, chair, and computer are at the right height. Don't hold the telephone between your neck and shoulder for long periods, which can cause the muscles along that side of your neck to cramp up.
- Keep your neck loose by performing gentle stretches—roll your head slowly in a circle, for instance—several times a day.
- Don't sleep on your stomach, because it puts your neck at an awkward angle, and use a supportive pillow that allows your neck to lie at a natural, comfortable angle.

Usually, neck pain goes away on its own in a week or two. If it doesn't, see your doctor. He or she will ask you about your symptoms, which may include pain in the neck only or pain that radiates down your shoulders and arms. Your doctor will also ask about any numbness in your arms or hands, because that could indicate nerve damage, a more serious problem. He or she may also want to perform an imaging technique, like X-rays, magnetic resonance imaging (MRI), or computerized tomography (CT) scans to get a look at the discs in the area *(see Back Pain on page 184)*.

For pain that doesn't go away on its own, your doctor will probably recommend you take nonsteroidal anti-inflammatories to relieve the pain. He or she may prescribe something stronger if the pain is severe. Other treatment options include heat or ice, stretching, and strengthening. More severe cases may require transcutaneous electric nerve stimulation, in which tiny electrical impulses are delivered to the area via electrodes placed on your skin, or oral or injectable steroids.

Runner's Knee

Chondromalacia patellae, or runner's knee, occurs when the cartilage underneath your kneecap becomes damaged due to overuse, a fall or a blow to the knee, or muscle weakness that pulls the bones out of alignment. It affects about 2 of every 10,000 people but is more common in runners (hence the name), skiers, cyclists, and soccer players.

You can keep your kneecaps healthy by taking the following precautions:

- Always warm up for five minutes before you begin exercising or stretching.
- Be sure to stretch the quadriceps muscles in the front of your thigh and the hamstrings at the back of your thigh for several minutes before and after each workout.
- Lift weights to build strength in your quadriceps and hamstrings.
- Increase the length and intensity of your workout slowly—no more than 10 percent in one week.

The most common symptom is a dull pain around or under your kneecap that gets worse when you walk down stairs or hills, both of which place increased pressure on the area. You also may feel a grating sensation when you extend your knee. Your doctor will diagnose the problem based on your symptoms and an X-ray of the area.

Usually, runner's knee will get better after a month or two if you do low-impact exercises, such as riding a stationary bicycle or swimming, instead of running or other high-impact activities. You can take nonsteroidal anti-inflammatories for the pain. You'll also need to do exercises to strengthen your quadriceps and hamstring muscles, which support the knee. Your doctor may also recommend electrical stimulation to strengthen the muscles. In more severe cases, your doctor may recommend arthroscopic surgery, in which a surgeon inserts a small instrument into the area to smooth the surface of the cartilage and remove any rough edges.

Shin Splints

When you run or do other types of exercise for too long or on a surface that is too hard, the muscles in the front of your lower leg can be overused, causing inflammation in the fibrous tissues that attach those muscles to the shin bone. The inflammation causes the area to become painful, resulting in the condition known as "shin splints." Although there aren't any reliable statistics on the problem, it's very common in active men.

To protect your shins, take these steps:

- Warm up for five minutes before you exercise or stretch.
- Stretch your muscles well, especially in the front of your leg, before and after exercise.
- If you have flat feet, wear arch supports to cushion the impact on your shins.
- Don't increase your exercise intensity more than 10 percent per week.
- Do exercises to strengthen the muscles around your ankles, which will help the rest of your leg hold up under the pressure of high-impact activities.

Shin splints cause a dull ache in your shins when you're at rest and more intense pain when you put weight on your legs. Your doctor may want to do an X-ray to rule out a stress fracture.

If you think you have shin splints, rest your legs for several weeks by substituting no-impact activities like swimming or bicycling for your usual high-impact ones. Apply ice to your shins for the first day or two to reduce the inflammation, then apply warm compresses to speed healing. Use nonsteroidal anti-inflammatories for pain. After the pain subsides, return to your regular routine gradually and avoid prolonged high-impact activities on hard surfaces. If your pain doesn't go away, is severe, or your shin is hot and inflamed, see your doctor.

Sprains and Strains

Ligaments hold your bones together in a joint area. A *sprain* occurs when you overstretch or tear one or more ligaments, usually during a fall or sudden twist to a joint. You can sprain ligaments in most parts of your body, but by far the most common sprain—indeed, the most common injury in the U.S.—is the ankle sprain. Knees and wrists also are fairly common sprain sites.

A *strain*, on the other hand, is an injury to a muscle or tendon. You can have an acute strain, which occurs as a result of lifting something heavy or moving too suddenly, or a chronic one, which is the result of overuse. Back and hamstring muscle strains are the most common, but people who play racquet sports often strain muscles and ligaments attached to their elbow bones.

There's no ironclad way to prevent strains or sprains, but you can decrease their likelihood by following a few simple rules. They include:

- Stretch—but do it correctly. Do some simple stretching exercises at least three times a week to keep your muscles and ligaments loose and limber. Just be sure to always warm up for five minutes before you stretch, and don't overstretch or bounce to push your body beyond a comfortable point. You should never stretch to the point of pain, only mild tension.
- Warm up and stretch, especially before exercise. Many strains and sprains occur because muscles aren't ready for vigorous activity.
- Maintain a healthy weight. Being overweight can put you off balance and places a greater strain on your muscles, tendons, and ligaments.
- Wear properly fitting shoes. Shoes that are too big or too small can increase the likelihood of a trip or fall, both of which can cause strains and sprains.
- Don't overdo it when you exercise. If you want to increase the intensity or duration of your workout, do it only by 10 percent a week. Being overly tired can increase your risk of injury, as can overworking your muscles.

Symptoms of a sprain vary depending on its severity, but they can include pain, swelling, bruising and sometimes loss of movement or use of the affected joint. Strain symptoms may include pain, muscle spasm, and muscle weakness, but you may also have some swelling. A serious sprain or strain can be very painful. Both are diagnosed based on your symptoms.

Working Out, As You Age

We all get older. We get creakier. We get more easily fatigued. But that doesn't mean we have to stop working out. In fact, regular physical exercise becomes even more important for men who are older than 30, because that's when our bodies start to lose muscle mass, cardiovascular endurance, and flexibility. After age 30, men who are not active tend to lose about 1 percent of their strength each year over the remainder of their lifetimes. Working out can stave off that decline until you're well into your 50s and can slow it down significantly after that as well. The same, incidentally, holds true for aerobic fitness. Inactive men experience an average 1 percent per year decline unless they do something to combat the decline.

Men older than 50 have a different set of fitness needs than younger men, so if you're older, you can't expect to perform the same fitness regimen you did in your 20s or 30s. This is the age when injuries, even minor ones, start to take a toll, so you have to pay closer attention than ever to what your body is telling you. Even minor aches and pains require a slightly longer recovery time, and if you don't give your body adequate time to heal, minor injuries can turn into major—or at least chronic—ones. That doesn't mean you have to become a couch potato the second your body starts balking. Just be sensible. If running is hurting your knees, switch to biking or swimming for several weeks. If heavy bench presses cause pain in your elbow, try chest flyes with straight arms until the pain goes away. At the very least, try to maintain a regular aerobic program. Almost anybody—even people with minor injuries—can swim or walk.

One in four men start to suffer from arthritis in their 50s. Weight training can help strengthen the muscles around your joints, reducing pain and helping you maintain greater mobility. Shorter workouts may be necessary. But by incorporating short bouts of activity into your daily routine, you may find the pain more tolerable, and you'll reap the traditional health benefits of exercise as well.

If you lifted weights properly in your 20s, 30s, and 40s, there's no reason you can't lift just as well in your 50s, even if you use lighter weights. But if you start lifting after age 50, you need to be especially conscious of using proper form. Poor technique increases your risk of injury and decreases the benefits of the exercise. When you're older, there's less margin for error. That said, if you've never lifted weights, there's no better time to start than middle age (or even old age—men in their 90s have doubled, tripled, and quadrupled their strength). Adding lean muscle tissue is one of the very best ways to keep you vital and active and help fend off the decrepitude that may begin to sideline many of your peers.

For the first 24 to 48 hours after a strain or sprain, reduce the pain and swelling by following the RICE strategy, which stands for:

- Rest for a day or two;
- Ice for 20 minutes four to eight times a day;
- Compression of the area with an elastic bandage; and
- Elevation—keeping the injured area above your heart level, if possible, which will help reduce the swelling. A nonsteroidal anti-inflammatory may help as well.

If an ankle sprain is severe, your doctor may want to put a cast on it. Other types of serious strains and sprains may require surgery to repair damaged tissue. No matter how serious the injury, you'll probably be put on an exercise regimen to strengthen the injured area. Rehabilitation is a key component of a complete recovery, but it's important to be patient and pay attention to how your body is feeling. You may need to take it easy for three to six weeks after a moderate ankle sprain, but a severe sprain can take up to a year to heal.

Stress Fractures

Bones are normally strong enough to withstand the everyday wear and tear we put on them. But if your physical activity rate has accelerated recently, you may be placing more strain on your bones than they can handle, which can cause tiny, hairline cracks, or stress fractures, to form. There are no good data on how many people suffer stress fractures each year, but the ailment is more likely to strike people who are extremely lean and active.

If you're starting an exercise program, don't increase the length or intensity of your workout too quickly, and make sure you're getting around 1,200 milligrams of calcium daily from a combination of diet and supplements. *(See page 245 for information on the possible dangers of too much calcium.)*

Since a stress fracture may not show up on an X-ray for up to six weeks after the injury, your doctor will probably diagnose the injury based on your symptoms—typically pain in the area that gets worse when you're active and better with rest—and a bone scan. In this procedure, a technician will inject you with a radioactive substance that is absorbed by bone. If you have an area that's trying to heal, it will absorb even more of the substance. After several hours, you'll be put in a machine called a scanner to look for areas that emit increased amounts of radiation, indicating that more of the substance has been absorbed.

Since stress fractures usually don't require a cast, your doctor will probably recommend that you take it easy for up to a month (you may be able to do no-impact activities, like swimming or bicycling) and try to keep weight off the injured area if it's painful. If the fracture is in your leg, ankle, or foot, you may need to use crutches or a cane to get around. You can probably resume high impact activities like running after three to six weeks.

Tendonitis

Tendons are thick cords of fiber that attach your muscles to your bones. When your tendons become inflamed or irritated as a result of overuse or injury, you have what's known as tendonitis, a condition that most commonly affects your shoulders, knees, and elbows (tennis or golfer's elbow is actually tendonitis) but can also affect your hips, wrists, and Achilles tendon at the back of your ankle. Tendonitis is one of the most common occupational and sports injuries.

There are certain factors that increase your risk of developing tendonitis. They include:

- Repetitive motion. If you do too much of any one activity—whether it's typing, hitting a golf ball or tennis ball, or running—you're placing your tendons under stress and increasing your risk of tendonitis. That's why it's a good idea for recreational athletes to cross train instead of focusing exclusively on one sport.
- Age. As your muscles and tendons become less flexible, your risk of tendonitis increases.

To prevent a bout of tendonitis, warm up for at least five minutes before beginning exercise, stretch well before and after exercise, vary your routine by cross training, and don't increase your intensity or duration more than 10 percent per week. If you're prone to Achilles tendonitis, avoid running on hills or hard surfaces.

Tendonitis is fairly easy to diagnose based on your symptoms, which usually include pain, tenderness, and stiffness, especially when you move near the affected area. Tennis elbow, for instance, affects the outside of your forearm near your elbow and worsens when you use your arm; you feel Achilles tendonitis in the thick tendon above your heel, especially when you walk or run.

Your doctor may perform several other tests, like an X-ray or magnetic resonance imaging (MRI) to rule out other potential causes of the pain.

You can treat tendonitis at home with the RICE method to decrease pain and inflammation. *(See page 61 for an explanation of this method.)*

After several days, start alternating ice with heat, which can speed healing by increasing blood flow to the area. Massage can help loosen and relax the area as well. Tendonitis can take several months to heal. If it doesn't seem to be getting better, your doctor may want to give you an injection of cortisone into the tissue surrounding the tendon to reduce the pain and inflammation. If you have actually ruptured a tendon, which can happen especially with your Achilles, you'll need surgery to repair it.

PART TWO

Common Health Problems

You're feeling tired and achy, or you get lightheaded every time you stand up quickly, or you have a nagging pain running down your leg that just won't go away. Getting to the bottom of common complaints such as these is the basis for most medical practice. Usually, minor symptoms are caused by minor problems that often go away on their own. But they can sometimes be the first clue to a more serious condition, which is why it's often so important to see a doctor when you're not feeling well.

Although men traditionally have not utilized the health care system as much as women, we're starting to show up in increasing numbers. There were 329 million doctor's office visits made by men in 1998, according to the National Center for Health Statistics. That means more and more of us are paying attention to the signals our bodies are sending us and taking action when those signals turn into distress signals. However, men are still too often reluctant to "bother the doctor" when they should.

In the upcoming pages, you'll find current, concise information on everything from cancer and heart disease to baldness and sleep problems. This is not meant as a substitute for hands-on medical care. Instead it is meant to help you decide when it makes sense to see the doctor—and when doing so might even save your life.

CHAPTER 3

Going to the Doctor

Now that we are ready to tackle some common general health problems in more detail, it is time to take on two tough questions, questions that men in particular often like to avoid.

The first is: How do you pick a doctor? We men often avoid thinking about significant relationships—and the relationship with our doctor can be one of the most important and significant in our lives. And the time to think about it—and actually pick a doctor—is before we really need one. An emergency is the worst time to scramble and find a doctor. In terms that men might understand, it is like trying to find a good car mechanic in the middle of the night when you are stranded on a highway.

But once you actually find a doctor you like and who is competent, further questions arise about how often you should go for regular checkups—and what kinds of symptoms should cause you to see your doctor right away.

Picking a Doctor

Assuming you have a choice—meaning that your insurance or health plan gives you a choice—how do you go about picking a competent doctor who is right for you? Notice that there are two very important components to your decision: finding a doctor who is both competent *and* good for *you*. Some men will put more emphasis on one or the other of those factors, but most of us would like a doctor who meets both criteria. And frankly, finding out about either competency or personality can be very difficult, unless you have some kind of inside track on such information. By "inside track," I mean someone—a relative, a friend, a friend of a friend, etc.—who is in a position to know about these things; someone like a nurse or doctor or physical therapist or lab technician who works in a hospital or clinic with various doctors. If you can, find such a person you can trust and ask them who they go to, or who they recommend for their family and friends; this may be the best way to at least get some names to check out.

Obviously, the range of your possibilities will vary considerably depending on what kind of community you live in. If you have a wide range of choices, you should narrow down the possibilities by making a couple of basic decisions first. For example, if you are in a large city with many hospitals, you might want to first pick the hospital you would want to go to for tests when necessary or, even more important, for actual care if you ever need to be hospitalized. In addition to geographical convenience, my own preference is to pick a hospital that is affiliated with a medical school and/or a major medical center—versus a small hospital that has no such affiliation. Indeed, I would recommend going extra miles for such a hospital if you have a choice. Being connected to a major medical institution obviously doesn't guarantee quality but it significantly increases the chances that you'll receive good care.

What kind of doctor?

Once you narrow down your choices of a doctor to a particular hospital, you then have to decide what kind of doctor you want to choose. Today, that usually involves picking a *primary care doctor,* meaning the kind of doctor who can take care of most of your general medical needs and refer you to specialists when necessary.

At this point, I need to first briefly explain how doctors are educated today. (You may know all of this, but I want to make sure we are all on the same page.) After completing four years of medical school, almost all newly graduated doctors will continue their training by specializing. That means completing a *residency*—

so-called because they go to a hospital or medical center in which they will basically be doctors "in residence" for three or more years (many more in the case of some specialists) to learn a particular area of medicine in much more detail than what was taught during medical school. Once they have completed such specialty or residency training, doctors are said to be "board eligible" because they are now eligible to take the exams prepared by the accrediting board in their specialty. Once they have actually passed the exams they are "board certified."

The various specialties can basically be grouped into two groups: the so-called "primary care specialties"; and the more narrowly focused specialties that do not deal with a broad range of everyday medical problems.

Today, for men there are basically two kinds of primary care doctors who have taken at least three additional years of residency training:

- Family physicians have at least three years of training after medical school in a mix of adult medicine, pediatrics, some obstetrics, and some minor surgery. (There are still a few older "family doctors," mainly in smaller towns or rural areas, who went to medical school before post-graduate training became the standard; they are the kind of doctors we used to call GPs or general practitioners).
- General internists, in contrast, have at least three years of training in just adult medicine and do not train in pediatrics, obstetrics, or surgery.

There is a third type of primary care specialist who does four years of training divided between internal (adult) medicine and pediatrics. They often call themselves family physicians even though they trained with a combination of internal medicine and pediatrics rather than in a specific family physician training program.

Is Your Doctor Board Certified?

If you want to find out if a given doctor is actually board certified, you can contact the American Board of Medical Specialties (ABMS) at their Web site (www.abms.org) or call them at 866-ASK-ABMS. The beauty of board certification is that it usually means you don't have to be too concerned about what kind of medical school or residency program the doctor went through; if they can pass the specialty exam, it usually means they learned what they need to know to be a competent doctor. If a doctor is not board certified, it means you have to do more checking about his or her competency.

By now, I imagine you are asking, *Does it really make any difference what kind of primary care doctor I pick?* And the answer is *Probably not,* as long as the doctor meets certain standards including two very basic ones:

Being either board eligible or board certified, as described above. All else being equal, it is best for your doctor to be board certified because that means he or she has actually passed the rigorous examination in his chosen specialty. A doctor who has been in practice many years and is still just board eligible has either chosen not to take the exam or has failed it.

Being on the staff of a recognized and accredited hospital (meaning one that has been accredited by the Joint Commission on Accreditation of Healthcare Organizations, or JCAHO for short). Before a hospital gives staff privileges to a doctor, they usually check very carefully on his or her background, training, malpractice claims, etc. However, this kind of checking is obviously done only for doctors who apply to them because they need to have hospital privileges—that is, they need to be able to order tests at or admit patients to a hospital. Some kinds of specialists—like dermatologists or cosmetic surgeons—may be able to practice entirely in their office or clinic setting and never have to apply to a hospital for staff privileges. That means that as long as they were able to get a state license to practice medicine, they can hang out a shingle and do whatever they want. And quite frankly, the difficulty of getting a state license can vary considerably from one state to another, though in general it is much more rigorous today than it was in the past.

Here's another word of caution: Once a doctor gets licensed to practice in a state, he or she can call themselves anything they want. That means, for example, that a doctor who has had no formal training in dermatology can call himself a dermatologist, or a doctor who was trained in gynecology can call herself a plastic surgeon even though she did not do her specialty training in plastic surgery. Again, if a doctor is on the staff of a recognized hospital, this kind of misleading labeling would be very unlikely—the hospital simply would not allow it. But if the doctor practices exclusively in an office or clinic setting without any hospital supervision, it's possible. A doctor's lack of hospital privileges does not automatically mean you should be suspicious of that doctor. But it does mean that you will have to do some more careful investigation, such as checking with your state medical society and/or state licensing board—the former being the professional organization of doctors in a state who choose to join, the latter being a state government agency charged with the licensing and disciplining of physicians in the state.

So we now come back to the question of what kind of primary care doctor is best for you. If you are looking for a single doctor who can service your entire family, you would pick a family physician, since they are trained in both adult medicine and pediatrics, as well as some gynecology for your spouse. However, if you are at a later stage in life where the kids are grown and gone and you are statistically more likely to develop potentially serious medical problems, then you might want to pick a general internist who focuses only on adult patients. General internists tend to have more in-depth knowledge about adult medicine than do family physicians.

At this point I will raise the question of "if and when" a man should also develop a relationship with a *urologist,* the specialist who is trained in both surgical and nonsurgical care of the urinary tract system (kidneys, bladder, and associated tubes) and the male reproductive system (prostate, penis, testicles, and associated tubes). As a man gets into middle age and beyond, the chance of being referred to a urologist for prostate problems goes up considerably. However, even younger men often end up being referred to a urologist for problems ranging from sexually transmitted diseases to male infertility.

In addition to checkups with their primary care physician, some men feel better also seeing a urologist regularly—much as a woman might see a gynecologist in addition to her primary care physician. But as urologists would be the first to admit, they do not have the training to provide the broad general care that family physicians or general internists do. So even if you see a urologist on a regular basis, you should not consider that a substitute for a good primary care physician.

Whichever type of primary care doctor you pick, you must still find out if that person is going to be good for you in terms of personality and style of communication: Some men like a doctor who is brief and to the point, while others want as much information as possible. And, even if you get good advice from people who should know, you will never know for sure if a given doctor is right for you until you actually meet and try out that doctor. For this reason, there is a sense in which the first visit with a new doctor should also be regarded by both the doctor and the patient as a "date"—a meeting to find out if you are compatible. There is absolutely nothing wrong with deciding after such a first visit that this particular doctor is not the right one for you. Indeed, in the long run, it will be better for both you and the doctor to make that decision right up front rather than at a later stage when a breakup would be more difficult.

Your money, your health

In this day of managed care, there is one other quality that you should look for in your physician—and that is the sense that your doctor is working on your behalf, not on behalf of the insurance company or HMO that actually pays the bill. As you well know, doctors are under a lot of pressure today to control the costs of medical care—and with good reason, given the spiraling rate of health care costs in this country. Actually, the most expensive care is not always the best care; sometimes too many tests or too many procedures or too many medications are ordered when fewer might be just as good and possibly safer. But you also want to be reassured

Immunizations

You may be surprised to find this section in a book aimed at adult men. And that tells you something about the problem: We have done a pretty good job of convincing the public that they should get their kids immunized, but we have done a terrible job of reminding adults about immunizations that can be lifesaving for them too. And I include us physicians in that indictment; while pediatricians are very conscious of their responsibility to get kids immunized, physicians who take care of adults seldom bring up the subject. So this is one of those areas where you may have to take the primary responsibility for being informed about immunizations that make sense for you. Here's what you need to know about some of the most important adult immunizations:

Flu Shot: I begin with this one because even though it is the most common adult immunization, it is still woefully underutilized by people at highest risk for getting influenza. On average, "the flu" kills about 20,000 Americans every year, most of them over age 65, especially nursing home residents, who develop complications such as pneumonia after being weakened by the flu. Other high risk groups include people over age 50; people of any age with serious chronic diseases, especially of the heart or lungs; people who work with people at high risk, such as health care and emergency workers; and pregnant women after the fourteenth week.

Pneumonia Vaccine: The more correct name for this vaccine would be the "Pneumococcal vaccine" because it protects against selected strains of the pneumococcus bacterium, which is one of the most common causes of pneumonia—but can also cause other serious infections like meningitis. The same groups at risk for the flu are usually at risk for these problems and should get this vaccine about every five years depending on your doctor's recommendation. (We don't know for sure how long the protection from a single shot can last; we are learning as we go about how long you can go between shots.) It can be given at the same time you get the flu shot but, as just mentioned, you don't have to get it every year.

that your doctor will never cut corners just to save money, that he or she will always do what is truly necessary and in your best interest. This is an item that I believe you should openly discuss with a new doctor, preferably at your first meeting so you know how the doctor feels about this very important issue.

Hepatitis Vaccines: There are vaccines for both hepatitis Type A and Type B. Since hepatitis B is usually much more serious and potentially fatal, I am more concerned that those at high risk for hepatitis B (very similar to the groups at risk for HIV infection and the health workers who take care of them) get the three-shot series needed for protection. *(For more information on hepatitis, see page 226.)*

Tetanus: Also known as "lockjaw" because of the way it "clamps down" the facial muscles, this often fatal bacterial disease can be easily prevented with proper immunization. Today, almost all children are immunized against tetanus as part of the DTP shots (the T stands for tetanus), but after infancy and childhood, a booster for tetanus is needed every 10 years to keep our resistance active. Unfortunately, most adults don't get such boosters—and most doctors don't ask about it—until they get a serious wound which makes them more susceptible.

Measles-Mumps-Rubella (MMR): People who got the MMR shots as kids are protected—as are people born in 1957 or earlier who may not have gotten these shots; that's because they were likely to have been exposed to the natural presence of these diseases. But anyone born after 1957 (by which time naturally occurring diseases were very rare) who did not get these shots needs to do so today because all three—mumps, measles, and rubella (German measles)—can cause serious problems if you get them as adults. For example, mumps can cause serious damage to the testicles. *(For more information on testicular problems, see page 283.)*

Chicken Pox: This disease can be more serious in adults than kids, so anyone who didn't have chicken pox as a kid should discuss this vaccine with their primary care doctor.

If you haven't done so, you should at least sit down with your doctor and talk about these vaccines and decide together which ones make sense for you.

When to Go to the Doctor

So now that you have a doctor, how do you decide when to go? Once again, this is often a particularly difficult question for men because we are prone to avoid doctors for several reasons. One reason is a foolish macho attitude that many of us more *mature* (read *older*) men were raised on: *We are strong enough to overcome our problems, even our pain, on our own—just give us time.* And a closely allied attitude is that *we don't like to bother anyone* with our troubles.

Sometimes those attitudes are admirable, but when it comes to our health they can be foolish and downright dangerous. So my general advice is always to err on the side of safety: When in doubt, check it out. But what about so-called "regular checkups," even when you feel fine? That phrase suggests that there is a firm understanding about how often you should see the doctor—and what you should have done when you go. In fact, that is *not* the case. However, there are some guidelines that are helpful in deciding when or how often you should go to your doctor for a checkup:

Age. The truth is that if you are young and healthy with no family history of serious disease and no current symptoms bothering you, a checkup or physical exam does not make much sense. But as you get older it begins to make more sense, simply because the statistical chance of finding something important increases with age. No one can give you an exact timetable proven to be the right one, so I will arbitrarily suggest that once you pass out of the hands of your childhood and adolescent doctors, you should consider a visit to your primary doctor every three years between age 20 and 40; every two years between 40 and 50; and yearly thereafter. Again, this would be for general checkups in the absence of any other problems. Chances are you will see your doctor more often than this because of temporary symptoms or passing problems.

Family history of serious medical problems. This can change the schedule dramatically. For example, if you have a family history of serious high blood pressure, you should be seeing your doctor (or company nurse) on a very regular basis to have your blood pressure checked. And in the following pages I will be discussing many medical conditions where a family history is a very important guide to deciding when to see a doctor.

Other risk factors. Aside from family history, there are other factors that can put you at higher risk for developing serious diseases and therefore require more regular checkups. Most of these risk factors are lifestyle choices like smoking or promiscuous sex. Other risks cannot be easily predicted or found except through regular testing, like high blood fats. If you develop a chronic medical problem, such as heart disease or diabetes, you will of course require more regular visits to your doctor to monitor your condition.

Beside the regular checkup, the *complete physical* is another sacred cow from past years that has been somewhat tarnished in more recent years, for two reasons. First, in the absence of actual symptoms, the complete head-to-toe physical seldom finds anything important. (When there are actual symptoms to guide the examining physician, the physical exam can be much more helpful.) And second, there are often tests that can more accurately pinpoint a problem than the physical exam.

Let me give you a somewhat controversial (and among doctors, sensitive) example. Listening to chest breathing sounds with a stethoscope can often be very helpful in sorting out breathing problems. But most physicians today are also going to want a chest X-ray if they have any doubts about what they are hearing or not hearing—and most physicians today would be very reluctant to make a firm diagnosis of serious pneumonia without a confirming chest X-ray. (Even when they are quite certain it is pneumonia they would want a chest X-ray to see just how extensive it might be.)

But even as the head-to-toe physical has come to be regarded as less valuable for general checkups, various screening tests have become more important and valuable. Therefore, today a checkup often revolves more around asking questions about various lifestyle issues or ordering certain screening tests than performing a complete physical. I take the time to point this out so you will not feel neglected by your doctor if he or she spends more time asking questions about your family and personal medical history and figuring out appropriate tests than in actually doing a long and thorough physical exam.

Common Diagnostic and Screening Tests

Throughout this book I will be referring to various tests that are useful in screening (looking for problems before they cause actual symptoms) or actual diagnosis (figuring out the cause of symptoms once they occur). I will usually say something about those tests in relation to a given topic, but I think it will be useful for you to have a general idea about various tests as you begin this section. Here are some of the kinds of tests commonly used today, arranged in alphabetical order.

Angiograms (angiography). Angiograms are pictures of blood vessels, either arteries or veins. Since blood vessels don't show up on ordinary X-rays, they have to be filled with something that will, and that "something" is called a contrast medium or "dye." (It is usually an iodine based dye, but in people known to be allergic to iodine or who have a history of allergies or asthma, other dyes can be tried and/or medicines taken to minimize any reaction.) Unfortunately, in order to get a good concentration of the dye in the blood vessels to be studied, a catheter (thin hollow tube) must be guided into or near the specific blood vessel and then the dye released. This involves considerable skill and complex equipment. Theoretically, almost any blood vessel can be studied this way as long as it can be reached by a catheter—which is usually inserted in a blood vessel near the skin in the leg or arm or neck and pushed to the area to be studied. In a coronary angiogram, for example, the catheter is inserted in an artery in the groin and then pushed up to the main artery coming from the heart and into the openings of the coronary arteries where the dye is injected. In order to avoid the need for X-rays, catheters, and dye, magnetic resonance technology (see below) can sometimes be used as an alternative to get pictures of blood vessels—the procedure is known as MRA, or magnetic resonance angiography. While the quality of MRA pictures is usually not as good as regular X-ray angiograms using dye, it is getting better and increasingly being used for some blood vessel studies.

Blood tests. Hundreds of tests can be done on samples of blood obtained from needle sticks into veins or arteries, or tubes inserted into blood vessels on a longer-term basis. (Some tests can also be done on blood obtained from skin punctures that don't go into an actual blood vessel, like finger sticks for checking sugar levels in persons with diabetes.) The most common "blood test" is the famous CBC, or complete blood count, which studies such basic information as the number of red, white, and platelet cells in the blood; the different kinds of white blood cells; and the amount of hemoglobin (which carries oxygen to our cells) in the red blood cells. This is the "blood test" usually done as part of any routine physical. Another common test checks for a dozen or so common chemicals or nutrients in the blood. Both of these kinds of "blood tests" can be done very quickly today with highly automated machines. Many other blood tests will be mentioned in the course of this book.

Biopsies. Biopsies mean tissue samples that are removed from the body to be studied under the microscope. These tissue samples can be obtained in many different ways—during surgery; from a needle inserted through the skin to a targeted organ, such as the liver; or with instruments inserted through endoscopes into various hollow organs or spaces (see below).

CT scans. These exams used to be known as CAT scans, short for computerized axial tomography. Today, the axial word is left out, and they are known as CT scans, for computerized tomography. Whatever the name, the technique involves passing hundreds of multiple narrow X-ray beams (known as tomograms) through your body; they are collected by a special large camera that rotates around the axis (hence the name axial) of your body. These images are then sent to a computer, where they can be manipulated (as we do in very elementary fashion with digital camera images in our computer) into various two and three dimensional images of the parts of the body examined. Contrast material (dye) can also be used during these exams to provide better images of certain tissues including blood vessels.

Endoscopy. This technology uses a thin, flexible fiber-optic tube with a camera at the tip that can be inserted into a body space for a direct look at that area—and often to remove tissue samples for biopsy study or even for a minor surgical procedure to remove abnormal tissue, like a polyp in the large intestine. These tubes can be inserted through the mouth (for a look inside the esophagus, stomach, and first part of the small intestine); through the anus (for a look at the large intestine and last part of the small intestine); down the windpipe (for a look at the breathing system); through the penis (to look at the inside of the prostate and bladder); through the nose (to look at the sinuses); or even through the skin into the abdominal cavity (to study and do procedures on various abdominal organs, in which case the procedure is referred to as laparoscopy).

MRI (magnetic resonance imaging). This technology does not use X-rays, as does the CT scan, but instead uses a magnetic field and radio waves to produce temporary changes in body cells that are translated into a computerized image of the area studied. As with plain X-rays and CT scans, contrast media (dyes) can be used to improve the images of various tissues. MRI technology is particularly good at visualizing tissues that are surrounded by bone, so it is often used for studies of so-called "soft tissues" (non-bony tissues) such as the brain, spinal cord, and muscles. And like CT scans, it can be used for more detailed pictures of blood vessels than a routine X-ray can provide. However, people with certain metal hardware in their bodies (like some heart pacemakers) may not be able to have an MRI scan because of the strong magnetic fields involved.

Radionuclide scans. Also known as nuclear medicine scans, these images are obtained by injecting substances that produce very small amounts of radioactivity that can be detected by special scanning cameras. (The radioactive substances are often known as radionuclides or radioisotopes.) This technology is most commonly used to examine the thyroid gland, the lungs, various bones, the liver, and the heart. Most of the time, a computer is used to improve the images obtained by the scanning camera.

Ultrasound. This technology uses sound waves that bounce off body tissues and structures to provide images; therefore these images are sometimes known as echograms. This technique is without risk or pain except for the mild pressure felt as the transducer (the handheld instrument that transmits the sound waves) is pressed on the area to be studied. Doppler ultrasound is a variation that can study the flow of blood in a blood vessel; it is routinely used today to study the flow of blood through the vessels in the neck leading to the brain *(see page 160)*.

Urinalysis. This very common study uses a urine sample to check for pus cells indicating infection and substances such as blood or sugar or protein that can be quickly identified by dipping special reagent strips into the urine and looking for color changes on the strips. When necessary, urine samples or collections of urine over a longer period of time can be used for many different and more sophisticated tests.

X-rays. This is still the most common "imaging" or "scanning" test used for medical diagnosis. A "plain" or "routine" X-ray uses electromagnetic radiation passed through the body onto a special film that is then "developed" to produce the classic black and white images we all have seen. This is still the fastest and easiest way to visualize bones and many other tissues, such as lung tissue. As with both CT and MRI scans, images can often be improved by using contrast media (dyes), such as barium, that can be swallowed or inserted through the anus. With modern equipment, the amount of radiation from a single plain X-ray is usually very small. For example, the amount of radiation exposure from watching TV is about 6 MREM (that's millirems, a standard unit of measuring radiation) per year. The exposure from living in Denver (the mile-high city) is about 50 MREM per year. In contrast, the amount of radiation from a chest X-ray is about 8 MREM, from a dental X-ray about 10 MREM, and from a hip X-ray about 80 to 90 MREM. However, the MREM from a CT scan of the head and body is about 1,100 MREM. (And remember that there is no radiation from the regular MRI scan.)

When to Seek Immmediate Medical Attention

Finally, in this discussion of when to see a doctor, I will highlight certain symptoms that should lead you to call your doctor immediately—or go to the emergency room. These symptoms require prompt attention to sort out whether they involve life-threatening emergencies or are simply worse than usual forms of non–life-threatening problems.

Sudden and severe headache

The vast majority of headaches are more of a nuisance than a life-threatening problem *(see page 212 for more on headaches)*. But if you ever experience a sudden and intense pain in your head—like nothing you have ever felt before—that could signify a serious bleeding problem in your head. The most common causes of this kind of "bleeding headache" are:

- Aneurysms (bulging and weakened bloods vessels) that are leaking or have burst open.
- Bleeding strokes (where brain blood vessels start to bleed from other kinds of damage, such as high blood pressure), in which case the pain is usually accompanied by other symptoms such as slurred speech.

I should also mention the headache that occurs if you come down with meningitis (inflammation of the linings around the brain and spinal cord), which is usually accompanied by nausea, vomiting, stiff neck, and a fever.

Sudden and severe chest pain

As is the case with headaches, most chest pain is not life threatening. Indeed, most pain in the outer chest wall (or rib cage) is caused by muscle strains in the small muscles between ribs or in some of the larger muscles overlying the front, back, and side areas of our chest. And most inner chest pain is caused by the phenomenon we call "heartburn" *(see page 217 for detailed information on heartburn)*. But what we all worry about when we are having persistent chest pain is whether or not we are having an actual heart attack.

I refer you to a much more thorough discussion of the pain associated with heart attacks *(see page 141)*, but at this point I want to stress the obvious: If there is any doubt in your mind about whether or not you are having a heart attack, you should get yourself to an emergency room as quickly as possible, preferably by calling 911. Chest pain that is associated with other worrisome symptoms, such as shortness of breath, sweating, nausea and vomiting, dizziness, etc., is obviously likely to be more serious. But the pain of a heart attack versus other kinds of chest pain is not always crystal clear initially. However, in an emergency room, where blood and other tests are readily available, chest pain can usually be quickly sorted out in terms of whether or not it is truly serious. And if the pain is caused by a developing heart attack, treatment within the first few hours of the onset of chest pain can often mean the difference between life and death. In fact, today about 90 percent of people having a heart attack who make it to the hospital alive will survive.

Sudden and severe abdominal pain

Same story—usually not life threatening but sometimes might be. Usually even severe abdominal pain is caused by gas or cramping from a viral illness. But if the pain is persistent or progressive, you should at least call your doctor. The most likely causes of more serious abdominal pain are appendicitis, gallstones *(see page 202),* pancreatitis (inflammation of the pancreas), diverticulitis *(see page 234),* or a perforated ulcer (an ulcer that has penetrated through the wall of the stomach or small intestine).

Sudden and severe shortness of breath

It's normal to feel "out of breath" after strenuous activity or even when you are excited about something. But that type of breathlessness subsides fairly quickly. However, shortness of breath that comes on without any apparent reason is obviously cause for concern. An "asthma attack" is the most common cause of sudden and severe shortness of breath, and I mention it at this point simply because there are too many unnecessary deaths every year in this country from asthma attacks. I say "unnecessary" because if the breathing problem had been recognized as potentially serious in its earliest stages and treatment had been started quickly, the death could have been prevented. One of the best ways for a person with known asthma to detect a developing problem early is with the use of a device known as a "peak flow meter." This simple and inexpensive device can detect a potentially serious problem early and therefore alert the person to take quick action. *(For more information on asthma, see page 171.)*

There are many other symptoms—such as blood in urine or stool—that may or may not signify serious disease. For example, blood in the urine could signal anything from a minor prostate infection to major bladder cancer. Similarly, blood in the stool could mean a bleeding hemorrhoid or colon cancer. Obviously you should report any new, persistent, or progressive symptoms to your doctor and let him or her be the one to decide whether they are significant—and what, if anything, needs to be done. I will be discussing many of these symptoms in the context of specific disease problems in the remainder of this book.

First-Aid Emergencies

I am including this brief section because I think everyone should know at least how to react to what appears to be a serious situation resulting either from someone collapsing or someone being injured. I also think it is still more likely that a man is going to be called on for "leadership" in such situations, though obviously women can be just as or even more effective than men.

Now, for those of you who would like to be at least more aware of what you should and should not do in serious situations, I will offer the following "way of thinking" about emergencies. It is no substitute for more extensive knowledge and training.

Collapse Situations

This category covers the most common of the potentially serious scenarios you are likely to encounter—namely a situation in which you actually see someone fall or collapse to the ground without any obvious reason or injury, or you come upon someone collapsed on the ground. This person may be conscious or unconscious but in either case he appears to be quite helpless. Fortunately, most of the time the cause of this situation is a simple fainting spell—not something more serious like a major heart attack or stroke. So the most basic task you can perform in this situation, aside from removing the person carefully from any truly life-threatening situation (like a nearby fire), is to quickly determine if he is breathing and if his heart is beating. That is not as difficult as it may sound. Even if someone appears "lifeless" you can usually determine if he is breathing by simply holding your hand very close over his mouth and nose: though his chest may not appear to be moving, you will often feel each breath as it is exhaled. And if he is breathing, his heart is still working, at least for the moment.

The reason this very basic determination is so important is that if the person is breathing, and his heart is beating, you can usually buy some time to call for more expert help and focus your attention on keeping the person safe and comfortable. And that will be the case in the vast majority of collapse situations. In fact, in most of these situations the person will slowly "wake up," and it will become more obvious that he is not in immediate danger, though he may well require further medical assessment by others more qualified.

One variation on this theme is the grand-mal seizure—a person who collapses because he is having a seizure. In that situation your first responsibility would once again be to keep the person away from any nearby danger; in this case you can be more comfortable about moving him because internal injuries are much less likely. Also it will be obvious that the person is breathing with a beating heart. You should try to roll the person on his side if possible to prevent any aspiration (swallowing any secretions or vomit into the windpipe) and put something firm but forgiving, like a wash cloth or towel, between his teeth to prevent injury to the tongue from severe clamping of the jaw. (Do not put your fingers in the mouth.)

If the person is not breathing, obviously it is a very different situation. This is where you would attempt CPR (cardiopulmonary resuscitation) and/or the use of a portable defibrillator machine for the heart (if you had one and knew what to do with it). It is way beyond the scope of this book to discuss these kinds of first aid, but I would personally urge you to learn more about these techniques. I would also urge you to think about buying a portable defibrillator for your workplace. These relatively new and very compact devices (which sell for $2,000 to $3,000) can be quickly and easily used on a person who has collapsed because of a serious rhythm problem in the heart, usually associated with an actual heart attack. Many public places (airports, stadiums, etc.) are buying these devices and training employees in their use, as are some families with high risk inhabitants.

Serious Injury

If a person is in a state of collapse because of an injury—either one that you have witnessed or one that is obvious, such as a car accident—you may well have additional things to respond to. It is beyond your scope to handle all possibilities in a serious injury, but there are a couple of situations that do demand action. If the victim is bleeding seriously, try to stop the bleeding as quickly as possible. For an untrained person who needs to act because no other help is available, direct pressure on the site of the bleeding—using anything available, like a piece of clothing—is the best way to help. Stopping or slowing the bleeding until more expert help arrives can be lifesaving. Moving an injured person is always questionable because you don't want to aggravate any serious internal or spinal cord injuries. However, if the person is in imminent danger, such as trapped in a car that is likely to explode, you may have no choice but to move him or her to safety.

If there appears to be a major fracture—a bone sticking out or a limb protruding at a very abnormal angle—you should be very careful about disturbing the involved limb. However, it is permissible to at least cover the limb or maybe even gently splint it with a carefully wrapped blanket, for example, in order to prevent further movement and damage. You should be especially careful about moving a person whose neck could be fractured, for fear of damaging the spinal cord and causing permanent paralysis.

Again, this discussion is designed only to make you aware of what you might consider in a situation that appears to be serious and in which you are the only person available to "do something." Obviously, unless you are appropriately trained, you should act with extreme caution in these situations.

CHAPTER 4

Cancer

Now that I have covered some general issues in your ongoing medical care, it is time to look at certain health problems in more detail. I will begin with the two disease categories that seriously affect more people than all others combined—major cancers and common heart conditions. Those chapters will be followed by a selected list of other common problems, arranged in alphabetical order.

There is good reason to begin this section about diseases that plague men with special chapters on cancer and heart disease. They are, quite simply, the biggest threats to your health. Cardiovascular (heart and blood vessel) disease killed more than 445,000 men in the U.S. in 1998, the most recent year for which reliable figures are available, making it the leading cause of death. Cancer was the second most common cause of death, taking the lives of 282,065 men. Furthermore, statistics tell us that one in three men can expect to develop some form of major cardiovascular disease before age 60, while fully half of all men will develop cancer during their lifetime. These figures are alarming, to be sure. But they carry with them a critical caveat: Today we can do a lot to prevent these diseases or at least detect them early enough so that they can be cured.

There are a number of lifestyle choices that we now know can increase or decrease your risk of cancer. Thanks to years of scientific research, it's been well established that factors like smoking, being overweight, and eating a high-fat diet increase the odds that you'll die of cancer. According to the American Cancer Society, about 172,000 cancer deaths in men and women in 2001 were directly attributable to tobacco use and, thus, were preventable. Another third of the cancer deaths in 2001 were related to lifestyle factors.

The silver lining, of course, is that there are plenty of ways to decrease your chances of falling prey to cancer. Many of them you've heard before. Stop smoking. Exercise regularly. Eat less saturated fat and at least five servings of fruits and vegetables a day. Wear sunscreen. But as scientists continue to tease out the causes of these common problems, we're getting new information almost daily on previously unknown preventive and early detection measures that have the potential to save even more lives—maybe even yours.

As a result of new tests and treatments, more people are surviving illnesses like prostate cancer and colon cancer—diseases that 50 years ago were almost certain to be death sentences. Meanwhile, the sooner a cancer is found and treated, the better will be your chance of beating it. With this in mind, here are the essential medical facts about the cancers that are most likely to affect you or someone you know.

A Word about the Disease Profiles

Note that beginning with this chapter, I will be discussing diseases and conditions according to a specific outline in the hopes that by breaking the information down, you'll be able to find what you're looking for quickly and easily. Essentially, "The Basics" provides an introduction to the condition, telling you what it is as well as offering pertinent information about the various organs of the body that may be involved. "Prevention & Risk Factors" emphasizes those factors you can take into your own hands in order to reduce your chances of suffering from a particular disease. Then "Diagnosis & Screening" explains the tests your doctor will usually perform in order to diagnose the condition. The "Treatment Options" section highlights standard medications, procedures, or other courses of treatment for that condition or which can used to screen for a problem before symptoms occur. I am usually intentionally brief in dealing with treatments, since this is the area where new medications and technology may render more specific information quickly obsolete. Furthermore, only your doctor—who is familiar with your medical history—is really qualified to recommend a course of treatment. And finally, for chronic conditions or those where the treatment means you'll be experiencing major lifestyle changes, I've included a section called "Living With," which outlines some of the issues you'll have to think about during and after your recovery.

Colon Cancer

The Basics: The colon, which consists of five to six feet of large intestine plus the rectum, is the last part of the body's digestive system. When you eat a meal, the food eventually passes through the colon, where solid waste products are formed. The waste products that the body doesn't need are stored until you defecate. Cancer of the colon occurs when cells lining its inner surface begin to divide uncontrollably, forming a tumor, or mass of abnormal cells. The mass eventually interferes with the normal functioning of the colon and, eventually, may spread, or metastasize, to other parts of the body, especially the liver.

Colorectal cancers are the third most common cancers in men, after prostate and lung cancers. In 2002, an estimated 72,600 men will be newly diagnosed with colorectal cancer and more than 27,000 men will die of the disease. The yearly rate of newly discovered colon cancer declined by more than 1.5 percent between 1985 to 1997, perhaps due to increased screening for polyps. Colorectal cancer accounts for about 10 percent of all cancer deaths, but mortality rates have declined over the past 20 years.

When colon cancer is detected at an early stage, the five-year survival rate is approximately 90 percent. Unfortunately, only 35 to 40 percent of people with colon cancer find it early, partly because there are usually few symptoms at the beginning. If the cancer has spread to local lymph nodes, the five-year survival rate drops to 65 percent, and if it spreads to more distant parts of the body, it plummets to 8 percent.

Prevention & Risk Factors: No one knows exactly what causes colon cancer, so there is no certain way to prevent the disease. Nearly three-quarters of all colon cancers occur in people without any known risk factors. Although some studies have found that people who regularly take aspirin (or other nonsteroidal anti-inflammatory drugs) are at decreased risk, the benefit is far from certain. Even so, it's worth making note of the things that may contribute to the likelihood of being struck by the illness and changing any behavior-related factors that can put you at increased risk:

Age. The risk of colon cancer becomes higher as you get older and is most common in people older than 50. It can occur at younger ages, however, sometimes even in boys in their teens.

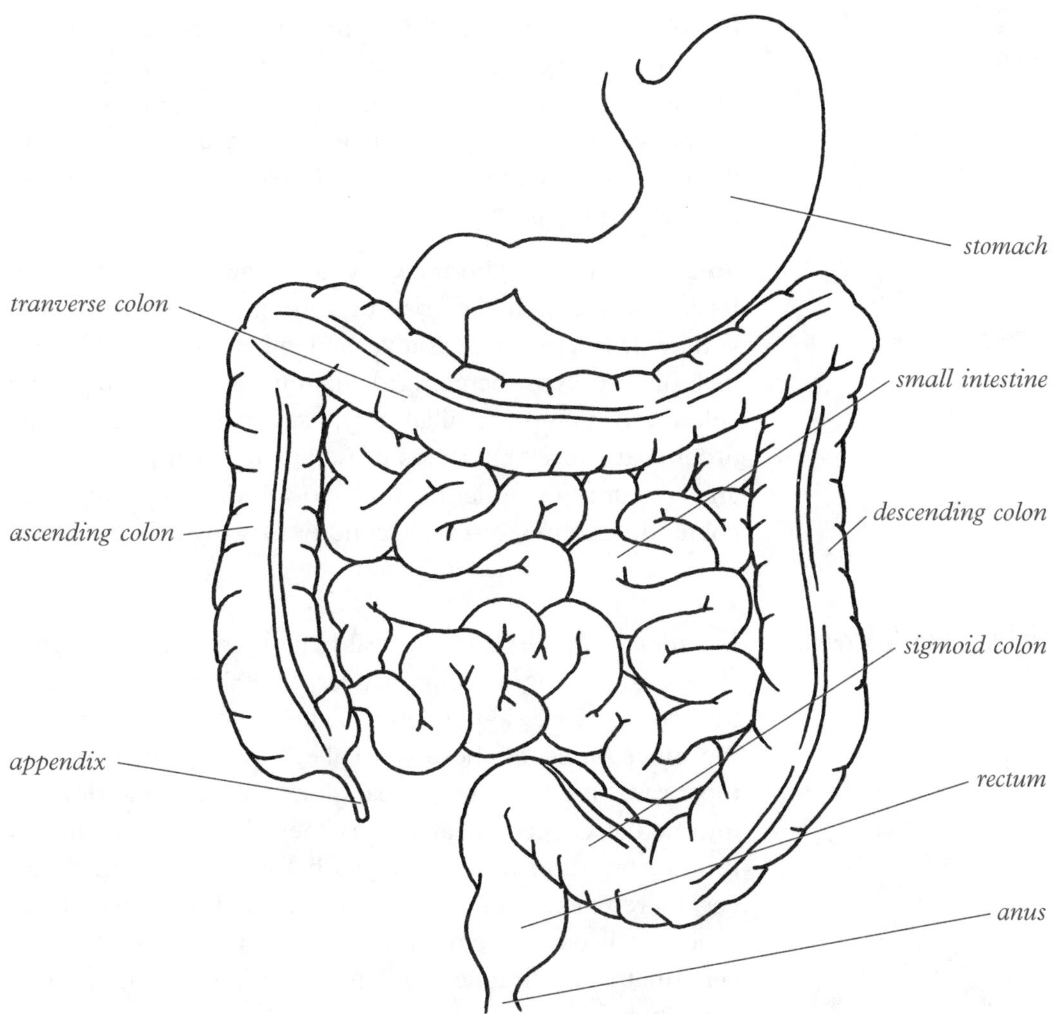

Diet. If you eat a high-fat, high-calorie diet that's low in fiber, you're at greater risk for the illness than if you're diligent about getting at least five servings of high-fiber fruits and vegetables every day. Scientists are still in the process of trying to understand how the things you eat affect your risk of colon cancer.

Obesity. The relative risk for colon cancer in men who are seriously overweight is 40 percent higher than in men of normal weight.

Family history. If one of your first-degree relatives (a parent, sibling, or child) had colon cancer, you're at a slightly increased risk for developing the disease, particularly if your relative was diagnosed before the age of 50. If more than one first-degree relative had colon cancer, your risk goes up significantly!

Your own medical history. If you've had colon cancer before, you are at higher risk of getting it again. Likewise, your risk is greater if you've had other bowel problems, including: polyps, benign growths on the inner wall of the colon and rectum; familial polyposis, a rare inherited disorder that causes hundreds of polyps to form in the colon and rectum; or inflammatory bowel disease (ulcerative colitis or Crohn's disease), conditions in which the lining of the colon becomes inflamed.

Diagnosis & Screening:

In order to understand the real benefit from early diagnosis and screening in colon cancer, you should understand that colon cancer almost always starts with a growth from the inner lining of the colon called a polyp—and that in most cases it takes 5 to 10 years for that growth to develop into actual cancer. That means there is usually plenty of time to find and remove polyps before they become cancer, thereby preventing colon cancer. And that's why there is so much current emphasis on screening for colon cancer—that is, finding polyps before they cause symptoms or actually become cancerous.

There are several different methods for trying to do this, including:

Testing for hidden (invisible, occult) blood in the stool. This method is based on the fact that sometimes a polyp or cancer will shed blood into the stool. If large amounts are shed, it will be visible in the stool or at the time of a bowel movement, and that is reason to call your doctor immediately. Testing for hidden blood is obviously designed to find blood you can't see.

Sigmoidoscopy. This test, which is usually done in a doctor's office, involves inserting a slender and flexible fiberoptic tube via the rectum up through the last one-third of the colon (often known as the sigmoid and descending portion of the colon) and looking for polyps or actual cancer. It has the advantage of not requiring sedation and is relatively easy to do as compared to a colonoscopy (see next test). However, it has the great disadvantage, in my view, of not examining the entire colon.

Colonoscopy. This procedure involves a tube similar to the one used in sigmoidoscopy, but the tube is larger and longer. Compared to sigmoidoscopy, it requires more skill on the part of the doctor and sedation to make it tolerable. That means more personnel and more expense. Actually, a colonoscopy is usually much less painful than a sigmoidoscopy because of the sedation; most patients do not remember the procedure or any pain during it. Unfortunately, the "cleaning out" of the colon the night before is often quite unpleasant. Colonoscopy has the great advantage of being able to examine the entire colon—and enables the removal of any polyps seen before they might become cancerous.

Barium enema. This time honored test involves inserting barium via the rectum to outline the colon before X-ray pictures are taken and then looking at the X-rays for defects suggesting a possible cancer or early growth. Today this exam is usually done also using a so-called "air contrast" technique to make it more effective. It is becoming increasingly clear that it is a less sensitive technique than colonoscopy, and I regard it as a second-line approach to screening for colon cancer.

At this point, I could present the various recommendations of different organizations regarding the pros and cons of the various screening tests described above. But I am going to save you all that reading by jumping to my own bottom line: As far as I am concerned, the only screening test to consider is the colonoscopy. It is the only one I have used for myself, and it is the only one I recommend to my family and friends. Several recent and major studies have indicated its superiority in finding early polyps or cancer compared to the other tests. And when a colonoscopy is perfectly normal—that is, when no abnormality is found—you can wait up to ten years before having another one done for screening purposes.

So why isn't everyone jumping on the colonoscopy bandwagon? The main reason is cost. Even though Medicare has now agreed to pay for this as a screening test every ten years, many private insurance companies are still not paying for it *for screening purposes* because it costs more than the other tests—and there is a very slight but real risk of more complications compared to sigmoidoscopy. The most worrisome complication is perforation of the colon—actually poking the tube through the wall of the colon and making a hole, which is obviously not a good idea. However, in the vast majority of cases, this can be repaired surgically with no long-term effects. And perforation is very uncommon in skilled hands. As it becomes clear that colonoscopy is better than sigmoidoscopy because it can examine the entire colon, and that it may save money in the long run by preventing actual cancer which is costly to treat, I believe more and more insurance companies will start paying for it for screening. (And someday colonoscopy *may* be replaced by the so-called "virtual colonoscopy"—a set of scan images that can be used to reconstruct a person's colon in visual form that can then be examined for abnormalities. This would have the advantage of avoiding the insertion of the colonscope into the colon, though it would have the disadvantage of not being able to remove any polyps seen.)

Because insurance companies will pay for colonoscopy for diagnostic purposes—looking for polyps or early cancer when there are actual symptoms or signs (see below for a rundown), some patients and doctors will "stretch the truth" by reporting some "blood in the stool" in order to get insurance companies to pay for what is really a screening test—that is, doing it to look for problems before any actual symptoms or signs develop. While I am opposed to such dishonesty, I am telling you what sometimes happens because I so strongly believe colonoscopy is the best way to screen for a potentially lethal disease. Indeed, I would recommend a person pay for it out of pocket if necessary because I think it such a valuable tool.

So now we come to the all-important question of when and how often you should have a colonoscopy. For men with no risk factors as described above, I would recommend a base-line (first time) colonoscopy screening at age 50. If you have risk factors, it should be done earlier in consultation with your primary care physician. If nothing is found during this base-line screening, you can probably wait 10 years before having another one. If one or more polyps are found, you will need more frequent follow-up exams.

A colonoscopy should also be scheduled immediately for any significant warning symptoms (abnormalities sensed by the patient) or signs (visible signals of possible disease). Unfortunately, in the case of possible warnings of colon cancer, it is sometimes difficult to decide what is significant. So I will discuss some of the possibilities in a little more detail:

Visible blood in the stool. If you can actually see blood in your stool or in the toilet bowl, you should regard that as a sign of colon cancer until proven otherwise. The problem is that usually such bleeding is due to something else less serious, most often hemorrhoids. However, I know too many tragic cases in which visible bleeding was ignored for months or even years until it was too late and a lethal cancer was finally discovered. That's why you should report any new or suspicious episode of visible blood to your doctor and let him or her decide whether and how it should be investigated.

Change in bowel habits. This one is even trickier than rectal bleeding because all of us have had the experience of a change in bowel habits from our normal pattern. But if those changes persist—I will arbitrarily say for more than two weeks—and especially if they are accompanied by other abdominal symptoms such as pain or a sense of fullness, then you should talk with your doctor about it. The one thing you should not do is wait until your next checkup to report any potential problems to your doctor. By then, it may literally be too late.

The reason I have spent so much time emphasizing the importance of screening and/or early diagnosis in the case of colon cancer is that it is one of the few cancers that we can really find early enough to cure routinely. *(The other one for men is prostate cancer—see page 103.)* In fact, I will go so far as to say that at least theoretically, colon cancer should be 100 percent curable given that there is so much time between the earliest polyp formation and the development of serious cancer. If this cancer can be found early and removed surgically, it can be cured—period!

Treatment Options:

If colon cancer is found, the course of treatment your doctor recommends will depend on the size and location of the tumor as well as how advanced it is and how good your overall health is. Following are the most common treatments, which may sometimes be used in combination to get the most effective results.

Surgery. A partial colectomy, in which the surgeon removes the tumor and an adjacent segment of the colon and nearby lymph nodes, is the most common strategy for people with colon cancer detected in early stages. Usually the surgeon can put the remaining colon back together so it works as well as before. Some people may need a temporary colostomy, in which an opening is made through the abdominal wall into the colon so waste can be emptied into a special bag attached to the outside of the body during healing. Today only about 15 percent of people who have surgery will need a permanent colostomy.

Chemotherapy. If the cancer has spread to your lymph nodes, chemotherapy will also be used to kill cancer cells that may have escaped the colon and spread to other parts of your body.

Radiation. Not used as often with colon cancer as with rectal cancer, this treatment kills cancer cells with high-energy X-rays.

Living with Colon Cancer: After surgery, you're likely to have a few weeks of abdominal tenderness, and you may have a tendency to diarrhea. Since chemotherapy affects all the cells in your body, not just cancerous ones, it can produce a number of side effects, including nausea and vomiting, hair loss, mouth sores, and fatigue. Common side effects of radiation include skin changes at the site of the radiation, loss of appetite, nausea, fatigue, diarrhea, and, in some cases, bloody stools.

Although there will undoubtedly be many things to cope with in post-cancer life, a big one for men is the presence of a colostomy, even if it's temporary. Becoming intimate with a partner can seem awkward and difficult, and you may be tempted to avoid sex entirely. But plenty of men in this situation continue having a normal sex life after colon cancer, according to the American Cancer Society, which has these tips on dealing with an "ostomy" appliance:

- Make sure your appliance fits correctly.
- Check the seal and empty your bag before starting any sexual activity.
- Try wearing one of the special, smaller ostomy bags during sex, or, if you can predict when your colostomy is active, plan sex for a time when it's inactive and just wear a stoma cover, which covers the hole in your abdomen.
- If you have an elastic support belt, tuck the pouch into the belt during sex. Two other options: Wear a sash around your waist to keep the pouch out of the way, or tape the pouch to your body.

Lung Cancer

The Basics: Your lungs are sponge-like, cone-shaped organs within each side of the chest that are the most critical part of your respiratory system. When you inhale, your lungs take in new supplies of oxygen, and when you exhale, your lungs get rid of carbon dioxide, a waste product of the body's cells. Lung cancer starts when something damages the tissue of the lungs, triggering cellular changes. The cells begin to divide uncontrollably, forming a tumor, or mass of abnormal cells.

There are two main types of lung cancer: *non–small cell* lung cancer, which is more common and usually grows and spreads more slowly, and *small cell* lung cancer. Doctors determine which type you have by looking at some of the cancerous cells from your lungs under a microscope.

An estimated 90,200 new cases of lung cancer will be diagnosed in men in 2002, and almost the same number of men will die of the illness. Fortunately, the incidence and number of deaths from lung cancer is declining in men. Experts attribute both declines to decreased smoking among men (unlike among women, who are smoking—and getting lung cancer—more). The five-year survival rate is about 60 percent when the disease is discovered before the cancer has spread, but only 15 percent of lung cancers are found that early. This means that 85 percent of people diagnosed with lung cancer are dead within five years!

Prevention & Risk Factors:

Unlike some types of cancer, experts know a fair amount about the causes of lung cancer. Following is a rundown of the factors that can put you at increased risk:

Smoking cigarettes. This is far and away the most dangerous thing you can do in general—and particularly as a risk for lung cancer. About 85 percent of lung cancer is caused by smoking! Tobacco contains harmful chemicals that damage the DNA of the cells of the lungs, and, over time, such cells can become cancerous. Factors like the number of cigarettes you smoke per day, the age at which you started smoking, and how deeply you inhale play a role as well. Research shows that after 10 to 15 years of not smoking, a former smoker's chance of developing lung cancer begins to approach that of a non-smoker. In other words, it pays to quit—at any time.

Secondhand smoke. Government surveys suggest that as many as 3,000 people develop lung cancer each year simply from inhaling smoke from other people's cigarettes.

Smoking cigars or pipes. Although usually not as deadly as cigarettes unless heavily inhaled, cigars and pipes contribute to the incidence of lung cancer. How long you've smoked, the number of cigars or pipes you smoke per day, and whether and how deeply you inhale all affect your risk. Even if you don't inhale, however, you're still at increased risk of developing lung cancer and at greatly increased risk for cancers of the mouth and throat.

Tobacco Troubles

Throughout this book I will be highlighting the dangers of tobacco at appropriate points. But at this point, early on, I would like to systematically explore the dangers of tobacco—and the benefits of quitting tobacco use at any age.

The Numbers

By any accounting, the deadly numbers associated with tobacco are staggering. Despite all the warnings, about 50 million Americans still smoke—still more men than women, although women are unfortunately "catching up."

Here are just a few of the consequences:

- It is the number one killer of men in this country.
- It causes over 400,000 deaths every year in this country.
- You lose about 5 to 6 minutes of life expectancy for every cigarette you smoke.
- One out of every two smokers will die of something caused by smoking.

The Poisons

Most people still think primarily of lung cancer when they consider the dangers of smoking. In fact, "only" about one-third of the deaths caused by smoking are due to lung cancer. Given that there are an estimated 4,000 different chemicals in cigarette smoke (many of them still secret because tobacco companies won't release this information and the government can't yet force them to do so), it is no surprise that tobacco has widespread effects in the human body. The "big three" are nicotine, tars, and carbon monoxide.

Nicotine is the primary addicting component of tobacco—now described by many experts as even more addicting than cocaine. Withdrawal symptoms are well known to smokers who try to quit—irritability, cravings, difficulty concentrating, etc. And switching to so-called "light" cigarettes with lower levels of nicotine and tars does not help; many studies now indicate that people who smoke such cigarettes quickly "learn" to smoke more and/or inhale more deeply to get their needed fix of nicotine. Nicotine also causes an increased heart rate and elevated blood pressure. *Tars* refers to the mix of sticky stuff that contains many known cancer causing chemicals. These are the substances primarily responsible for lung damage. *Carbon monoxide* is the same odorless gas that kills people in their homes because it decreases the amount of oxygen that can be carried by red blood cells to the cells of the body, including brain cells. Other toxic chemicals found in cigarette smoke include arsenic, formaldehyde, ammonia, lead, benzene, hydrogen cyanide, and vinyl choride.

The Effects

Another way to examine the dangers is to look at specific effects on different body systems. Here are a few "lowlights":

In the lungs tobacco smoke causes the destruction of cells in the alveoli, the tiny air sacs that are so critical to oxygen exchange from the air we breath into the bloodstream. (When enough of these cells get destroyed, you can be officially diagnosed with emphysema.) Tobacco smoke also damages cilia (the hairlike structures that line the passageways into the lungs) which are responsible for removing toxic substances and germs that get into our lungs. (That's why smokers have a much higher risk for chronic bronchitis.) And, of course, most cases of actual lung cancer (about 85 percent) are caused by smoking. *(For more information on emphysema and bronchitis, see page 199.)*

In the heart and blood vessels the effects of the chemicals in tobacco smoke are many, including a narrowing of coronary arteries, a decrease in good (HDL) cholesterol, and direct damage to arteries throughout the body that can increase the risk for high blood pressure and strokes. In addition, increased levels of carbon monoxide in the blood can be enough to kill oxygen deprived heart cells. No wonder that a smoker has up to three times greater risk for a heart attack than a non-smoker!

There are many other effects throughout the body—including: an increased risk for cancers of the mouth, tongue, throat, voicebox, esophagus, stomach, bladder, pancreas, and kidney; an increased risk for colds, asthma, bronchitis in yourself and your children; and an increased risk for wrinkles, ulcers, cataracts, and macular degeneration.

Finally, I should stress that smoking pipes and cigars is usually no safer. Many people who do so claim they do not inhale. But if they are regular cigar or pipe smokers, they almost always inhale far more than they realize. And if they have switched over from cigarettes, they usually inhale a lot.

Smokeless Tobacco. Smokeless is not safe—period. While it is true that direct damage to the lungs is less, almost all of the other dangers from inhaled smoke are still possible because the chemicals in tobacco—ncluding nicotine—are easily absorbed through the linings of the mouth and throat. And that, of course, greatly increases the risk for oral and throat cancers compared to regular smokers. (The same increased risk is true for cigar and pipe smokers even if they don't inhale.) And despite the obvious cosmetic downside of stained teeth and dripping, dirty mouths, smokeless tobacco advertisers have been very effective in hooking young boys on their products: sales of smokeless tobacco products have increased by over 50 percent since 1980!

Benefits of Quitting

Time for some good news: no matter how long you have smoked, no matter how old you are, it ALWAYS pays to quit. It is true that the earlier in life you quit, the greater the benefits. But some are almost immediate. Here is a "timetable of improvement" to encourage you:

Within Minutes	Very quickly, your heart rate and blood pressure will lower. (If you don't believe me, try taking your pulse right after smoking a cigarette and then take it twenty minutes later.)
Within Several Hours	The nicotine is starting to leave your body.
Within 8 to 12 Hours	Your blood levels of oxygen go up and carbon monoxide levels go down and are now back to normal.
Within 24 Hours	Your risk of having a heart attack is starting to drop.
Within 1 Week	You will notice you can breath easier (especially during exercise or climbing stairs), your sense of smell and taste will have improved, and your clothes and breath will smell better.
Within 1 Month	Your cilia (those hairlike structures in your airways I mentioned above) will have recovered and you will therefore probably notice an increase in the mucus being "raised" from your lungs. You may also cough more as a result. But any increased coughing should decrease over the next several months.
Within Years	The risk of having a heart attack or stroke should return to that of non-smokers within about five years. And the risk of getting lung cancer should return to that of non-smokers in about ten years. Since it takes a while to get over the increased risk of these "big ones" it is important to quit as soon as possible.

How to Quit

So how do you quit? Most experts say that the actual details or strategy of quitting are usually less important than the timing of the decision to quit. In fact, most people who quit do so "cold-turkey" without any medications or nicotine replacement gum or patches. But here are some time-honored tips about improving your chances of quitting when you decide to do so:

- Pick a time (and if possible, a place) when and where you will be under less stress. Sounds obvious, but you would be surprised at how many people give so little thought to this issue. For example, many people pick January 1 as part of a "New Year's resolution." But that may be the worst time for some people because it is when they are getting ready to go back to work, which is stressful. For many, a planned vacation is a better time because they can arrange many unusual and diverting activities rather than be stuck in their usual routine.
- If you haven't already, start a regular exercise program *(see Chapter 2, page 36)*. Studies show that all else being equal, exercise definitely increases your chances of quitting.
- Cut down on alcohol and caffeine drinks, which can increase the desire for nicotine and are often associated with "having a cigarette." Alcohol can also reduce the ability to resist temptation, especially in the first few months after quitting.
- Plan ahead for oral substitutes (healthy snacks or even hard candy) and drink lots of water.

Now what about the nicotine patches and gum that are available without prescription? (Nicotine inhalers and nasal sprays are available only by prescription.) I know many people for whom these aids have made the difference after trying other ways of quitting. Studies indicate they almost double your chances of success. The problem is that you should not smoke or use any other tobacco product at the same time because you may get too much nicotine into your system, even to the point where you can increase your risk of a heart attack or stroke. If you are going to use these products, read the directions very carefully – and follow them. You might also talk with your doctor about using the antidepressant medication Bupropion which is available only by prescription; because it does not contain nicotine, you can use it along with nicotine aids. Finally, I should stress that most people don't quit the first time so don't be discouraged if you don't.

Radon exposure. This colorless, odorless, tasteless radioactive gas occurs naturally in soil and rocks, and, when you inhale it, it can damage the lungs, predisposing the cells to becoming cancerous. The people at greatest risk are those who work in mines. Even though the risk of radon has been overblown, research has shown that some homes (some estimate about 10 percent) contain dangerously high levels. Hardware stores carry inexpensive, easy-to-use kits that allow you to test the radon level in your home. Smokers are most likely to develop lung cancer due to radon exposure.

Asbestos. This natural material is made up of tiny fibers which break easily and can float through the air. When you inhale the particles, they can lodge in your lungs, damaging cells and increasing your risk of lung cancer. People who have been exposed to large amounts of asbestos at work (in industries like shipbuilding, asbestos mining, insulation work, and brake repair) have a three to four times greater risk of developing lung cancer than people who haven't been exposed to the substance. If you smoke, the risk from asbestos exposure is much greater.

Air pollution. Although no one has been able to pin down a precise connection, many experts believe that the exhaust from diesel and other fossil fuels can increase your risk of lung cancer.

Radiation exposure. Some evidence suggests that being exposed to radiation from occupational, medical, and environmental sources increases your risk of lung cancer.

History of lung disease. If you've had tuberculosis or another disease that scars the lungs, you're at increased risk of developing lung cancer. Likewise, if you've had lung cancer in the past, you're more likely to develop it again than someone who's never had the disease.

Diagnosis & Screening: Unlike colon cancer, there's no routine or proven screening test for lung cancer, but if you're a long-time smoker it might be worth talking to your doctor about instituting an individual program of testing every year or two. Screening tests include:

Sputum exam. For this test, you'll be asked to provide a sputum sample so a pathologist can examine lung cells under a microscope.

Chest X-ray. There is no solid evidence that routine chest X-rays or newer CT scans make a difference in finding lung cancer early, but many doctors will order them for heavy smokers.

Biopsy. If a suspicious area is found, in order to diagnose lung cancer definitively, your doctor will need to examine a sample of lung tissue under a microscope. To retrieve the tissue, he or she will use one of the following methods: bronchoscopy, in which the doctor inserts a thin lighted tube through the mouth or nose and down the windpipe; needle aspiration, in which the doctor inserts a needle through your chest and into your lungs; thoracentesis, in which the doctor inserts a needle through your chest to obtain a sample of the fluid that surrounds your lungs; or thoracotomy, a type of major surgery in which the doctor actually opens up the chest to get at the lung tissue.

Researchers are currently working to find screening tests that can help identify the illness in its early stages. Until then, it's important to be aware of the symptoms—especially if you're a smoker or have smoked regularly in the past—and see your doctor if anything crops up. Symptoms can include: a persisitent (chronic) cough that gets worse instead of better; chronic chest pain near or under the ribs; coughing up blood; painful or difficult swallowing; breathlessness or wheezing; chronic pneumonia or bronchitis; a hoarse voice; fatigue; facial and neck swelling; and weight loss.

Treatment Options: The approach your doctor takes toward treatment depends in large part on whether you have non–small cell or small cell lung cancer as well as the location, size, and extent of the tumor and your general health. The options:

Surgery. The type of surgery the doctor performs depends on where the tumor is located. For instance, in a segmental or wedge resection, he or she removes just a small part of the lung; in a lobectomy, he or she removes an entire lobe or section of a lung; and in a pneumonectomy, he or she removes the entire lung on the affected side. Often, people with small cell lung cancer are in such an advanced stage that surgery isn't an option, so the doctor will use a combination of other treatments to control the cancer or reduce the symptoms.

Chemotherapy. Unfortunately, chemotherapy for lung cancer is usually not effective in preventing death, though it may provide temporary improvement in symptoms in some cases.

Radiation. This treatment kills cancer cells with high-energy X-rays, and it also may be used in lung cancer to relieve symptoms like shortness of breath. Although radiation is typically administered with an external machine, with lung cancer the doctor can insert a radioactive implant near your tumor to deliver radiation internally.

Photodynamic therapy. Most often used to relieve symptoms like breathlessness and bleeding, this therapy involves injecting a chemical, such as Photofrin (porfimer sodium), into the bloodstream, from which it is absorbed by cells all over your body. Because the chemical lingers in cancer cells longer than normal cells, doctors then use a laser to activate the chemical, which kills the cancerous cells.

Cryosurgery. Used primarily for non–small cell lung cancer, this treatment involves freezing and destroying cancer tissue.

Prophylactic head irradiation. Designed to prevent cancerous metastases from growing in the brain, this treatment is sometimes used for people with small cell lung cancer.

Living with Lung Cancer: If you have surgery, recovery can take several months. During that time, air and fluid may collect in your lungs, and you may have pain in your chest and arm and shortness of breath. Since chemotherapy affects all the cells in your body, not just cancerous ones, it produces a number of side effects, including nausea and vomiting, hair loss, mouth sores, and fatigue. Common side effects of radiation include sore throat, difficulty swallowing, loss of appetite, and fatigue. If the radiation is directed at the brain, you may have headaches, nausea and vomiting, hair loss, problems with memory, and fatigue. If you receive photodynamic therapy, you may need to avoid direct sunlight and bright indoor light for six weeks or more after treatment, because the therapy makes your skin and eyes sensitive to light. It also may cause difficulty swallowing, breathlessness, coughing, or painful breathing.

Prostate Cancer

The Basics: The prostate is a walnut-size gland located below the bladder in front of the rectum. It surrounds the upper part of the urethra, the tube from the bladder through which urine and semen flow. It contains gland cells that produce seminal fluid, a milky substance that protects and nourishes sperm cells in semen. More than 99 percent of prostate cancer develops from these glandular cells. (Most prostate cancer is called adenocarcinoma, meaning it starts in glandular cells.)

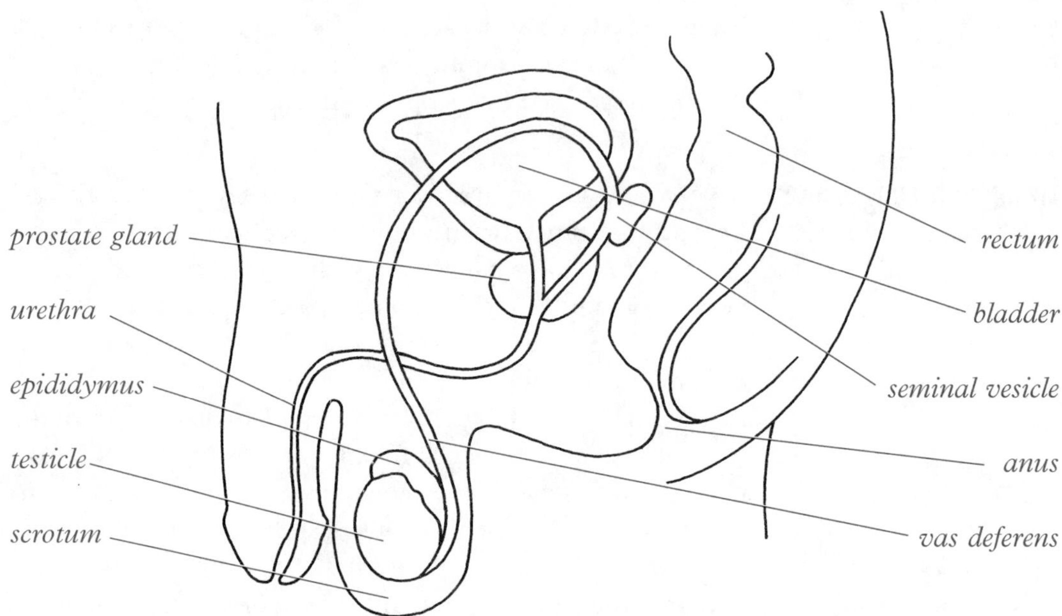

Most experts believe that prostate cancer begins with a condition called prostatic intraepithelial neoplasia (PIN), in which prostate gland cells undergo precancerous changes. The condition typically starts early—in men as young as 20. By age 50, almost 50 percent of men have PIN. The cellular changes are classified as low grade or high grade. About 30 percent of men who have high-grade PIN will develop prostate cancer.

When cells begin to divide uncontrollably, the precancerous condition has become cancerous. The rapidly dividing cells form a tumor, or mass of abnormal cells, which eventually interferes with the normal functioning of the prostate, sometimes enlarging the prostate so much that it can obstruct the flow of urine. The cancer may spread, or metastasize, to other parts of the body. Prostate cancer typically invades the nearby seminal vesicles, then metastasizes to the lymph nodes, bones, lungs, liver, or kidneys. Fortunately, most prostate cancers grow very slowly, but some can grow and spread quickly.

Prostate cancer is the second most common type of cancer found in American men, after skin cancer. An estimated 189,000 new cases will be diagnosed in 2002, and about 30,200 men will die of the illness. It is also the second leading cause of cancer death in men, exceeded only by lung cancer. Between 1988 and 1992, the diagnosed rates of this disease increased dramatically, thanks to increased use of the prostate-specific antigen (PSA) blood test, which allows doctors to detect prostate cancer early in men who have not yet developed any symptoms. Since then, diagnostic rates have leveled off.

While more men now have the disease, the survival rate has increased, because about 80 percent of prostate cancers are found before they've spread. Another way to put the numbers in perspective is to point out that while the overall lifetime risk of developing prostate cancer for American men is about 30 percent, 60 to 70 percent of cases will be the kind that spreads. Thus, the lifetime risk of actually dying from prostate cancer is about 3 percent. Which is to say that most men who are diagnosed with prostate cancer, especially those in later life, will actually die of something else.

Prevention & Risk Factors: Experts haven't uncovered a specific cause of prostate cancer, but they have identified certain risk factors—some of which you can change, some of which you can't—that increase the likelihood of developing the illness.

Age. Your risk for developing the illness increases with age. Although men of any age can develop prostate cancer, it is found most often in men over 50. The average age at the time of diagnosis is 70, and more than 80 percent of the men diagnosed with prostate cancer are over the age of 65.

Race. Prostate cancer is about twice as common among African-American men as it is among white American men, although no one knows why.

Family history. Your risk is two times higher if your father, uncle, or brother had the disease.

Diet. Some research suggests that a diet high in animal fat or calcium may play a role in the development of prostate cancer. *(See page 245 for more information on calcium.)*

Meanwhile, researchers are beginning to suggest ways you might protect yourself from the illness. For instance, eating a diet high in fruits and vegetables may reduce your risk. Because of promising preliminary studies, a large study on the potential protective benefits of vitamin E and selenium is currently underway. Both substances are antioxidants that are known to neutralize so-called "free radicals" that can damage genetic material and lead to cancer. A study sponsored in part by the National Cancer Institute showed that vitamin E may reduce prostate cancer risk by 30 percent, but the group didn't go so far as to recommend taking dietary supplements. Tomatoes, grapefruit, and watermelon contain lycopenes, a substance that helps prevent DNA damage and may help lower prostate cancer risk.

Getting regular physical activity and maintaining a healthy weight also may help reduce the risk of prostate cancer.

Diagnosis & Screening:

Because prostate cancer is usually very slow growing, it is possible in many cases to detect it before it spreads beyond the gland. Sometimes there are early warning symptoms, such as: difficulty starting urination, even with the feeling of a full bladder; more frequent urination, both day and night; or a less forceful stream during urination. These kinds of symptoms are caused by gland growth that pinches the urethra, the tube that carries urine from the bladder through the penis to the outside world. The urethra runs through the center of the prostate gland and can be partially, or in worst case scenarios, completely blocked when the gland enlarges. Obviously these symptoms can occur with enlargement from any cause, and indeed most of the time they are due to benign enlargement of the gland, so-called BPH (benign prostatic hypertrophy). That means that we must use various tests to decide whether prostate enlargement is due to cancer or some other less serious condition. *(For more on BPH, see page 292.)*

One time-honored test is the digital (finger) rectal exam, in which the examining physician inserts a lubricated and gloved finger into the rectum, where the posterior surface of the prostate gland can be felt through the front wall of the rectum. The doctor is trying to feel for any lumps or hard areas that might signify cancer. This exam can also allow the doctor to feel for any tumors in the rectum and to take a stool sample to test for hidden blood *(see screening for colon cancer on page 88)*. Because it can uncover several different problems, I think that a digital rectal exam should be done routinely as part of any physical exam in a man and routinely on a yearly basis in men starting at age 50.

The Controvesial PSA Test

Today, the most common test used for screening (looking for prostate enlargement even before symptoms develop) is a blood test measuring levels of PSA—prostate-specific antigen, a protein produced exclusively by prostate gland cells. (The results are reported in a number that means nanograms per milliliter; obviously you don't have to remember that, only the actual number.) Most of this protein is released into semen during ejaculation, but some enters the bloodstream, where it can easily be measured. Testing for this protein has revolutionized screening for prostate cancer—and produced a lot of controversy.

There is no doubt that blood screening for PSA has detected many cases of prostate cancer earlier than would have otherwise occurred and therefore probably saved many lives. The reason I use the word "probably" is that we can never know for sure in an individual case in which cancer has been detected by the PSA test if that person's cancer would have been detected early enough without the test to still have resulted in a curative treatment or if the cancer that was detected would ever spread to become life threatening. Overall numbers strongly suggest that screening with PSA testing has resulted in a reduction in the death rate from prostate cancer because of early detection. And I personally believe that to be the case even though I understand how hard this is to prove in rigorous scientific fashion.

The other reason that PSA testing is still controversial is the problem of "false negative" and "false positive" results. It is estimated that in about 30 percent of PSA tests, the results are reported as "normal" even though the man has early cancer, a so-called "false negative" result. Obviously that could lead to a false sense of security—nothing to worry about when in fact there might be reason to worry. (I use the word "might" here because as I will explain more fully in the treatment section, finding cancer cells in the prostate does not necessarily mean it will spread and cause death.) Even more dramatic, about 75 percent of men who have a "positive" PSA result will turn out *not* to have cancer, a so-called "false positive" result. In this case, the "false" word is less accurate because these results are "correct" in that the amount of PSA is indeed elevated but the elevation is caused by infection or enlargement of the prostate gland for reasons other than cancer—usually benign enlargement. Thus the "false" result is the implication that the PSA is up because of cancer when in fact it is elevated because of something else.

And that leads to the biggest problem with PSA testing: When you get an abnormally high number, you are usually forced to do more testing, such as ultrasound guided biopsies of the prostate (see below), to find out for sure what is going on in the gland. And those tests can be painful and expensive. But when they do find cancer and that early diagnosis leads to a curative treatment, most everyone would agree, at least in retrospect, that it was all worth it.

By now I hope you can understand that the controversy about PSA testing is not whether it does what it claims to do—measure levels of PSA in the blood—but whether finding out those levels is really "worth it."

There are several ways to try and increase the chances of getting a more accurate PSA test. One is to use some guidelines to help interpret the meaning of a given PSA number. For example, we now know that PSA is transported in the blood in two ways—"bound" to other proteins or "free" from other proteins. We can find out how much of each is occurring by doing a more sophisticated test than the usual "total" PSA done in screening. It turns out that when the amount of free PSA compared to total PSA is less than 25 percent, the chances that the PSA signifies cancer increases. Another way to make more sense out of a single PSA test is to see how much it differs from previous results, one reason to do these tests on a yearly basis. If the increase over several years is more than 0.75 per year (see below for an explanation of numbers), then it may be more significant. Finally, many doctors think it is important to take a man's age into consideration in interpreting a given PSA test result; the basic idea is that the older the man, the more liberal we should be in allowing a higher number to be interpreted as "normal" simply because the prostate gland enlarges in benign fashion in most of us as we get older.

What do the PSA numbers mean? I have finally come to the point where I need to talk about what number from a PSA test is "normal" and what kinds of numbers should cause concern. As many of you know, the usual number given as the upper limit of normal is 4.0 (again, this means 4.0 nanograms per milliliter). Anything below 4.0 is usually not cause for concern, unless, as I pointed out above, the number is significantly larger than a previous PSA test. But does that mean that anything over 4.0 is abnormal and should be investigated? Not automatically. For example, in a man in his late 60s or early 70s, a result of 5.0 might be considered normal–whereas in a 50-year-old man it would be cause for concern. As you are beginning to understand, I hope, this business of interpreting a single PSA number can be tricky.

Another controversial question regarding PSA testing is how often it should be done and at what ages. If you look at recommendations from different official organizations, you will find various guidelines, including some that don't recommend any routine PSA screening because of the problems mentioned above. But once again, I will state my opinion which is that it should be done yearly starting at age 50 and even sooner in African-American men or men with a family history of prostate cancer. It is what I have done for myself since age 50, and what I recommend to my friends and family. However, I also believe it makes little sense to continue such testing after age 75, because any cancer found at that time is not likely to be treated aggressively anyway (see below). The actual age at which to stop screening is a decision that should be made on an individual basis between each man and his doctor.

When a given PSA number is finally determined to be "abnormal," the next step is to take multiple small biopsy specimens from the prostate gland for examination under the microscope, the only way to make a definitive diagnosis. This is almost always done through the rectum under the guidance of ultrasound to find any particularly suspicious areas that should be biopsied. If the biopsies come back indicating cancer, there are many more decisions—and controversies—to face.

Treatment Options: Unfortunately, when a man is diagnosed with cancer cells in the prostate he will usually face a bewildering array of possible treatment options. I say "usually" because if the man is elderly and/or in poor health, the various options described below are less likely to be considered. Indeed, in a man over age 75, screening for prostate cancer makes little sense. That's because it is unlikely that any treatment would be recommended given the fact that cancers first discovered at that age are likely to be very slow growing, almost dormant, making it highly unlikely that the cancer will be lethal.

Before surveying various treatment options, I should

point out that it is important to try and determine the stage of the prostate cancer—that is, whether or not it is still confined to the gland itself or has spread beyond the gland. The doctor will order various imaging studies and other tests to try to make this determination, but sometimes the only way to find out for sure is at the time of surgery, if that option is chosen.

One of the most important decisions a man must make is where and how to gather information about the various treatment options. In an ideal world, the man (and his family) should be given a full range of information in unbiased form by his own doctor. Unfortunately, this is often not the case. If the doctor is a urologist, he or she will more likely favor surgery. It the man consults radiologists, they will more likely favor radiation—and even a specific kind of radiation (either external beam or implanted "seeds"), depending on their special interests. Sometimes an oncologist (the medical specialist in cancer who is neither a surgeon or radiologist) can be the best source of unbiased advice.

Today there are many excellent sources of information in print and on the internet. Unfortunately there is also a lot of bad stuff scattered on the information superhighway. I personally think that some of the information provided by major medical schools (Harvard, Johns Hopkins, or the Mayo Clinic, for example) is the most unbiased. However you do it, you should take the time to gather various opinions. Prostate cancer is not an emergency, though a decision about treatment should be made within weeks rather than months.

One of the most intriguing options today is so-called "watchful waiting"—meaning doing nothing while you are continually monitored using PSA and other tests to see if the cancer appears to be growing and needs treatment. This option is being chosen increasingly by men in their 70s and 80s, again because they believe their cancer will be slow growing and not likely to cause their eventual death. However, men in their 40s and 50s are more likely to consider surgery because of its long track record of proven cure if the gland can be removed before the cancer has spread. The follow-up data on radiation is now reaching a point where long-term outcomes can be compared to those of surgery. If they continue to compare favorably, many men will consider choosing radiation because of the somewhat lower risk for the complications of treatment men most dread—impotence (inability to have an erection) and incontinence (difficulty in controlling urination). But currently, many men in their 50s and early 60s will favor surgery because of its record of cure.

Having offered this overview of the difficulty in choosing how to treat prostate cancer, I will list very briefly the various options:

Surgery. Called a prostatectomy, the surgery in which the doctor removes all prostate tissue (radical prostatectomy) is the most common approach. Newer nerve-sparing techniques allow the doctor to increase the chances of saving the nerves that control erection and urination, trying to spare men the most dreaded side effects of surgery—impotence and incontinence. If you have a large tumor or one that lies close to the nerves, however, you may not be a candidate for this nerve-sparing surgery. Obviously the skill and experience level of the surgeon can make a big difference in this type of surgery. You should ask about numbers of cases done—and complication rates. Specific types of surgery include:

Retropubic prostatectomy, in which the doctor removes the entire prostate and nearby lymph nodes through an incision in the abdomen.

Perineal prostatectomy, in which the doctor removes the entire prostate through an incision between the scrotum and anus and sometimes the lymph nodes through another incision.

Cryosurgery, a much more controversial approach, used to treat localized prostate cancer by inserting a metal probe through an incision between the anus and scrotum and freezing the cancer cells.

Radiation. This approach uses high-energy X-rays to kill cancer cells. It can be delivered via an external radiation machine or may come from tiny radioactive pellets about the size of a grain of rice that are placed inside and/or near the tumor. Although both approaches may be used together, the latter approach is typically used on its own only in men with small tumors.

Anti-hormone therapy. This treatment is typically used for men who aren't good candidates for surgery or radiation or for men whose cancer has spread to other parts of the body. It doesn't eliminate the cancer, but it can arrest the spread of tumor and provide relief from some of the symptoms. The idea behind anti-hormone therapy is to prevent the cancer cells from getting the male hormones, or androgens, they need to grow. There are several different approaches to accomplish this goal. Orchiectomy is surgery to remove the testicles, which are the main source of male hormones. Although it's a fairly simple procedure and is the surest way to reduce male hormone levels, it can be emotionally difficult and isn't an option most men want to pursue. There are also many different medicines available to either reduce the production of male hormones or block their action in prostate cancer cells.

Living with Prostate Cancer:

During or after treatment, your doctor will most likely put you on a follow-up protocol to make sure the cancer does not return or spread. You'll receive regular PSA monitoring and digital rectal exams if your PSA goes up. Although prostate cancer itself is fairly curable, the treatments may cause problems that last a lifetime. That's why it's so important to weigh your options and to get a second (or third) opinion before choosing a course of treatment.

The main side effects of radical prostatectomy and cryosurgery are lack of bladder control and the inability to get an erection. For most men, normal bladder control returns within several months of the surgery. But one study found that two years after radical prostatectomy, 10 percent of men still had poor urine control; 14 percent leaked more than twice a day; and 28 percent wore pads to keep dry. Cryosurgery seems to have about the same results.

Most men who have a radical prostatectomy won't be able to get an erection without medication or some other treatment for at least a year. Depending on one's age and the quality and type of surgery that was done, erections may never return. If sex does become possible, orgasms will be dry because semen production requires a prostate gland.

Radiation therapy can cause fatigue, diarrhea, rectal leakage, frequent urination, burning during urination, and blood in the urine. Symptoms can linger even after treatment stops. Within two years of external beam radiation, between 30 and 60 percent of men become impotent.

Hormone treatment has serious side effects as well. For instance, roughly 90 percent of men who have orchiectomy are left with impotence and decreased or no sexual desire. Meanwhile, anti-hormone drugs can cause nausea, vomiting, diarrhea, or breast growth or tenderness. The low testosterone level caused by hormonal therapy can cause infertility, low libido, and difficulty having an erection.

Because coping with the diagnosis and treatment of prostate cancer is often especially difficult for men and their families, it's important to make sure you receive emotional support. Since your loved ones may be struggling with their own fears, it can help to join a support group, where you can share your thoughts about what's happening with people who are going through the same process. Men often find prostate cancer particularly difficult to deal with because of the sexual implications.

Skin Cancer

Melanoma

The Basics: Your skin is your largest "organ." It protects the rest of your body from infection, regulates your temperature, and produces vitamin D. It has two main layers. The outer layer is called the epidermis, the inner layer is called the dermis. In the inner part of the dermis are cells called melanocytes, which produce melanin, the substance that gives your skin its color. These cells are where melanoma, the deadliest form of skin cancer, begins.

Moles are actually normal, benign clusters of melanocytes. Most people have between 10 and 40 moles on their bodies. In people with melanoma, the DNA in normal melanocytes has undergone a transformation. Instead of telling the cells to divide in an orderly manner, it instructs them to keep dividing endlessly, forming cancer that may spread to other parts of the body.

In 2002, an estimated 30,100 men will be diagnosed with melanoma, and 4,000 men will die of the illness. But the incidence of this disease is on the rise. In the past 20 years, melanoma rates have increased about 3 percent a year. The disease is about 10 times more common in white American men than in African-American men.

About 80 percent of melanomas are found early, at a stage when they are highly treatable. The five-year survival rate for all people with melanoma is 88 percent; if you find one when it's still localized, it's almost 100 percent. But melanoma can spread to other parts of the body quickly, and the survival rate drops precipitously—to just over 10 percent—when this occurs.

Prevention & Risk Factors: Researchers are still trying to uncover the causes of melanoma. They know it is not contagious, but they still are uncertain of the exact cause or causes. There are, however, certain risk factors that seem to predispose people to melanomas.

Sun exposure. The increased incidence of melanoma over the past 20 years can probably be blamed in large part on the fact that people spend more time in the sun and therefore are exposed to greater amounts of the sun's ultraviolet radiation, which can cause skin changes that set you up for melanoma. One reason researchers have come to that conclusion is that people who live in warm parts of the country (and, as a result, spend more time outdoors) are more likely to develop melanoma. To help prevent sun-induced melanoma, it's important to avoid prolonged exposure to the sun between the hours when it's most intense, from 10 A.M. to 3 P.M.; wear a hat and long-sleeve shirt when you're going to be in the sun for a long time; and apply sunscreen with a sun protection factor (SPF) of at least 15 to your exposed skin every day. Most dermatologists I knew are "religious" about using sunscreen.

Sunlamps and tanning booths. Artificial sources of ultraviolet radiation can damage skin in the same way the sun's rays can, putting you at increased risk of developing this disease.

Sunburns that blister. If you had a severe sunburn that actually developed blisters, even if it happened as a child, you're at increased risk of melanoma for the rest of your life. The damage such intense burns does to the skin may trigger cancerous changes in the cells.

Dysplastic nevi. These atypical moles look different than most moles. They're usually larger and have irregular or indistinct borders, and they may have a range of colors in them, from pink to dark brown. They're usually flat, but parts of them may be raised above the skin's surface. The risk of developing melanoma is greater in people who have lots of dysplastic nevi.

More than 50 ordinary moles. If you have lots of moles on your body, you're at increased risk for melanoma simply because the disease begins in the melanocytes of an existing mole. Many moles provide more opportunities for the illness to start.

Fair skin. If you're fair and your skin burns or freckles easily, you're more likely to develop melanoma than a person with darker skin, because your skin is more easily damaged by the sun.

Family history. If you have two or more close relatives who have had this disease, you're at greater risk of developing it yourself, because melanoma seems to run in families. About 10 percent of people with melanoma have family members who also have had it. Of course, that means that the vast majority of people who develop melanoma have no such family history.

Personal history of melanoma. If you've had melanoma in the past, you're at increased risk of developing it again.

Age. Melanoma rates increase as you age, even more so in men than in women. Researchers at the University of California Irvine College of Medicine recently found that, starting at about age 40, men are more likely to develop melanoma than women. Up to that age, women are slightly more vulnerable.

Diagnosis & Screening: Some doctors will conduct a thorough skin exam as part of a routine physical. But there are no specific recommendations for annual screening for skin cancer. As a result, finding skin cancer requires a certain amount of vigilance on your part; it helps to have a family member or friend check parts of your body you cannot easily see.

Because the first sign of melanoma is often a change in the size, shape, color, or feel of an existing mole, it's important that you do regular skin checks—monthly, if you can—examining moles for subtle changes and keeping an eye out for new growths. The best time to do a skin exam is after a bath or shower, so your skin is clean, using a full-length or a hand-held mirror. Be thorough. Look not only at your arms, legs, trunk, and face but under your arms, at your fingernails and palms, between your buttocks and in your genital area, between your toes, under your toenails, on the soles of your feet, and on your neck, ears, and scalp. In men, melanoma is often located on the trunk, head, or neck. In dark-skinned people, it tends to turn up under the fingernails or toenails or on the palms of the hands or soles of the feet.

It helps to think of your mole check in terms of the letters ABCD:

- A for asymmetrical shape.
- B for uneven, notched, or blurred borders.
- C for uneven color.
- D for an increase in diameter.

Melanomas are typically larger than the diameter of a pencil eraser. Be particularly on the lookout for moles with a black or bluish-black area, a red flag for the existence of melanoma.

Other things to watch for: scaliness in a preexisting mole; an itchy feeling in a mole; oozing or bleeding moles; and hard or lumpy moles. Even if you've seen dozens of pictures of worrisome moles, don't rely on your own judgment to determine if you should be concerned about a suspicious-looking one. Get anything suspicious checked out by a dermatologist, a doctor who specializes in skin disorders.

If your doctor believes you have melanoma, he or she will do a biopsy to confirm the diagnosis. In this procedure, the doctor either removes the whole growth, if it's not too large, or a portion of it, then sends the tissue to a pathologist, who will examine it under a microscope to determine if it is indeed cancerous.

Treatment Options: Melanoma treatment depends on the location and thickness of the tumor, how deep the melanoma extends into the skin, whether the cancer has spread to lymph nodes or other parts of the body, and your age and general health. Before starting treatment for this often deadly cancer, it's always a good idea to get a second opinion to make sure the recommended course is the one that makes the most sense for you. Following are the most common treatments:

Surgery. The most common approach is to remove the melanoma as well as some of the normal tissue around the mole to be sure that all the cancerous cells are actually excised. If the mole is large and deep and the surgeon removes a large amount of skin and underlying tissue, you may need a skin graft, using skin taken from another part of your body to cover the open area. Your surgeon may also remove lymph nodes to learn if they contain cancerous cells. If they do, it could mean the cancer has spread to other parts of your body, in which case you'll need one or a combination of the following additional treatments.

Chemotherapy. This approach uses drugs such as hydroxyurea (Hydrea) and dacarbazine (DTIC-Dome) to kill the cancerous cells. A version of chemotherapy currently under development is limb perfusion, in which doctors place a tourniquet on the arm or leg in which the melanoma was found to stop the flow of blood to and from the limb. Then, they inject high doses of anticancer drugs into the limb. The advantage is that this therapy is more directed and focused than general chemotherapy, in which even healthy parts of your body may be damaged by the drugs.

Immunotherapy. This treatment uses drugs such as interferon-alfa and interleukin-2 to rev up your body's immune system and make it better at finding and fighting cancer cells.

Radiation. This approach, which uses high-energy X-rays to kill the cancer cells, is most often used to help control melanoma that has spread to the brain, bones, or other parts of the body.

Living with Melanoma: Side effects of surgery depend mainly on the size and location of the tumor and the extent of the operation. The scar to remove an early stage melanoma is usually a small, one- to two-inch line that fades with time. With larger, thicker tumors, the scars will be larger and more noticeable. If you have lymph nodes removed as well, limb swelling may be a problem, because the lymph fluid will no longer drain as easily. It also may be more difficult to fight infection in the affected arm or leg, because you don't have as many lymph nodes. Also—be on the lookout for any new melanomas!

Common side effects of chemotherapy include hair loss, fatigue, nausea and vomiting, and mouth or lip sores. Radiation can cause fatigue and hair loss and well, and immunotherapy may cause flu-like symptoms, including fever, chills, muscle aches, loss of appetite, nausea, vomiting, and diarrhea.

Basal Cell and Squamous Cell Carcinomas

The Basics: These two cancers form in the outer of the skin's two layers, the epidermis. The epidermis itself is composed of two kinds of cells. At its surface there are flat cells called squamous cells. Beneath these are round cells known as basal cells.

Almost half of all people in the U.S. will have epidermal cancer at least once by the age of 65. More than 90 percent of those skin cancers will be basal cell carcinomas, a slow-growing cancer that is highly curable, especially when detected early. Squamous cell carcinoma is only slightly more likely to spread than basal cell carcinoma, but it's important to find both types early so the cancer doesn't invade and destroy the surrounding tissue. There are about a million new cases of basal cell and squamous cell carcinomas every year, and 2,000 people died from them in 2001.

Prevention & Risk Factors: The same risk factors for melanoma (sun exposure and fair skin) apply to epidermal skin cancers. However, instead of moles, there are different skin abnormalities that can turn into squamous cell cancers. They are called *actinic keratoses*. These rough, red or brown, scaly patches on the skin typically appear on parts of your skin that receive the greatest exposure to the sun, like the head, face, neck, hands, and arms. These are the lesions that President George W. Bush has had removed from his face.

History of skin cancer. If you've had any skin cancer before, you're at increased risk of developing it again, either in the same place or somewhere else on your body.

Age. Your chances of developing skin cancer increase as you get older. Most epidermal skin cancers appear after age 50.

Diagnosis & Screening: Because the first sign of basal cell or squamous cell carcinoma is often a new growth or a sore that doesn't heal, it's important that you do regular skin checks—monthly, if you can—examining your skin for subtle changes and keeping an eye out for new growths. There's no single, uniform appearance to these skin cancers. They can start as a smooth, pale waxy lump, a firm red lump, or a flat red spot that is rough, dry, or scaly. Sometimes the spot bleeds or develops a crust. You should examine your skin for epidermal skin cancers in the same way you look for melanomas.

Treatment Options: The treatment plan depends on a number of factors, including the location and size of the cancer, the risk of scarring, and your age and general health. To make sure you're making the right choice, it's a good idea to know of all your options. Following are the most common treatments:

Surgery. Many basal cell and squamous cell carcinomas are fairly easy to remove, because they tend to be more superficial than melanoma. Sometimes the entire cancer is removed during the biopsy. A commonly used type of surgery is known as curettage and electrodesiccation. After numbing the area with a local anesthetic, the doctor scoops out the cancer with a spoon-shaped instrument called a curette, then runs an electrical current over the area to control bleeding and kill any remaining cancer cells. Another option for larger cancers is called Moh's surgery, in which the doctor gradually shaves off the cancer layer by layer, checking each layer under a microscope to see if it contains cancerous cells.

Cryosurgery. In this method, which is typically used for precancerous conditions like actinic keratosis, the doctor applies liquid nitrogen to the growth to freeze and kill the abnormal cells. When the area thaws, the dead tissue falls off.

Laser therapy. If the cancer is quite superficial, involving just the outer layer of skin, your doctor may opt to remove it with a laser, training a highly-focused beam of light on the area.

Topical chemotherapy. Superficial cancers and precancerous conditions like actinic keratosis can also be treated by applying an anticancer cream or lotion to the skin. One such drug is called fluorouracil (Efudex, Flouroplex).

Radiation. Most skin cancer responds well to radiation, in which high-energy X-rays are used to kill cancer cells. It's especially useful for carcinomas located on difficult-to-treat areas like the eyelid, the tip of the nose, and the ear.

Living with Skin Cancer:

Most types of surgery will leave a scar, which can range in size and visibility depending on how deep and extensive the tumor was. Radiation therapy can cause a rash or make your skin dry and red. Changes in the color and texture of the skin may become noticeable even years later.

CHAPTER 5

Cardiovascular Conditions

For most of us, the beating of our hearts signifies life itself, so any health problem connected to this powerful organ cuts to the very core of our fears about our own mortality. Fear alone will hardly keep this killer at bay. A better approach lies in the number of steps you can take to protect yourself. Some, like eating more fruits and vegetables, are fairly simple. Others, like maintaining a regular workout routine or managing stress, take a little more time and effort.

But one of the easiest things you can do is get informed. Read through the following sections so you understand the symptoms of some of the most common heart problems, and contact your doctor if you think something is wrong. Get to know the lifestyle changes that can make a difference. Most of them will not only keep you healthier in the long term, they'll make you feel better right now.

Coronary Artery Disease

The Basics: Coronary artery disease is the most common health problem in both American men and women. It can lead to actual heart attacks, which is the number one killer for both sexes, causing about a quarter million deaths in American men alone every year.

Researchers have identified many risk factors that contribute to this process (such as smoking, elevated blood fats, and high blood pressure) and are beginning to better understand what happens at the cellular level to initiate the clogging of our coronary arteries. *Atherosclerosis*, the major cause of coronary artery disease, usually begins with damage to the innermost lining of the arteries, the endothelium. When this lining is damaged, various substances like fat and sometimes calcium start to collect and form plaques. These plaques can break apart (rupture), leading to the sudden formation of blood clots which can block the flow of blood to heart muscle. In order to better understand what happens when plaques form and sometimes rupture, it is helpful to understand some of the terms that we doctors sometimes casually toss around. Specifically, I want to take the time to discuss the process that can lead to an actual heart attack so that you can better understand the discussions about screening, diagnosis, and treatment that will follow.

Coronary Arteries in Cross Section

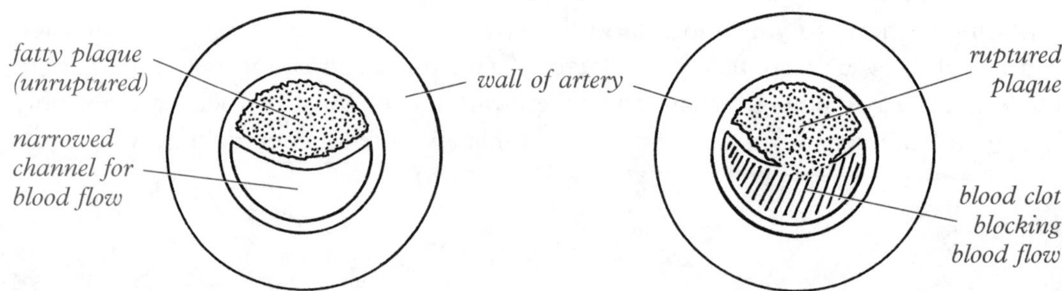

First I should explain that heart muscle cells must get their oxygen and nutrients from blood brought to them by the coronary arteries. They cannot get these essentials by simply extracting them from the blood flowing through the chambers of the heart. The coronary arteries that supply blood to heart muscle cells arise from the aorta, the major artery emerging from the heart's main pumping chamber (the left ventricle). Every time the heart beats, it pushes blood out through the aorta to all parts of the body. And just above the heart there are two coronary arteries that branch off the aorta, carrying blood directly back to the heart muscle cells through a branching system of arteries that run over the surface of the heart. Blockages to the flow of blood to heart muscle can occur anywhere in this system of coronary arteries; obviously, the larger the blocks and/or the larger the artery blocked, the more likely it is to be dangerous since it will affect a larger area of heart muscle. (I should also point out that besides actual blockages in the arteries from plaques and/or blood clots, coronary arteries can sometimes go into spasms when the muscle cells in the artery wall contract; these spasms can also interfere with blood flow through the arteries, but this is a much less common cause of decreased blood flow than blockages from plaques and clots.)

Coronary Artery System

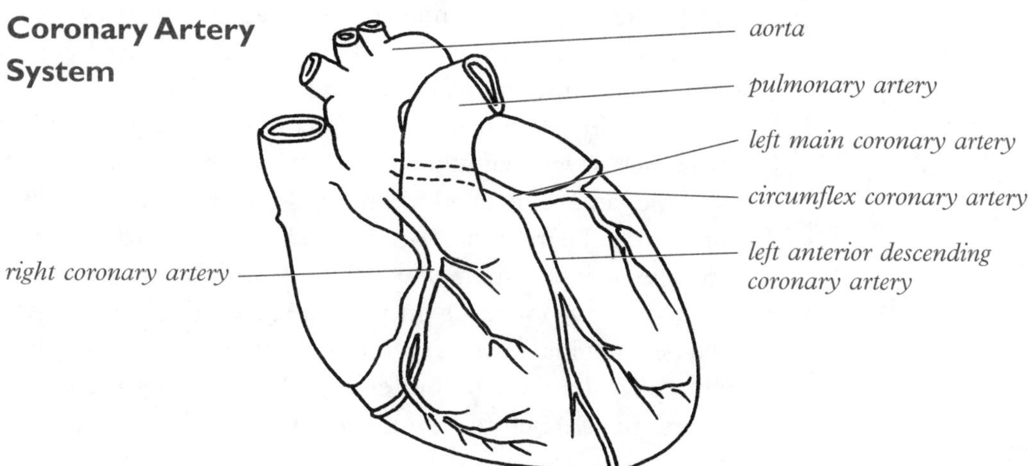

Angina Versus Infarction

When blood flow is decreased below what is needed by the heart muscle to do its job, various symptoms can result. That means that either a decrease in flow or an increase in demand—or both—can lead to a problem. In other words, it is a matter of balance between coronary blood supply and heart muscle demand from moment to moment. For example, even though there may be no change in blood flow through the coronary arteries, if a middle-aged man goes out to shovel snow, thereby suddenly increasing the demand on his heart to pump more blood to meet his new energy needs, he can quickly be in big trouble. Or if a man sleeping in bed suddenly has a blood clot form in his coronary artery system, he can also be in big trouble from a sudden decrease in blood supply to his heart muscle, even though the demand on his heart has not changed. And if a man has a sudden blood clot form in a major coronary artery while he is running a marathon, he is likely to be in very big trouble because supply is decreasing and demand is increasing at the same time!

When the balance between supply and demand changes, various symptoms can result. The most common is the chest pain or discomfort called angina, which is the kind of pain that develops because muscle cells (in this case of the heart itself) don't get enough oxygen. Angina and other symptoms may be brief and temporary, but if the imbalance between blood supply and demand continues, the symptoms will continue. If the decreased supply of blood in relation to demand continues long enough or becomes severe enough, the deprived heart muscle cells will die, an event called infarction. This is what happens in an actual heart attack—permanent damage to the heart muscle—versus angina, which is simply a symptom that may or may not result in permanent damage. Some have likened angina to a "cry for help" from heart muscle; if you pay attention to the cry, you can often rescue your heart muscle before permanent damage occurs. And one reason I am taking the time to explain the difference between angina and actual infarction is that a lot of men have had some chest pain that did not evolve to permanent heart muscle damage, and yet they think they have had a "heart attack." In fact, the only time that label should be used is when permanent damage to the muscle has been accurately diagnosed. (Because the infarction occurs in heart muscle, which is also known as myocardium, you will sometimes hear a heart attack called a myocardial infarction, or an "MI.")

Stable Versus Unstable Plaques

I want to describe one other concept that is currently the "hot stuff" in the study of coronary artery disease. For many years our focus has been on the kind of plaques that grow as a bulge into the center (lumen) of the coronary artery, where the blood flows. These kinds of plaques can eventually get large enough to interfere with blood flow and produce symptoms such as angina. They are the kinds of plaques that can usually be detected with various tests, such as a stress test or angiogram (see below). And they are the kind of plaques that are often treated with angioplasty or bypass surgery to relieve symptoms. However, because they usually have a thick covering, these are not the kind of plaques that are most likely to suddenly rupture and cause a blood clot that can lead to a massive, fatal heart attack from major obstruction of blood flow.

Rather, what we have been learning in the last 10 to 15 years is that plaques that are often smaller or that lie "hidden" in the wall of the coronary artery—as opposed to those that project into its center or lumen—are the ones that are more likely to rupture and cause sudden death. Because these plaques usually have a thin covering, they are often called "vulnerable" or "unstable" plaques. The big problem is that they often do not produce warning symptoms before they rupture—and they are often not detected by our standard tests, including the so-called "gold standard" test, the angiogram (see below).

I am not describing all this to scare you—although it is scary. The good news is that the standard advice we have been giving for years to reduce the risk for thick coronary artery plaques also seems to decrease the risk for unstable plaques. So it becomes even more important than we once thought to pay attention to these risk factors.

Prevention & Risk Factors: There are three major risk factors for coronary artery disease that we can't do anything about—our sex, our family history, and our age (the older we get, the more likely statistically we are to have a heart attack). It is true that until about age 50, men are much more likely to have heart attacks than women. That's because women are somewhat protected by the supply of female hormones produced by their ovaries until menopause. However, after the age of menopause, women start to rapidly catch up to men in terms of heart attack risk, and by about age 70 they are at the same risk as men. I should also point out that "family history" can be misleading. Having a family history of distant relatives who died of "heart failure" in their old age does not increase your risk for serious heart attacks. Rather, the kind of family history you should worry about are close relatives (parents, siblings, uncles) who had serious coronary artery disease before the age of 60. (The phrase "heart failure" refers to a heart so weakened it cannot pump vigorously enough to get blood out to the body; this is a condition that can have many underlying causes, one of them being damage done to heart muscle by heart attacks from coronary artery disease.)

The big three risk factors that we can do something about are high levels of fats in our blood (hyperlipidemia), high blood pressure (hypertension), and smoking. As I stressed in my earlier tobacco discussion *(see page 96)*, the message about smoking is real simple—don't! In fact, while most people think mostly about lung cancer when they worry about smoking, smoking actually causes more deaths due to heart disease. If you smoke, there is no single better decision you could make to improve your health than to quit smoking! In fact, I would personally say that if you continue to smoke, it doesn't make much sense to worry about a better diet and more exercise because any benefits are likely to be overridden by the dangers of smoking. The messages about high blood fats and hypertension are more complicated so I am going to take more time to discuss them at this point.

High Blood Cholesterol (Hypercholesterolemia)

By now, most of you know that "high cholesterol" is bad for your heart. However, you may still be confused by the different types of cholesterol and the meaning of their different numbers, so I am going to offer a brief primer. (Triglycerides are another kind of blood fat which may also increase your risk for coronary heart disease, but they are generally not as important as cholesterol.)

The cholesterol in our bodies is actually carried around in combinations with proteins called lipoproteins ("lipo" means fat). These lipoproteins differ in several ways, including density. The ones that have low density are logically called low density lipoproteins, or LDL for short; since these are the ones that deposit cholesterol in our coronary arteries and lead to the fatty blockages called plaques, they are usually referred to as "bad cholesterol." The ones that have high density are called high density lipoproteins, or HDL for short; since these are the ones that remove cholesterol from the plaques in our coronary arteries, they are usually referred to as "good cholesterol." When you have your blood cholesterol levels measured, you are usually given several numbers, including a total cholesterol (which includes both HDL and LDL, plus some other less important lipoproteins) plus separate numbers for HDL and LDL. The question then arises as to which numbers are most important and what numbers you should be striving for.

For years, most physicians and patients paid most attention to the total cholesterol number. However, as we have come to better understand these numbers, we now realize that all of them are important—and that the most useful single number may be the so-called ratio of total cholesterol to HDL (good) cholesterol. Let's take two men, both of whom have total cholesterols of 200 (that's milligrams per deciliter, or mg/dl—which is the way cholesterol numbers are reported). That sounds pretty good for both of them at first blush. However, when we look at the separate numbers that make up the total, we find that one man has an HDL level of only 25, which would give him a ratio of eight (200 divided by 25), while the other has an HDL of 50, which would give him a ratio of four (200 divided by 50). So while their total cholesterols are the same, their actual "cholesterol status" is very different. Since the goal is to have a ratio of four or under (the lower the better), one of our men is OK while the other has a dangerously high ratio.

Another approach is to focus on just the HDL and LDL numbers. The most recent guidelines from the National Cholesterol Education Program urge getting the HDL to or above 40 (the higher the better) and the LDL down as low as 100. Many physicians still use 130 as the goal for LDL, but in people with other known risk factors like diabetes and/or a history of CAD, the goal of 100 may be worthwhile. Quite frankly, I don't really care whether you use the ratio or the individual numbers for HDL and LDL as your goal as long as you understand that the more HDL the better, the less LDL the better.

Treatment of High Cholesterol

The new guidelines also call for every adult to get a full lipid (blood fats) profile blood test (total cholesterol, HDL, LDL, and triglycerides) done every five years. But that is really the bare minimum. Many adults will have more frequent testing either because they have a diagnosed cholesterol problem that needs monitoring or because they have other risk factors for CAD. I would certainly recommend a lipid profile as part of any comprehensive health checkup. Finding and treating a cholesterol problem is one of the best preventive health measures available today.

Now the really important question is: *What can we do to increase the good cholesterol and lower the bad cholesterol?* Dietary changes and an increase in exercise can help in many cases, and I would urge them as the first line of defense. Certainly it pays to reduce saturated fats in the diet because they are readily converted in the body to cholesterol. They are usually a much larger source of increased cholesterol in the blood than actual cholesterol-rich foods like eggs. And regular exercise can often raise good cholesterol levels in modest fashion. But when you are facing serious cholesterol problems (too little good and/or too much bad), it is quite likely that you are going to need medicine in addition to lifestyle changes.

At this point I could run through the list of medicines which can help lower bad cholesterol and, usually to a much lesser degree, raise good cholesterol. But once again I am going to save you a lot of time by getting to this bottom line: If you have a serious cholesterol problem, your doctor is very likely to go straight to the newest and best medicines available, a class of medicines known as statins. These are drugs which block the action of an enzyme in the liver that helps make cholesterol; blocking this enzyme usually dramatically reduces the level of bad cholesterol and modestly raises the level of good cholesterol. There are several of these drugs currently approved in the U.S. and several more in the pipeline; you have undoubtedly heard of them by their trade names—for example, Lipitor, Lescol, Mevacor, Pravachol, Zocor—because they are heavily advertised directly to the public, often using celebrities with testimonials. And while the different manufacturers would like you to think that their particular brand is best, most experts think they are more or less the same. Sometimes, one particular statin drug will produce some side effects such as nausea in a given person, whereas another one will not—so trying different statins may sometimes be necessary.

The two most serious side effects that can occur with the statins are liver damage and muscle damage. Both are rare, but anyone taking statins needs to be monitored periodically with blood tests, especially when first taking them, to check for such damage. (You may recall that one statin drug, Baycol, was recently removed from the market because it caused far more cases of muscle damage than any of the other statins.) Fortunately, when evidence of liver or muscle damage is found with blood tests, the drugs can be lowered in dose or stopped if necessary, and there will be no lasting damage. Indeed, given the wide use of statins (over 12 million people in the U.S. alone are taking them) they have proven to be remarkably safe and very effective—so effective that most doctors today will turn to them as the first drugs to try for serious cholesterol problems.

In fact, statins have proven to be so effective and safe that they are often described as a "miracle" for people who have very serious cholesterol problems. Again, I stress that they must be monitored carefully by a competent physician. But I believe they can mean the difference between prolonged life and early death for people with a serious cholesterol problem that cannot be corrected any other way.

We are now learning that these drugs may have benefits for coronary arteries besides lowering cholesterol, such as making unstable plaques more stable by reducing inflammation in them. The statins may even have benefits elsewhere in the body, possibly reducing the risk for Alzheimer's disease and osteoporosis (bone thinning).

Unfortunately, statin drugs are still very expensive and may be unaffordable for people without good health insurance. (This is a problem in general—effective drugs that too many of our citizens cannot afford—that must be addressed by our politicians, by either putting pressure on drug companies to lower prices when appropriate or helping with funds to buy them—or both.) There are other cholesterol-lowering drugs available, like resins, niacin, and fibrates, but in general they are less effective and have more annoying side effects. However, they may be considered in the relatively rare person who cannot afford or tolerate a statin drug—and in those whose major problem is a very low HDL and/or high triglyceride level. Sometimes a statin will be used in combination with one of these other drugs.

Finally, what about two popular OTC (meaning you can buy them "over-the-counter" without a prescription) supplements advocated for high cholesterol—garlic and soy? Garlic oils have become very popular for this purpose but some recent studies suggest they aren't very effective for lowering cholesterol. The studies on soy are more encouraging but suggest that soy is not potent enough for people with serious cholesterol problems—and that large amounts of soy every day might be potentially dangerous.

High Blood Pressure (Hypertension)

As with cholesterol, there is often a lot of confusion about blood pressure numbers—what they mean and which ones are important. So once again, I am going to explain them in very simple terms.

As you know, your blood pressure is typically measured using two numbers—a first number called the *systolic* pressure and a second number called the *diastolic* pressure. They are usually expressed as the systolic number "over" the diastolic number—for example "120 over 80," or written as 120/80. (The unit for these numbers is millimeters of mercury or mm Hg, which stems from the classic way of measuring blood pressure—using a column of mercury to see how high it is raised by a given blood pressure.) The first number, the systolic pressure, reflects that very brief moment of pressure that occurs when the heart is actually contracting and forcing the blood through our arteries as the wave of pressure we feel as the "pulse." (Each pulse wave reflects a single heart beat, which is why we can determine our heart rate by counting our pulse rate.) The diastolic pressure reflects the "resting" pressure in our arteries when the heart is not contracting. For many years, physicians debated about which number is more important in terms of reflecting the dangers of high blood pressure. We now know that both numbers are important and that an elevation in either one can be dangerous.

Which brings us to the important question: *What numbers are too high?* As with cholesterol values, there is no exact number at which you switch from "normal" to "abnormal." But in general, we doctors like to see people get their systolic blood pressure under 140 and their diastolic pressure under 90. In fact, we much prefer the systolic to be under 130 and the diastolic under 80. And to put it even more dramatically, the lower the blood pressure the better, as long as you feel OK. For example, many women of small size have blood pressures where the systolic is under 100 and the diastolic is around 60—and they feel perfectly fine. In general, blood pressures under 80/50 are very unusual in people who are healthy.

However, as most of you also know, it is sometimes hard to determine what a person's blood pressure really is day in and day out under normal circumstances. That's because our blood pressure numbers can often go up temporarily when we are nervous—such as when our blood pressure is being taken in a doctor's office! (That seems to be especially true for men who don't like going to the doctor.) In fact, so common is this phenomenon that it has been given a name—"white coat hypertension"—meaning high blood pressure that seems to be brought on by nervousness in seeing a doctor. All of which is to make the point that before we label someone as having the disease of hypertension—persistently elevated blood pressure that might be dangerous—we need to make sure we are getting numbers that accurately reflect what the person's pressure is most of the time. That's why we often ask a person to take their own pressure several times during the day at home (or at work) using some of the excellent home devices now available. Having said this, I must also point out that a person whose blood pressure often goes up under circumstances of stress—so-called labile blood pressure—may be at more risk for eventually developing permanent high blood pressure.

Once you are diagnosed with hypertension, it is important to look for any underlying causes that can be corrected. This kind of hypertension—so-called "secondary hypertension" because it is secondary to other problems—is relatively rare. The vast majority of hypertension has no known cause—and contrary to what the name implies, it is not caused by "tension" or "nerves." Indeed, you cannot tell what a person's blood pressure is by whether or not they seem high strung or nervous; perfectly calm people can have very high blood pressures and vice versa. In fact, most people with high blood pressure who are not diagnosed by screening checks have no warning symptoms until it has already caused serious damage to the heart (in the form of a heart attack), the brain (a stroke) or the kidneys (kidney failure) or until it causes a truly catastrophic event like the rupture of a weakened artery in the brain (a burst aneurysm). That's why we rightly label hypertension as a "silent killer" and why we stress the importance of having your blood pressure checked regularly. This is especially true if you have a family history of hypertension or if you are African-American and therefore at greater risk for developing high blood pressure and its complications.

Treatment of High Blood Pressure

So what is the best treatment for hypertension? Again a complicated question—considerably more complicated than figuring out the best treatment for high cholesterol where, as I pointed out, there is a class of drugs that is clearly superior for most people with the problem. In the case of hypertension, lifestyle measures are often more helpful than they are in treating high cholesterol. For people with borderline high blood pressure—meaning in the 130 to 140 range for systolic numbers and/or the 80 to 90 range for diastolic numbers—the following measures can often lower the blood pressure into a normal range without taking medication:

Lose weight. For someone who is overweight, losing as little as 10 pounds can sometimes make a big difference in blood pressure, and losing more can make an even bigger difference.

Exercise regularly. As with weight, a relatively modest change in exercise habits can often make a significant difference.

Reduce salt in your diet. While there is considerable debate about the role of salt in actually causing high blood pressure, there is wide agreement that if you have high blood pressure it often pays to cut down on the salt in your diet.

Increase the fruits and vegetables in your diet. A recent major study once again demonstrated the value of this kind of diet in lowering blood pressure. Fruits and vegetables contain potassium, magnesium, and calcium, all of which may help bring down high blood pressure.

Decrease excessive alcohol intake. More than two standard-size alcoholic drinks a day tends to raise blood pressure (while one such drink a day may actually lower it). This is definitely a case where more is *not* better.

Consider meditation techniques. While I think the benefits of various meditation techniques are sometimes overstated in terms of actual physical benefits, there is no doubt they can be useful in modestly lowering blood pressure. And they may well improve your emotional and spiritual outlook!

Stop smoking. Always the best health advice I can give.

Again, I would point out that the above, especially in combination, can sometimes make a real difference in lowering borderline high blood pressure. However, when blood pressure numbers are truly high—over 150 systolic and 100 diastolic—medication is usually required along with lifestyle changes to effectively treat the problem. But unlike the situation with high cholesterol medications where one class of drugs clearly stands out, there are many different classes of medications to choose from in treating high blood pressure. In fact, again unlike high cholesterol treatment, it often requires a combination of different medications to effectively treat seriously high blood pressure. And that means that it may pay to go to a true specialist in hypertension treatment to find the right drug or drugs to treat the problem. Usually, a good primary care doctor can do the job, but you should not hesitate to seek out a specialist in high blood pressure treatment if you are having trouble controlling your pressure—or if you are having trouble with side effects from the medicines you are taking. There are literally dozens of different blood pressure medications available today and all of them can be effective for the right person, but they can all also cause significant side effects. So again I stress that this is one disease—serious high blood pressure—where real expertise can often make a big difference.

At this point I am going to list and briefly describe the major categories of drugs used to treat high blood pressure. Remember that within each of these categories, there are many choices and that combinations of drugs from different categories are very common today. (Many of these drugs are used to treat other conditions such as coronary artery disease and heart failure so I will often refer to these groups of drugs.)

Diuretics. As their popular name "water pills" suggests, these are drugs that promote increased urination and fluid loss from the body, thus reducing fluid pressure in our arteries. They have been used for decades and have a proven track record of safety and effectiveness. Examples include chlorothiazide and furosemide.

Beta blockers. These drugs act to block so-called beta receptors in various body cells—hence their name. These drugs have also been used for decades and are prescribed for many other problems ranging from headache prevention to the prevention of the physical signs of anxiety. By blocking beta receptors, these drugs have many effects, including lowering blood pressure and heart rate. They are also widely used to protect the heart after a heart attack or during heart failure. Examples include atenolol and propranolol.

ACE inhibitors. These drugs get their name not from the hardware stores but from the fact that they inhibit a body chemical called angiotensin converting enzyme (ACE for short) that causes narrowing of blood vessels. These drugs also help protect the kidneys in people with diabetes and kidney problems. Along with beta blockers, they are very effective in protecting the heart after a heart attack or in heart failure *(see page 147)*. Another newer and related category of drugs are called angiotensin receptor blockers. They act directly on angiotensin receptors to prevent blood vessel narrowing. Examples include captopril (ACE inhibitor) and losartan (receptor blocker).

Calcium channel blockers. As the name suggests, these drugs block cellular structures called calcium channels and therefore affect the flow of calcium in cells. That, in turn, can prevent narrowing of blood vessels. Examples include diltiazem and verapamil.

There are several other categories of high blood pressure drugs but the above are the ones most physicians will start with—either individually or in combination—in treating high blood pressure. Again, I stress that all of them have potential side effects and must be monitored for any potential problems.

Other Risk Factors for Coronary Artery Disease

There are several other important risk factors for coronary artery disease that are also discussed elsewhere, including obesity, physical inactivity, and diabetes *(see pages 28 and 196)*. And there is one other relatively new risk factor that I would like to at least briefly discuss at this point—namely homocysteine.

Homocysteine is a naturally occurring amino acid in our blood that has been increasingly linked as a risk factor to coronary artery disease—the higher the homocysteine blood level, the higher the risk of coronary artery disease. There is still a lot of debate about why it might be dangerous, what levels are dangerous, and who exactly should be tested. However, there is a growing consensus that until we get answers, it might be prudent to take supplements of folic acid and vitamins B-6 and B-12 if you have high levels of homocysteine, especially if you have other risk factors for coronary artery disease. All these help lower the homocysteine level. *(See page 175 for a discussion of homocysteine and Alzheimer's Disease.)*

I have been deliberately vague about what levels of homocysteine are "high" and about how much of these vitamins you should take because I would much prefer that you make these decisions with your doctor as part of an overall strategy in reducing your risk of heart disease. Similarly, you should talk to your doctor about taking supplements of vitamin E (anywhere from 100 to 400 IU daily) to help prevent coronary artery disease. There is considerable controversy about the use of vitamin E in preventing coronary disease. Some recent studies suggest that antioxidant vitamins may even interfere with the benefits of statin drug therapy for high cholesterol. Having said this, I will also tell you that many doctors I know are taking 200 to 400 units of vitamin E just to hedge their bets.

And I am going to mention one other preventive approach that you are likely to be hearing more about—namely that of combatting infection and/or inflammation in vulnerable arterial plaques to forestall their growth and rupture. Researchers are looking especially close at a microorganism called chlamydia, which is a common cause of other human infections, such as pneumonia and sexually transmitted disease (STD). There is some evidence that this microorganism can increase the risk of plaque rupture in coronary arteries—and that treatment with antibiotics might reduce that risk. Researchers are investigating a blood test for a substance called C-reactive protein, which is a signal of inflammation in the body, as a way of determining who might benefit from antibiotic therapy. But, again, this is an area of research that is evolving and is not ready yet for prime time in terms of firm recommendations for testing and treatment.

Finally, I want to underscore the known benefit of taking a daily aspirin to prevent the formation of blood clots, in this case those clots that can form suddenly and block blood flow in a coronary artery. I have long advocated a daily aspirin in people who are not allergic to aspirin (rare) and who are not likely to develop internal bleeding problems (something you ought to discuss with your own doctor). Initially, we were recommending a single adult aspirin tablet (325 mg) because that is what was tested in various large scale studies. However, more recent studies suggest that just a baby aspirin (81 mg) a day is sufficient to prevent clotting, so that is what I am now doing for myself. Again, you should discuss this with your doctor, but I am convinced that the majority of adults over age 50 would benefit from this practice. *(See page 182 for a discussion regarding the interaction of aspirin and other similar anti-inflammatory drugs.)*

Diagnosis & Screening: Now that you have some understanding of the basics of coronary artery disease, hereafter referred to as CAD, it will be easier to understand the possibilities and problems in figuring out what might be happening in your coronary arteries.

Symptoms of Coronary Artery Disease

Obviously, you should report to your doctor any symptoms that suggest you might already have significant CAD. Most important, you should seek immediate emergency attention (which usually means calling 911) if you develop angina. The big question, of course, is how you can tell if chest pain is actually angina caused by coronary artery disease—versus the many other possible causes of chest discomfort, including heartburn caused by stomach contents backing up into the lower end of your foodpipe.

And the honest truth is that often a lay person can't tell the difference—which is why you should play it safe and have it checked out by your doctor or in the emergency room if there is any doubt. However, there are usually some pretty good clues that chest pain or discomfort might be angina, including:

- It occurs with physical exertion (and, less certainly, with mental stress) and gets better when you stop and rest.
- It radiates up into your neck, jaw, shoulders, and/or arms (usually on the left side but not always).
- It is not related to body position or taking a deep breath.
- It is accompanied by shortness of breath, sweatiness, general anxiety, or light-headedness.

I must also stress that the "pain" of angina is usually not sharp but more likely to be dull or aching or a sensation of pressure in the chest. Again, when in doubt, check it out.

There are many other possible symptoms of coronary artery disease ranging from abnormal heart rhythms to significant and repeated dizzy spells. But they are often much harder to recognize as CAD than the chest discomfort we call angina. However, the real goal is to diagnose CAD before it causes any symptoms—and certainly before the development of an actual heart attack. In fact, there are many tests designed to do so, but they all have their pros and cons as screening tests (finding the problem before symptoms arise) even though they are routinely used for diagnosis once symptoms appear. I am going to discuss them one by one and describe their use as both screening and diagnostic tests.

Resting electrocardiogram. This is the familiar test done as you lie down while wires are attached to your body to record electrical activity from the heart on a strip of moving paper. (It is often referred to in shorthand as either an

ECG or EKG.) If this test shows something, it can be very helpful. However, seeing changes on an ECG is more likely to happen in the midst of an actual episode of angina—which is why it is often the first test done in the emergency room—than when it is used as a screening test in a person with no symptoms. In other words, having a "normal" ECG as part of a routine physical in your doctor's office doesn't tell you much; we have all heard of someone who had a normal ECG and then dropped dead of a heart attack a week later. So the question is how to increase the likelihood of finding an existing problem using the ECG.

Stress electrocardiogram. Commonly known as a "stress test," the usual way of doing this is to conduct the ECG while you are exercising on either a bicycle or, most likely today, on a treadmill. By increasing the demand for heart pumping during exercise, we are more likely to "unmask" existing blockages that would not show up on an ECG taken during rest. It is pretty much a waste of time to do a resting ECG for screening even though, as I said above, it can be very useful during an episode of actual chest pain. The down side of a stress ECG is that it requires more personnel and equipment than the resting ECG and is therefore more costly. For this reason it should not be done regularly without some reason, such as spells of chest discomfort or a history of significant risk factors. However, as I did for myself, I would recommend a stress test as a base-line exam for most men at about age 50, even thought I know many experts disagree with this suggestion. (By the way, a resting ECG is completely safe, but there is a slight risk of having a heart attack during a stress test—about a 1 in 10,000 chance. However, if you are going to have a heart attack, it's a good time to have one, since doctors and emergency equipment are immediately available.)

Radioisotope test. We can increase the likelihood of finding coronary artery disease even further by injecting a radioisotope (usually thallium or technetium) into a vein just as the stress test is ending—at the most intense level of exercise you can do. We then take pictures of the heart with a scanning machine to see how the isotope travels through the coronary arteries to heart muscle. If there are blocks in the coronary arteries, there will be corresponding "cold" spots in the pictures of the heart muscle—meaning blood carrying the isotope cannot get through to that area. Radioisotope scanning adds considerable cost to the stress test (often several thousands of dollars), so it is usually reserved for those who are considered to be at higher risk or who have equivocal results from a stress test.

Coronary angiography. This test is still considered to be the "gold standard" for the diagnosis of coronary artery disease because it allows us to look at actual pictures of blood flow through the coronary arteries. The test is done by inserting a thin tube (catheter) through the body's arterial system from a leg artery up to the heart and into the openings of the coronary arteries, where a "contrast dye" which shows up as white on X-ray pictures is injected. The X-ray pictures can thus show where the dye is blocked by plaques bulging into the lumen of the artery, the center area where blood flows. This test is very good at showing bulging plaques, but it may not show the more vulnerable plaques hidden in the wall of the artery. That's why somebody can have a normal angiogram and still have hidden CAD. (There are some newer experimental tests that aim to look for these hidden plaques—such as a small ultrasound camera inserted into the coronary arteries.) Since angiograms require very skilled doctors and sophisticated equipment, they are quite expensive. They also carry a slight risk of causing a stroke or an actual heart attack (about 1 in 5,000 cases). However, this test is extremely valuable in finding standard blockages that might need treatment with either angioplasty or bypass surgery (see below).

Finally, I want to mention one screening test that is

being widely promoted directly to the general public as something you can obtain without a doctor's prescription—so-called heart scans. They are sometimes advertised as part of a total body scan or, at other times, just as a separate scan for the heart. In either case, what is usually being promoted is a so-called "fast scan," which is a rapid computed tomography (CT) scan to provide an image of the heart. What the scanner is looking for is evidence of calcium deposits in the walls of the coronary arteries. These scanners are in fact very good at finding calcium in artery walls. But the big question is, what does it mean if calcium is found? Unfortunately, the only way to find out is to do some of the tests described above. In other words, you can't tell by looking at the scan whether any calcium found is in plaques that are actually dangerous or causing a problem. For that, you have to have more tests done—and therein lies the rub. (I should also mention that your insurance will not pay for heart or body scans done without a physician's order—and may even balk at paying for follow-up tests!)

There is no doubt that sometimes such a scan will lead you to tests that will find coronary artery disease you did not know you had, but at least in retrospect it might have been easier and cheaper to have had those tests in the first place and skip the scan. And a negative test—no calcium—doesn't mean you don't have significant CAD. All of which is why most experts today say they would rather have their patients go through their usual evaluation process of determining risk level and deciding which if any tests are really necessary. However, these experts also acknowledge that many people find it empowering to get their own testing done—and that sometimes it can lead to important information. The great hope is that someday these tests can be so precise and revealing as to determine more than just the presence of calcium, which may or may not be significant.

Treatment Options: Obviously, the treatment of CAD depends on the stage at which it is discovered. If it is diagnosed before any symptoms or an actual heart attack has occurred, CAD may often be treated with changes in lifestyle and relatively simple medications. However, if CAD is first diagnosed during an actual heart attack, various emergency treatments are needed, often including so-called clotbusters or balloon surgery (see the next page) that can be used in the early stages of a heart attack to break up the blood clots that are blocking the flow of blood. That's why it is so important to seek emergency care as quickly as possible when you think you are having a heart attack: If the doctors can restore blood flow within the first few hours, it might be possible to prevent any actual infarction (death of heart muscle). I'll repeat a statistic I cited earlier: Today about 90 percent of those having a heart attack who make it to a hospital alive will survive!

In between these two extremes—no symptoms and emergency symptoms—is the common scenario in which a person is having suggestive symptoms which lead to either a stress test or angiogram, with the discovery of some blockages in the coronary artery system. The treatment options for this situation can involve any or all of the following:

Lifestyle changes and medications. The good news is that the majority of people who are diagnosed with CAD can be treated without any of the procedures mentioned below. Lifestyle changes (such as stopping smoking, changing your diet, and getting more exercise) and treatment of risk factors (treating high blood fats, hypertension, and obesity) can often bring about dramatic improvement. And today, a wide range of medications can also help control symptoms. The use of drugs like statins and beta blockers can make an enormous difference even after CAD is discovered—or an actual heart attack has occurred. The most important advice I can give regarding treatment is to make sure you are going to a competent physician—which may mean a cardiologist versus a general internist or family physician—who is skilled and wise in the use of the various drugs currently available. The potential downside of going to a cardiologist who also does interventional procedures (angiograms and angioplasty, as described below) is that he or she may be more biased toward performing such procedures versus a more conservative approach. One of the best ways to find the "right" cardiologist if you need one is to have your primary care doctor recommend one who is balanced in his or her approach to the treatment of CAD.

Angioplasty. This procedure, often known as "balloon surgery," is now widely used to open up serious blockages seen during angiography. The procedure involves pushing a catheter with a small balloon at the end into the blockage and inflating the balloon to push the blockage against the wall of the artery, thereby opening up a channel for blood flow to resume. And today, a wire mesh called a stent is usually left in place to help keep the channel open. Without stents, the reclosure rate is about 40 percent; with stents, it is about 25 percent. However, recent research with a new type of stent, coated with a special medication to prevent inflammation and cell growth, demonstrated that reclosure rates could be reduced to near zero. If these studies hold up, such stents will be a huge improvement. The great advantage of angioplasty over bypass surgery is obvious—the chest does not have to be opened and there is virtually no time out needed to heal and recover.

Bypass surgery. This now very common operation (about a half million are done each year in the U.S. alone) involves a chest incision to expose the heart. Veins from the leg or arteries from the chest are then sewn onto one or more blocked coronary arteries to literally "bypass" the blockage. (This surgery should be described as "open-chest" rather than "open-heart" since the heart itself is not actually opened. Because the coronary arteries run along the surface of the heart, they can be bypassed without actually opening the heart itself.) When veins from the leg are used to form the bypasses, there is a significant risk of new blockages forming in the veins during the following

10 years; when arteries from the chest (the so-called mammary arteries) are used, that risk is greatly reduced. Obviously, the more experienced your surgeon and hospital, the more likely you are to have a successful outcome; smaller hospitals that do less bypass surgery typically have much poorer outcomes.

There is also growing concern about the long-term effects on the brain from bypass surgery, particularly when it is done using the heart-lung machine to circulate and oxygenate the blood so the heart can be stopped to make the surgery technically easier. For example, one recent study showed that 42 percent of patients who had bypass surgery demonstrated slower thinking even five years after their surgery. That's why more bypass surgery is being done "off-pump"—operating on the beating heart and not using the heart-lung machine to circulate the blood—in an attempt to eliminate any brain damage from pump use.

Obviously the best "treatment" for CAD is to prevent it in the first place. That's why it is important to start thinking about this disease in your young adult years when you can still influence the course of your life and the condition of your coronary arteries.

Heart Failure

I am including a separate section on heart failure both because it is so common and because it is so often misunderstood. In fact, heart failure is now the leading cause of hospitalization in people over age 65. It kills about 40,000 people a year and afflicts about 5 million Americans. One recent estimate suggests the direct and indirect costs of heart failure in this country are about $21 billion a year.

The Basics: Heart failure is not a specific disease but rather usually a chronic condition that can be caused by many underlying diseases. Whatever the specific cause or causes, the result is a heart so damaged that it cannot pump vigorously enough to meet the body's needs. Therefore, blood coming into the heart tends to "back up" in the lungs, producing congestion in the lungs. (That's why the condition is often known as "congestive heart failure," or CHF for short.) The typical symptom of CHF is shortness of breath, even with mild exertion or in worst cases even at rest. Symptoms elsewhere in the body depend on which organs or tissues are most affected, but swelling in the legs is very characteristic of heart failure.

Prevention & Risk Factors: Since heart failure is really a condition resulting from specific diseases, the prevention of heart failure usually means the prevention of the diseases most likely to lead to heart failure, including:

Coronary artery disease. When blockages in the coronary arteries are big enough to cause actual heart attacks *(see page 124)*, heart muscle is permanently damaged and replaced by scar tissue that cannot contract and contribute to the heart's pumping ability. If enough heart muscle is damaged, heart failure can result.

Hypertension. High blood pressure *(see page 133)* can put so much strain on the heart that the organ eventually enlarges in an attempt to compensate. This enlargement may in turn lead to damage to the heart muscle and, eventually, to heart failure.

Cardiomyopathy. This word covers a wide range of possible problems, all of which result in weakened heart muscle. Some of these problems cannot be prevented—including infections of heart muscle by various viruses or genetic disorders that can cause abnormal thickening of heart muscle. (This is the condition that often causes sudden death in young athletes.) However, one condition we do have possible control over is excessive alcohol, which can result in a weakened heart.

Heart valve disease. When the valves that regulate the flow of blood through the chambers of the heart do not function normally, blood can back up in the heart, causing heart failure.

Since severe heart failure can dramatically compromise quality of life, basically making a person a housebound invalid, it is important to prevent the condition whenever possible by preventing the diseases that cause it. That's why I spent so much time discussing conditions like high blood fats and hypertension, which can lead to coronary artery disease that can seriously damage heart muscle.

Diagnosis & Screening:

Usually a combination of the symptoms and a person's medical history will point to the underlying problem of heart failure. However, there are many tests that can be used when necessary, including:

◆ Chest X-ray (which can show the backup of blood in the lungs).

◆ Echocardiogram (an ultrasound exam of the heart that can show how it is beating and how the valves are working).

◆ Angiographic and radioisotope studies of heart function (*see Diagnosis & Screening of CAD on page 140.*)

◆ Heart biopsy (which takes a sample of heart muscle for examination under the microscope).

Treatment Options:

Obviously the treatment for heart failure is directed at the underlying cause or causes whenever possible. However, when those causes are unknown or when permanent damage has already resulted, the goal of treatment is to help the heart to pump better and/or to reduce the strain on the damaged heart.

There are many different medicines that can be used today to help people with heart failure lead longer and more normal lives. Two categories of drugs—beta blockers and ACE inhibitors—have proven to be especially helpful.

However, this is one of those conditions in which the expertise of a specialist can often make an enormous difference. Quite frankly, most primary care physicians are not equipped to effectively treat the most severe forms of heart failure; experts in heart failure are more likely to be found in major medical centers that have a lot of experience with this condition.

In the most extreme cases of heart failure, the only answer may be a heart transplant—or one of the artificial heart devices now being developed. Those devices fall into two main categories:

- So-called assist devices, which basically help the failing heart without replacing it.
- So-called artificial hearts, which replace the heart.

It is beyond the scope of this book to describe the various devices available today, but all of them should still be regarded as experimental and are available only through major medical centers.

Arrhythmias
(Abnormal Heart Rhythms)

The Basics: The heart is a muscular pump divided into four chambers. The two atria are on the top and the two ventricles are on the bottom. A normal heart beats as a result of an electrical impulse that originates in a special group of pacemaker-like cells located in the right atrium. This electrical signal travels along a specific pathway throughout the other parts of the heart, causing the heart to contract in coordinated fashion to pump blood out to your body. The signal must follow this exact route in order for the heart to pump properly. Your heart normally contracts, or beats, 60 to 100 times a minute.

A heart arrhythmia is any abnormal change in the regular beating of the heart. Arrhythmias can include skipping heart beats, beating at an erratic rhythm, or beating too quickly (called tachycardia) or too slowly (called bradycardia)—any of which can cause the heart to pump less effectively. Arrhythmias can be caused by many underlying problems: the heart's natural pacemaker can develop an abnormal rate or rhythm; the normal pathway of the electrical current can be interrupted; or another area of the heart can take over as the pacemaker. Although many arrhythmias aren't serious, they can be life threatening if left untreated.

Arrhythmias are often divided into two main categories—atrial (sometimes referred to as supraventricular because they begin in the chambers above the ventricles) and ventricular. In general, arrhythmias that occur in the atria are much less serious than those that occur in the ventricles. Atrial arrhythmias include such common ones as atrial fibrillation (an irregular beating of the upper chambers) and atrial tachycardia (a regular but rapid beating of the upper chambers). Because these upper chambers do not pump blood from the heart to all parts of the body, these arrhythmias are usually not life threatening, though they may produce symptoms such as fatigue and light-headedness. If atrial fibrillation, the most common atrial arrhythmia, continues for long periods of time, it can increase the risk of having a stroke secondary to blood clots that are more likely to form when the blood in the atrial chambers is not pumped efficiently into the lower chambers; such clots can be carried in the bloodstream to smaller vessels in the brain, where they can block blood flow and cause a stroke *(see page 156)*. That's one reason why it is important to convert atrial fibrillation into so-called sinus rhythm, the normal rhythm of the heart, as soon as possible with medications or an electric shock when necessary. Experts are also increasingly using so-called ablation treatment, in which a catheter is inserted into the heart system (as in an angiogram procedure) and the atrial tissue causing the arrhythmia is found and destroyed. However, there are many people for whom these treatments don't work and who therefore have to live with continuing atrial arrhythmias; usually they can lead very normal lives with medications to keep the pumping rate in the lower chambers within normal range and to help prevent blood clots from forming.

Ventricular arrhythmias include the most serious of all arrhythmias, ventricular fibrillation, in which the two lower chambers of the heart quiver in chaotic fashion rather than pump with regular contractions. Because this results in very poor, if any, blood flow out of the heart to the body (including the brain), ventricular fibrillation can lead to death within minutes unless stopped with an electrical shock. (This is the arrhythmia that is so often portrayed in the frantic hospital resuscitation scenes on TV.) And this is the arrhythmia that causes 90 percent of the cases of so-called cardiac arrest, which results in roughly 250,000 deaths a year in this country alone. Most cases of cardiac arrest from ventricular fibrillation are caused by damage to the heart's electrical system secondary to coronary artery disease *(see page 124)*.

Obviously it is important to make a distinction between atrial fibrillation, which is very common (afflicting roughly two million Americans) but not usually life threatening—and ventricular fibrillation, which is almost always fatal unless quickly stopped by electrical shock using a defibrillator. Defibrillator devices used to be available only in hospitals, but newer portable and automatic models are now becoming available for use by emergency personnel and even by lay people trained to use them in public settings like airports or sports stadiums. And in people with a higher risk of developing ventricular fibrillation, miniature defibrillators can be implanted under the skin below the collarbone with wires extended through a large vein under the collarbone into the heart itself, as was done on Vice President Cheney in the fall of 2001. This device then monitors the rhythm of the heart and automatically delivers an appropriate electric shock to stop any developing ventricular rhythm problems.

Prevention & Risk Factors: Many times, there is no discernible cause for a heart rhythm problem, but any condition that affects the structure of the heart or that changes the electrical activity of the heart can upset the regular heart rhythm. As a result, a number of underlying medical conditions can cause arrhythmia, including an overactive thyroid gland *(see page 261)*, coronary artery disease that blocks flow of blood to the heart's electrical system, an imbalance of potassium or magnesium in the blood, changes in heart muscle due to a cardiomyopathy, actual heart attacks, or heart surgery.

Certain environmental factors can increase the likelihood of a heart arrhythmia as well, and if your doctor determines that your arrhythmia is caused by any of them, you should take steps to reduce or eliminate them from your life. They include:

- Stress.
- Caffeine.
- Tobacco.
- Alcohol.
- Certain over-the-counter medications, including diet pills and cough or cold remedies.
- Illegal drugs like cocaine.

Diagnosis & Screening: You may not notice any symptoms of an arrhythmia, or it may cause a number of symptoms, including palpitations (a fluttering or pounding feeling in your chest), dizziness, light-headedness, fainting, shortness of breath, vague chest discomfort, or fatigue and weakness.

Sometimes your doctor may be able to detect an arrhythmia simply by listening to your heart through a stethoscope. More often, he or she will have to perform a diagnostic test or two to figure out what's happening. Some commonly used tests to detect a heart arrhythmia include:

Electrocardiogram (ECG or EKG). In this test, your doctor will place wires on your body connected to a recording machine. The heart's electrical signals cause a pen to draw lines across a strip of graph paper in the machine, and the doctor can study these lines to look for changes in your normal heart rhythm. An ECG is only useful if taken while you are experiencing an arrhythmia. For this reason, your doctor may need to perform a number of other tests to get a better sense of what's happening in your heart. A stress test is essentially an ECG performed while you're exercising, either on a treadmill or stationary bicycle. It can sometimes tell your doctor whether increasing your heart rate through exercise instigates and/or exacerbates the problem.

Ambulatory monitors. With a 24-hour Holter monitor, you wear a small, portable tape recorder that's connected to wires on your chest and it performs a continuous ECG. This test can show changes in your heart rhythm over the course of a typical day and is much more sensitive to revealing the type of rhythm disturbance than any other test. You can also wear a tape recorder over a longer period of time—anywhere from several days to several weeks. When you have symptoms or feel your heartbeat go "out of rhythm," you can start the tape recording. This method can help keep track of arrhythmias that occur sporadically.

Echocardiogram. This test is an ultrasound of the heart, and it is used if the doctor suspects that the arrhythmia is being caused by structural problems in the heart or its valves.

Electrophysiology study. This testing method involves cardiac catheterization, in which thin, flexible tubes called catheters are placed in a vein in your arm or leg and fed through the vein to different parts of your heart, where they can stimulate and record arrhythmias. The test is designed to help doctors pinpoint the site of the arrhythmia and determine how well it responds to certain treatments.

Coronary angiogram. If your doctor thinks your arrhythmia is caused by coronary artery disease, he or she may order this test. *(See page 143 for a more thorough discussion of this test.)*

Treatment Options:

Treatment depends on the type, location, and severity of your arrhythmia. In some cases, no treatment is necessary, but more often, your doctor will recommend one of the following approaches.

Medications. There are a large variety of drugs designed to treat various arrhythmias. They tend to be quite potent, and some can cause serious side effects. At times they may be used in conjunction with electrophysiologic testing to determine the effect they're having.

Pacemaker. If your heart's natural pacemaker is malfunctioning, this electrical device can be placed under the skin below your collarbone. It is then wired to your heart (through the veins leading to the heart) so that it can keep your heart beating at a steady pace.

Implantable defibrillators. These devices, which are also surgically implanted under the skin of your chest with wires into the heart, are used when your arrhythmia is serious enough that your doctor believes it is life threatening. (See above.)

Radio wave ablation. This treatment, which is increasingly used for atrial arrhythmias, involves inserting a catheter into the heart to identify the area responsible for a rhythm problem. The problem area is then destroyed (ablated) with radio waves. This technique obviously involves complex equipment and considerable expertise but can provide a permanent solution to a continuing arrhythmia that is not responding to medication.

Relaxation techniques. To reduce stress, which often causes or exacerbates arrhythmias, you can try a number of proven relaxation methods, including progressive relaxation (in which you lie down and consciously try to relax specific muscles, starting with your feet and working your way up to your head), meditation (in which you try to focus your mind on one thing, like your breath or a special word or a candle flame), or yoga (in which specific body postures can quiet and strengthen your body).

Lifestyle changes. If you notice that your arrhythmia is connected to certain dietary factors, like caffeine or alcohol, you should obviously limit your use of them. If smoking causes problems, it is still another reason to stop. Finally, as pointed out in the chapter on nutrition, omega-3 fatty acids found in fatty fish can help reduce the risk of sudden death from cardiac arrest. There is good evidence that men who eat almost any kind of fish at least once a week reduce their risk of sudden death by about half as compared to men who eat fish less often. (This effect has not been as easy to study in women, who have less heart disease at an early age.)

Strokes

The Basics: The word "stroke" refers to the brain damage that occurs when blood flow to the brain becomes interrupted enough to cause permanent destruction of brain cells. In this sense, a stroke is the counterpart of a heart attack (where permanent destruction or infarction of heart muscle occurs). Indeed, many experts now advocate calling strokes "brain attacks" to indicate the similarity and to stimulate the same sense of urgency about strokes that we have about heart attacks. Approximately 600,000 Americans have strokes every year; it is now the third leading cause of death in this country. About one-third die from the stroke, and about 40 percent end up in some kind of health care facility to obtain rehabilitation and help with daily living. Strokes are therefore a huge health problem requiring a lot of costly care and often robbing people of their normal life.

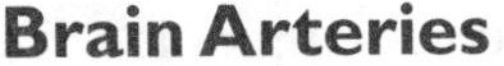

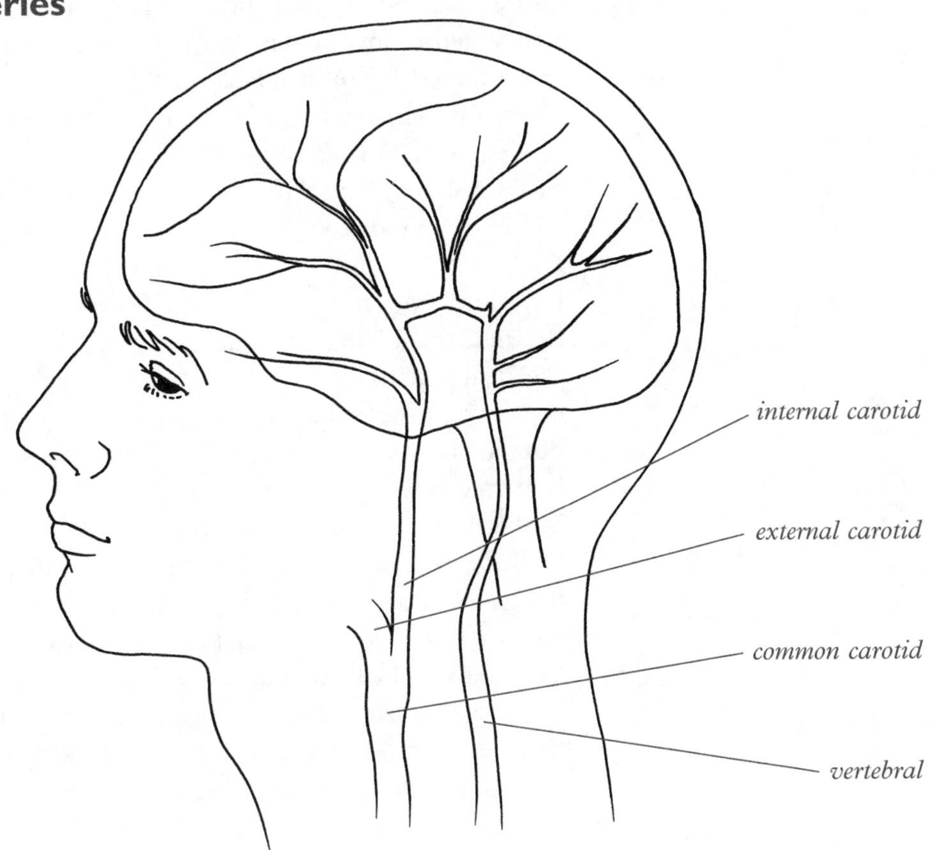

Ischemic Strokes

About 80 percent of all strokes are so-called "ischemic strokes." (The other major kind of strokes are called "hemorrhagic strokes" and are caused by ruptured blood vessels in the brain; I will say more about these later.) Ischemic strokes are caused by gradual or sudden blockages in arteries leading to the brain. These blockages cut down on blood flow, which is what the word "ischemia" means—reduced blood flow. When that happens in coronary arteries it can lead to angina, the pain signifying that heart muscle cells are not getting enough oxygen. In the case of brain cells, however, reduced blood flow does not cause pain, but it can produce many other symptoms. The actual symptoms depend on which part of the brain is being affected by reduced blood flow. Symptoms can range from problems with arm or leg movement to difficulty with speech or vision problems, again depending on which brain cells are being affected.

As with reduced blood flow in coronary arteries, the results may be temporary or permanent, depending on how long and how much the blood flow is diminished. When the reduced blood flow causes permanent damage (that is the death of brain cells), we call it an actual stroke. However, when the reduced blood causes temporary symptoms but not permanent damage, we call the event a "transient ischemic attack," or a TIA. And as with temporary angina in the heart, we must look upon a TIA as a very important warning that there may be big trouble in the arteries—in this case, those carrying blood to our brain. In fact, about half of those who have a permanent ischemic stroke will have had a TIA sometime during the months before the stroke. Therefore, I am going to spend some time in further defining TIAs and, more importantly, describing what you should do if you ever have one.

Transient Ischemic Attacks

By definition, these events are attacks that come on suddenly. They are caused by ischemia that leads to symptoms that are transient, meaning that they last less than 24 hours (often just hours or even minutes). As I explained above, the actual symptoms will depend on which part of the brain is being affected by the temporary decrease in blood flow.

The possible causes of TIAs are many—basically anything that can temporarily decrease blood flow to the brain. But the most common cause are tiny emboli (singular is embolus), which can best be described as pieces of clot or cholesterol plaque that flow in the blood until they get lodged in a blood vessel small enough to trap them and cause blockage. An embolus can come from anywhere "downstream," but often it comes from larger fatty blockages in the major arteries on either side of the neck—the carotids—which carry blood to the brain. Other sources of emboli can be blood clots that build up in the heart because of arrhythmias or damaged heart valves (see below).

Whatever the underlying cause of decreased blood flow, the symptoms will vary enormously depending on the area of brain tissue affected. Sometimes the symptoms are so obvious that everyone will notice—the inability to move an arm or a leg, or severely garbled speech. But other times the symptoms might be so subtle that only the person himself or a spouse might notice, such as a very slight change in speech, the inability to add numbers easily, or a change in vision. The message: Whenever you or anyone else notices a symptom (or cluster of symptoms) that might suggest a stroke, you should report it immediately to your doctor—and let him or her decide whether it is worth worrying about. And of course if the symptoms are severe or serious enough, you should get to an emergency room very quickly because it may be possible to stop a stroke in progress (see below), just as we can often stop a heart attack in progress before significant permanent damage is done.

Screening & Diagnosis: If your doctor suspects a TIA, or an actual stroke in progress, he or she has several ways of sorting out what might be going on. Sometimes, another cause for the symptoms, such as a seizure or low blood sugar, can be quickly found and treated. Sometimes a heart problem will be discovered as a cause—anything ranging from an infected heart valve to certain heart rhythm problems, most commonly atrial fibrillation, that increase the risk for blood clot formation in the heart's chambers. (The reason such arrhythmias can cause blood clots is that the blood pools in the upper chambers of the heart and such "stagnant" blood is more likely to form clots.) But in addition to other causes, the doctor will usually have to investigate possible problems in the neck arteries leading to the brain—and at this point you may well be referred to a neurologist. The following are among the tests that might be considered in trying to pinpoint possible problems in the neck (carotid) arteries:

Listening to neck arteries with a stethoscope. I mention this because you may have wondered what your doctor is doing when he or she places a stethoscope on the side of your neck during a routine physical exam—or after your complaining of worrisome symptoms. He is listening for so-called bruits (pronounced brew-ees), which are abnormal sounds that occur when blood flow is being disturbed by blockages such as fatty material protruding into the center of the artery. This "test" is far from foolproof, but it is simple and risk free and might signal a potential problem.

Image studies. If there is any degree of suspicion, the physician will quickly turn to various studies that can look inside the neck arteries to see what is going on. These may range from ultrasound to MRIs (magnetic resonance imaging), CT scans, or actual angiograms of the neck arteries where, as with heart angiograms, contrast dye is injected before X-ray pictures are taken to outline any blockages. Any or all of these tests can be helpful if done correctly and interpreted by an expert. I raise this warning especially in relation to ultrasound exams because they are too often done in office settings where the equipment might be inferior, the person performing the test might not be well trained, and the doctor interpreting the images might not be experienced. Such problems can lead to false positives—which usually get corrected with further testing—or even more frightening, false negatives, in which a person is told there is nothing wrong when in fact there is a problem. Quite frankly, if I were going to have an ultrasound exam of my neck arteries looking for potentially serious problems, I would have it done in the ultrasound department of a major hospital or a major clinic where I could be more certain of expertise.

Hemorrhagic Strokes

These types of strokes are less common than ischemic strokes but usually more devastating, with more destruction of brain tissue and a higher risk of death. They occur when a blood vessel on or in the brain ruptures, causing both interruption of blood flow beyond the point of rupture and, with large amounts of bleeding, direct destruction of brain tissue. Sometimes ruptures occur in vessels that have been congenitally weak since birth (aneurysm) or in otherwise deformed tangles of vessels called arteriovenous malformations that some people are born with. Most occur in blood vessels weakened by high blood pressure. Whatever the cause, a hemorrhagic stroke is usually signaled by a very severe headache, unlike anything you have experienced before. Sometimes this headache comes on very suddenly, sometimes more slowly. Thus, any unusually severe headache that is new for you should be regarded as an absolute emergency needing immediate attention. Sometimes the source of bleeding can be quickly identified and corrected enough to prevent extensive damage. The bottom line: Both ischemic and hemorrhagic strokes should be regarded as brain attacks that can be every bit as serious as a heart attack.

Prevention & Risk Factors: Since the underlying process—fatty plaques in artery walls—is very much the same for ischemic strokes as for coronary artery disease, the same risk factors apply to both. Indeed, the big three—smoking, high blood fats, and high blood pressure—dramatically increases the risk for both strokes and heart attacks. However, when it comes to strokes, high blood pressure is especially important. Not only does it increase the risk of ischemic strokes, but it dramatically increases the risk for hemorrhagic strokes caused by rupture of blood vessels weakened by high blood pressure. In fact, untreated high blood pressure is the leading cause of strokes in the U.S. So I refer you back to the discussion of high blood pressure in the section on coronary artery disease *(see page 133)* with a special emphasis on the phrase "silent killer." High blood pressure is really a ticking time bomb when it comes to strokes!

Once it is determined that your symptoms are in fact due to a TIA or an actual stroke in progress, there are several options available to prevent recurrence and/or an actual stroke from occurring. If the symptoms are persisting and/or obviously indicative of a major stroke in progress and blood clots in arteries leading to the brain are thought to be a factor, emergency treatment with clot busters might be tried, just as they often are in treating heart attacks in progress. As with heart attacks, they must be used within the first several hours after the onset of symptoms to be most effective. In fact, a recent study suggests that treatment *within 90 minutes* after symptoms have started is the most effective. That is one of several reasons why we stress the importance of reporting serious symptoms to your doctor immediately or, even better, going to the nearest major emergency room. However, in a true TIA, by definition the symptoms disappear within 24 hours, and then the question becomes how to prevent further attacks. Very often your physician will prescribe medications to reduce the risk of further blood clot formation. Aspirin, which blocks the clotting action of the platelets in our blood, is most commonly prescribed, but other more powerful drugs, such as the "anticoagulant" coumadin (Warfarin) might be employed.

Treatment Options: The best treatment for stroke is to prevent it in the first place by reducing risk factors, and paying perticular attention to any symptoms of transient ischemic attacks. Once an actual stroke occurs, treatment options are usually very limited, although I stress again that clot busters can sometimes be dramatically helpful in the first few hours after stroke symptoms start. (Such treatment obviously should not be used in hemorrhagic strokes, which are caused by bleeding and where clot formation could actually be useful.) Angioplasty (balloon surgery) is also being tried experimentally in some medical centers. There are also several experimental medicines that are being tested to see if they can reduce the damage in the brain caused by a stroke. All of this means that it makes sense to get to a good stroke center—which usually means a major medical center—as quickly as possible after suspicious stroke symptoms start.

If imaging tests have demonstrated fatty plaques in a neck artery that is blocking more than 70 percent of the area for blood flow, your doctors might recommend an operation on the artery called a carotid endarterectomy. In this surgery, the neck artery is actually opened and the blockage removed. In the past, many experts felt that this operation was being done too often and for the wrong reasons. But with more recent studies clarifying which patients might benefit from this preventive surgery, such operations can now be recommended with more certainty about when the benefits outweigh the risks (the risks of surgery include, paradoxically, a stroke—or even death). Once again, these risks are much less likely in the hands of surgeons and hospitals that do the surgery often. You should not hesitate to ask about the track record for a given person and place—and to seek a second opinion if you have any doubts.

Living with Strokes: Rehabilitation is one of the main focuses of stroke care. Although some people may improve to a certain degree on their own in the first month, long-term improvement often depends on the concerted effort of a team of caregivers. The process isn't an easy one. It requires the cooperation of family and friends as well as a fair amount of grit and determination to become as independent and productive as possible.

Keeping a positive attitude toward your recovery can be difficult at times, but it may play an important role in how you fare. Researchers in Scotland recently found that stroke survivors with a fatalistic attitude—who feel they can't do anything to help themselves or improve their situation—were nearly 60 percent more likely to die in the year or two after their stroke than their more upbeat counterparts.

CHAPTER 6

An A to Z Guide to Common Health Issues

While the following alphabetical guide to common diseases and conditions is by no means comprehensive, it does include essential information on the prevention, diagnosis, and treatment of many ailments common in men. You will not find more obscure diseases, or those (such as lupus) that are rare in men. Although you may use this as a reference—looking up a particular condition if you're experiencing symptoms—it would be wise to flip through this chapter before you're feeling sick, since I've tried to emphasize prevention and screening for early detection rather than treatment.

Addictions

The Basics: When you take a drug, whether it's legal or illegal, cocaine or caffeine, it affects your body chemistry, sometimes changing the way you think, act, and perceive the world. Over time, your brain tends to adapt to the substance, a situation that actually alters your brain chemistry and makes you develop a tolerance for the drug, meaning you need more of it to get the same effect. When you start feeling compelled to use the substance to get that feeling again and again, when you feel ill if you don't have the substance in your system, or when it starts taking more and more of the substance to make you feel good, you've probably become addicted to the drug.

Although scientists don't have a clear understanding of how your body becomes addicted to certain substances, they know that it involves your individual chemical makeup and that drugs can change your brain chemistry in such a way that you crave them when they're out of your system. Although addiction happens at least partially in the brain, experts agree that it's not usually simply a chemical problem. Social and economic problems can also contribute significantly to an increased risk for addiction.

In 1999, an estimated 3.6 million people in the U.S. were dependent on illicit drugs and another 8.2 million were dependent on alcohol, according to the Substance Abuse and Mental Health Services Administration's National Household Survey on Drug Abuse. Most studies show that men are more susceptible to addictions of all types than women. About 9.3 percent of men are heavy drinkers and 22.8 percent are binge drinkers, while about 25 million men in the U.S. smoke cigarettes.

Prevention & Risk Factors: Although the only sure way to prevent addiction is to abstain from drugs in the first place, many people are able to use potentially addicting substances in moderation. Some drugs are more addictive than others—one cigarette probably won't set you on the path to a life of smoking, but a puff or two of crack cocaine can make some people want more almost immediately. However, many experts feel that nicotine addiction is as difficult to break as any addiction, including cocaine.

Certain risk factors make it more likely that you'll become addicted to any substance.

Family history. Research has shown that people with a family history of drug or alcohol abuse are more likely to abuse the substances themselves. For instance, the risk of alcoholism in sons of alcoholic fathers is 25 percent, versus 10 percent in the general population.

Emotional disorders. Depression and anxiety increase your risk of alcoholism, smoking, and other forms of addiction. In fact, about one-third of all alcoholics also suffer from depression.

Personality traits. Alcoholics tend to be impulsive and excitable and to crave new experiences and sensations.

Lack of coping skills to deal with stress. Many people who succumb to drug addiction are under stress, but researchers believe that one factor that separates them from those who don't become addicted is an inability to handle the stress effectively.

Impaired decision-making. Studies have shown that some drug-dependent people perform poorly on a test designed to measure their ability to make decisions, indicating a malfunction in the part of their brains called the prefrontal cortex.

Experimenting with drugs at an early age. If you use drugs when you're young, you're more likely to be addicted when you're older. Among adults who first tried marijuana at age 14 or younger, nearly 9 percent were dependent on drugs as adults, as opposed to just 1.7 percent of adults who had first tried marijuana when they were 18 or older.

How Recreational Drugs Affect Your Body

CENTRAL NERVOUS SYSTEM DEPRESSANTS

Examples: Benzodiazepines, barbiturates, paraldehyde, chloral hydrate.
Effects: They depress and sedate your body, resulting in uncoordinated movements, slurred speech, impaired judgment and attention span, mood swings, dizziness, and sometimes suicidal behavior.

CENTRAL NERVOUS SYSTEM STIMULANTS

Examples: Cocaine, amphetamines, dextroamphetamine, methamphetamine.
Effects: They stimulate your body, causing euphoria, dilated pupils, rapid heart beat, anxiety, restlessness, and sometimes convulsions or stroke.

HALLUCINOGENS

Examples: Psilocybin, LSD, PCP, mescaline.
Effects: In addition to visual effects, hallucinogens can cause anxiety, depression, and, sometimes, schizophrenic behavior.

OPIOIDS

Examples: Heroin, opium, codeine, Demerol, Dilaudid, methadone.
Effects: They have a sedative effect, but they also can make you feel euphoric. Symptoms of use include rapid heart rate and constricted pupils. High doses can cause coma or respiratory arrest.

Diagnosis & Screening: Symptoms of drug addiction vary depending on the substance involved, but they almost universally include one key component: craving. If you wake up in the morning and crave a cigarette, a shot of tequila, a line of cocaine, a hit of marijuana, or even a cup of coffee, chances are you have some level of addiction. If you've experienced three or more of the following problems in the past 12 months, you should seek professional help for your addiction:

- You've developed a tolerance to the substance, so it requires more to achieve the desired effect.
- You feel sick, both physically and mentally, if you cut back or stop taking the drug.
- You find yourself using the substance in larger amounts or for a longer period of time than you intended to and feel unable to control it.
- You've tried unsuccessfully to cut back or control your consumption of the substance.
- You've had problems with your relationships with your family, friends, or coworkers as a result of the substance.
- You've given up doing things you would normally do, whether they're social, professional, or recreational, because of substance abuse.

Treatment Options: Treatment approaches vary depending on the drug you're addicted to, but in general, they should include a biological component, to address your physical addiction; a psychological component, to help you cope emotionally; and a social component, to help you stay away from situations that make it difficult to say no. A number of medications can be helpful for different sorts of addictions. Following is a sampling:

Naltrexone. This medication blocks the effects of narcotics like heroin, but it has been shown to be helpful for alcoholics as well.

Clonidine. A blood pressure medication, this drug can alleviate some of the withdrawal symptoms from opioid drugs like heroin and codeine.

Methadone. Although its use is controversial, this drug is probably the most effective therapeutic intervention available for certain people addicted to opiates.

Nicotine replacement products. Designed for smokers,

these products deliver small, steady doses of nicotine to your body to help relieve the withdrawal symptoms. They generally are available in four forms: patches, gum, nasal spray, and inhaler, and they've been shown to double your chances of quitting. For highly addicted smokers, a program of gradually reduced doses of nicotine via patches may be best.

Zyban (bupropion hydrochloride). First approved by the Food and Drug Administration as an antidepressant, this medication helps some people stop smoking by reducing nicotine withdrawal symptoms and decreasing the desire to smoke.

In certain instances, you may be best off entering a residential treatment program so you're in a controlled, medically supervised environment when you go through withdrawal and try to stay clean. Others may just need to enlist the help of an outside support group, like Alcoholics Anonymous or Narcotics Anonymous.

Do You Have a Drinking Problem?

Consider the following four questions:

- Have you ever felt that you should cut down on your drinking?
- Have other people annoyed you by criticizing your drinking?
- Have you ever felt bad or guilty about your drinking?
- Have you ever had a drink first thing in the morning (as an "eye opener") to steady your nerves or get rid of a hangover?

If you responded "yes" to any one of these questions, it is possible that you have a drinking problem. If you answered "yes" to more than one question, it is highly likely that a problem exists. In either case, it is important that you address your concerns right away. There are many excellent facilities and programs for people with addictions. For alcohol abuse, I feel that Alcoholics Anonymous (AA) has the best track record for availability and results—and the price is right.

Living with an Addiction: Like many other chronic illnesses, addictions often come back, so once you've quit using the substance you were dependent on, you'll need to be vigilant and aware of how easy it is to start up again. That's why it's a good idea to stay involved in a long-term relapse prevention program or support group that can help you through tough times.

Allergies and Asthma

The Basics: Asthma and other allergic reactions are among the most common health problems in the U.S. People with allergies are hypersensitive to certain otherwise harmless substances, including cat dander, pollen, mold, and dust. There are actually hundreds of everyday substances that can trigger allergies. When people with allergies are exposed to an allergen, their immune systems begin producing antibodies as if the substance were a bacteria or virus, and their bodies' tissues release chemicals such as histamine that cause itching, swelling, rashes, hives, mucus production, and breathing problems.

Asthma, a chronic inflammatory disease that affects the breathing passages in your lungs, is often caused by an allergy, but it also can come on for no apparent reason. As many as 50 million people in the U.S. have allergies, 17 million of whom suffer from asthma. The number of people with asthma is on the rise. Although it's usually a controllable illness, about 5,000 people die of asthma every year.

Prevention & Risk Factors: The precise cause of allergies and asthma remains a mystery, but years of experience with these common illnesses has shown that people who have a family history of the problem are at increased risk and that stress often exacerbates the problem. Obviously the best prevention is avoidance of triggering allergens when that is possible.

Diagnosis & Screening: Your doctor will suspect an allergy or asthma based on your symptoms. In addition to those mentioned above, common allergy symptoms include a runny nose, watery and itchy eyes, sneezing, and coughing.

Asthma is the name we give to the wheezing and shortness of breath due to allergic reactions that narrow the airways in our lungs. The narrowing is due not only to spasms of the muscles that line these airways, but to inflammation of their walls.

In order to diagnose an allergy, your doctor may do a blood test to check for elevated immunoglobulin levels and may perform one of several types of skin tests to see if your skin responds to a small amount of different types of common allergens. If you suspect that you have a food allergy, he or she might also suggest that you try an elimination diet, in which you eliminate the suspected allergen (yeast or dairy, for example) from your diet to see if your symptoms get better.

To diagnose asthma, your doctor will listen to your chest for signs of wheezing or impaired breathing and may also order breathing tests to measure your lung function, as well as a chest X-ray.

Treatment Options: Treatment for allergies often involves avoiding the suspected trigger. Often this is not possible or will not prove successful. For instance, if you're allergic to pollen, certain times of the year are going to be difficult no matter what. For non-asthma allergies, over-the-counter antihistamines can provide relief for mild to moderate symptoms, and decongestants can reduce nasal congestion. For severe symptoms, your doctor may prescribe corticosteroids to lessen your immune response and symptoms. In some instances, your doctor may recommend immunotherapy, or allergy shots, in which he or she injects you with gradually increased dosages of an allergen over a period of months or years to get your immune system used to the substance.

If you have asthma, you'll need to try to avoid allergens that trigger attacks when they can be identified. In addition, your doctor will probably prescribe various inhaled asthma medications, which you may take every day or only on an as-needed basis. "Beta2-agonists" are bronchodilators, which open up your narrow breathing passages. Anti-inflammatory drugs, such as inhaled or oral corticosteroids and cromolyn, can prevent swelling and inflammation of the airways. *Today asthma is regarded primarily as an inflammatory disease for which inhaled steroids are almost always the most important medications.*

Living with Allergies and Asthma: Understanding your triggers and sticking to a prescribed medication schedule can go a long way toward reducing symptoms of these illnesses. If you have asthma, it's particularly important to stop an attack in its initial stages, because it can gain momentum quickly. One device that can help enormously is a peak flow meter, which can quickly measure your breathing capacity and help you determine if you need medication; if you are asthmatic, you should have the device with you at all times to help you decide when your breathing problem might be a true emergency. If your breathing is really bad and an attack is hard to break, you should get to an emergency room quickly. Deaths from asthma are increasing—and almost all are due to not seeking help soon enough. I would also emphasize the importance of going to a true expert in asthma (usually an allergy specialist) if you are having problems managing your asthma.

Alzheimer's Disease

The Basics: Named for Dr. Alois Alzheimer, a German doctor who first identified the brain changes that characterize the illness, Alzheimer's is a progressive, degenerative brain disorder that causes impairment in your thinking, reasoning, and memory. It is characterized by specific anatomical changes in the brain's structure, including abnormal clumps of protein (amyloid), tangled bundles of nerve fibers, a loss of nerve cells in the parts of the brain that control memory and other mental functions, and decreased levels of certain brain chemicals that are critical for clear thinking. The combination of structural and chemical problems seems to disconnect parts of the brain that normally would work harmoniously, resulting in the decline in the cognitive abilities so characteristic of Alzheimer's.

The disease usually begins after age 65. About 3 percent of people between the ages of 65 and 74 have the disorder, while as many as half of people 85 and older may be afflicted. Because it is degenerative, Alzheimer's is typically fatal within 15 years, sometimes very quickly.

Prevention & Risk Factors: Although everything from viral infections to serious head injuries has been proposed as a potential cause of Alzheimer's, the cause of the illness largely remains a mystery. Age is certainly a risk factor for the disease. Other possible contributors:

Family history. If you had a parent or sibling with Alzheimer's, your chance of developing the disease is somewhat greater than someone without a family history. In fact, there may be a genetic susceptibility (not a certainty) in as many as 50 percent of Alzheimer's cases. About 10 percent of people with Alzheimer's have an "early onset" form (appearing when they are in their 40s or 50s), which is almost always inherited.

Environmental influences. Because scientists have found metals such as aluminum and zinc in the brain tissue of people with Alzheimer's, they have suspected that exposure to these substances could somehow be involved in the development of the illness, but no one has been able to find a direct link.

There's currently no known way to prevent Alzheimer's, but researchers are looking at a number of possibilities, including nonsteroidal anti-inflammatory drugs like ibuprofen and naproxen sodium, antioxidants such as vitamin E, the herb gingko biloba, and even a vaccine to attack the amyloid deposits that are characteristic of the disease. The statin drugs used to treat high cholesterol may also reduce the risk for Alzheimer's. In addition, so-called "brain exercises"—using your brain to learn new tasks—may be helpful.

A recent study suggests that high levels of homocysteine in the blood are also linked with a greater risk of Alzheimer's. Whether lowering homocysteine levels reduces that risk remains to be proven. However, I have come to believe that lowering high levels may be prudent while we await such studies given that the treatment involves usually modest amounts of vitamins B-6, B-12, and folic acid.

Diagnosis & Screening: There's no specific test (other than a brain biopsy) for Alzheimer's, so your doctor will diagnose the illness based on whether or not you exhibit serious cognitive decline. In general, people with Alzheimer's show a gradual decline in memory and the ability to communicate, and they may have trouble completing mundane tasks, become lost in familiar surroundings, and exhibit personality changes, including paranoia and depression.

Although lots of people become concerned that they have Alzheimer's, it's usually fairly easy to distinguish from the normal memory loss of aging. For instance, if you are constantly forgetting where you left your sunglasses or you can't remember the name of your new colleague at work, you probably don't have Alzheimer's, but if you can't remember a conversation you had recently or are confused about what your car keys are used for, you should consult your doctor. Likewise, if your mind is sharp but you have repeated trouble remembering recently acquired information, like dates, appointments, and other important events, it could spell trouble. Research has shown that 80 percent of people with this type of "mild cognitive impairment" develop Alzheimer's within 10 years.

Your doctor also may want to run tests to rule out

other possible problems, such as a thyroid problem or other brain problems. To test specifically for Alzheimer's Disease, he or she may order:

Neuropsychological tests. This battery of tests can help your doctor assess your memory, language, and problem-solving skills.

Brain scan. Several types of scanners can produce a picture of your brain, allowing your doctor to look for abnormal areas. Your doctor can order a picture of your brain taken by a magnetic resonance imaging (MRI) scan, a computerized tomography (CT) scan, or a positron emission tomography (PET) scan. This latter test is being used in many research settings to look for early changes in Alzheimer's. However, some doctors are inappropriately promoting it as a proven screening test.

Treatment Options: There is no cure for Alzheimer's, but drugs such as tacrine (Cognex), donepezil (Aricept), rivastigmine (Exelon), and galantamine (Reminyl) may help to temporarily improve memory or retard its decline in people with early disease. There also are a number of treatments available to relieve symptoms like sleeplessness, anxiety, depression, and agitation.

The herb gingko biloba has received a lot of recent attention. Germany recently approved gingko extracts to treat Alzheimer's disease, but it has never received a full-fledged endorsement from the medical community in the U.S. because studies have conflicting results. While it's probably safe to try the herb (240 milligrams a day is the approved dose in Germany), you must tell your doctor you're taking it, because ginkgo may cause side effects, including excessive bleeding, especially when used in conjunction with daily aspirin therapy. *(See also Memory Loss on page 243.)*

Arthritis

The Basics: Arthritis refers to anything that can cause pain and/or inflammation in one or more of our joints. There are over 100 possible causes of arthritis but the vast majority fall into one of two categories.

Osteoarthritis, the most common type, is a degenerative joint disease rather than an inflammatory one. In people with osteoarthritis, the cartilage in the joints—the rubbery material that serves as your joints' shock absorbers—stiffens up and eventually begins to erode, losing some of its ability to cushion the impact between the bones on either side of the joint. The disease can be especially disabling when it affects the spine, knees, or hips, all areas where men are most likely to get it. Osteoarthritis affects about 16 million people in the U.S., about half of whom are men.

Rheumatoid arthritis (RA), the other main type, is characterized by inflammation. It attacks the synovium, or lining, of your joints, causing pain, stiffness, swelling, redness, deformity, and loss of joint function. RA affects the hands and feet most often, and it tends to be symmetrical, striking both sides of the body—a characteristic that helps distinguish it from other types of arthritis. It can vary in severity as well. In some people, it lasts only a few months or a year and then goes away without causing any lasting damage. In others, it comes in fits and starts, flaring up for a period of time, then calming down again. And in some people it's a progressive and debilitating chronic illness. About 2.5 million people in the U.S. suffer from rheumatoid arthritis. It's about three times more common in women than in men.

Prevention & Risk Factors: Osteoarthritis is in large part a result of the wear and tear placed on your joints over years of activity. Some factors may increase the likelihood of developing the problem, including:

Previous injury to ligaments or cartilage. Early injuries can set you on the road to osteoarthritis.

Intense athletic activity. Extreme stress on your body's weight-bearing joints may cause your cartilage to break down faster than other people's, resulting in osteoarthritis. Non–weight-bearing exercise, on the other hand, such as swimming or bike riding, can strengthen your muscles and take some of the burden off overloaded joints.

Family history. You're at increased risk of developing the illness if one of your parents had it.

Age. The likelihood of osteoarthritis increases as you age, because your body becomes less able to regenerate cartilage cells as you get older and the years of wear and tear take their toll.

Rheumatoid arthritis, on the other hand, is actually an autoimmune disease—meaning the immune system attacks your own cells that line the joints. Scientists don't know what causes the problem, but they believe there are a number of contributing factors, such as:

Genetic factors. Some people with rheumatoid arthritis have similar genetic profiles, leading scientists to believe that there can be a genetic predisposition to the illness.

Environmental factors. Sometimes, the illness may be triggered by a virus or bacteria.

Hormonal factors. Because the illness occurs more frequently in women, some doctors believe that hormones may play a role in the development of the illness.

Diagnosis & Screening:

Symptoms of arthritis include:

- Achiness and soreness in your joints, especially when you move.
- Morning joint stiffness that lasts longer than 30 minutes.
- Swelling, warmth, and/or redness in one or more joints.
- Difficulty using or moving a joint.

In addition, people with rheumatoid arthritis may have fatigue or a general malaise, and the pain tends to occur in a symmetrical pattern, affecting both hands, say, or both feet.

In order to diagnose arthritis, your doctor will take a complete medical history and ask you a series of questions about your symptoms, including where and when it hurts, if anything makes the pain worse or better, how long the pain lasts, and if you're taking any medication. Your doctor also will perform a physical exam, looking for areas of redness and swelling, tenderness, or pain with movement.

Besides regular X-rays, your doctor also may want to get a look at what's going on inside your joint by doing one of the following imaging tests:

Computerized tomography (CT or CAT) scan. This test uses X-rays to produce an image of your joint, showing areas that are worn or damaged.

Magnetic resonance imaging (MRI) scan. In this procedure, you'll be placed in a machine that has a strong magnetic field and can produce a picture of your joint that shows soft tissue in a more detailed way than CT scans.

Arthrography. This is a special type of X-ray designed to show your whole joint after a special dye has been injected into the joint.

Rheumatoid arthritis can be difficult to diagnose in its early stages, because there's no single test for the illness, and it's often so similar to other types of arthritis that doctors must rule those out first. As a result, your doctor may take awhile to make a definitive diagnosis. He or she will need to have your medical history and do a thorough physical examination. Your doctor will probably also test your blood for rheumatoid factor, an antibody that is present in some (but not all) people with the illness, and for sedimentation rate, which can indicate inflammation in your body.

Treatment Options: Depending on the severity of your condition, your doctor will likely take a combination approach to treatment, recommending a variety of the following approaches as well as medications (see below).

Non–weight-bearing exercise. Activities like swimming and cycling strengthen your muscles and help take the strain off painful joints.

Range-of-motion exercises. Your doctor may recommend one or several of these light stretching exercises to keep your joints moving without overstressing them.

Maintaining a healthy weight. Being overweight places more of a burden on your joints, exacerbating the symptoms of arthritis. Lose weight if you need to.

Rest. When rheumatoid arthritis is in an active phase, it can help to take it easy. Rest reduces joint inflammation and helps fight the fatigue.

Exercise. Staying physically active will keep your muscles strong, which will preserve the mobility of your joints. Stretching can keep your muscles limber and flexible. Regular exercise also can improve the quality of your sleep and help you cope with pain.

Splinting the joint. A splint can provide support for an affected joint, which can reduce the pain and swelling.

Surgery. Common surgeries for rheumatoid arthritis include joint replacement surgery, tendon reconstruction, and synovectomy, in which the surgeon actually removes the inflamed tissue in your joint. It may eventually grow back. Joint replacement surgery for knee and hip joints is becoming very common for severe osteoarthritis.

Medications for Arthritis

At this point, I am going to take some time for an extended discussion of the various over-the-counter (OTC) and prescription medications that are constantly being advertised for the treatment of arthritis and other common pain problems.

Acetaminophen. This very popular OTC drug (best known under the brand name Tylenol) is effective in reducing pain and fever but not in treating inflammation. Therefore it is often used for osteoarthritis but is not usually effective for rheumatoid arthritis.

NSAIDs. The other commonly used drugs for joint pain (and other common pain problems like headaches, sprains, and muscle pain) fall into a category known as nonsteroidal anti-inflammatory drugs—or NSAIDs for short. As their name suggests, these are drugs that fight inflammation but are not steroids. That is an important distinction, because while steroids (see below) are powerful anti-inflammatory drugs, they are also likely to cause serious side effects when taken over a long period of time. There are many different NSAIDs available both OTC (aspirin, ibuprofen products such as Motrin and Advil, and naproxen products such as Aleve) and by prescription. The beauty of NSAIDs is that they are quite effective in fighting inflammation but usually without serious side effects.

However, there is one quite common and potentially serious side effect from NSAIDs and that is damage to the stomach lining that can lead to ulcers and bleeding. Actually, the percent of people taking NSAIDs who develop serious bleeding and other gastrointestinal (GI) complications is quite small—about 2 to 3 percent. And the majority of those complications occur in people over age 65 and/or in people with a previous history of ulcers.

However, this possibility has resulted in the development of a new category of NSAID known as "COX-2 inhibitors." I am not going to bore you with a long explanation of the difference between these newer NSAIDs and the older ones mentioned above except to say that by selectively inhibiting the COX-2 enzyme, they reduce the risk of serious GI bleeding. These are the arthritis drugs you see being highly promoted under trade names like Celebrex and Vioxx. These ads usually imply that these new drugs are much safer and more effective than the older NSAIDs. (The ads usually fail to mention that they are much more expensive.) Actually, such claims are only about half-true: There is no good evidence that the COX-2 inhibitors are any more effective than the older NSAIDs but there is evidence that they reduce the risk of developing serious GI bleeding by about 50 percent. Therefore they may be a good choice for people who need NSAIDs but are at high risk for GI bleeding. However, some highly respected physicians at the Cleveland Clinic recently raised the possibility that COX-2 inhibitors might raise the risk for heart attacks; this certainly has not been proven but is a possibility that needs further investigation.

The bottom line is that most people who need NSAIDs will do just fine with the older—and much cheaper—ones. And both groups of NSAIDs can cause serious GI bleeding, so people taking either kind should be aware of any suggestive symptoms of such bleeding like weakness, fatigue, vomiting blood, or black stools. It is also important to know that serious bleeding from ulcers can occur without any pain as a warning signal.

Recent research has also raised the question of whether certain non-aspirin NSAIDs (like ibuprofen) could interfere with the protective effects of aspirin against heart disease *(see page 124 for more on coronary artery disease)*. Because this was a laboratory study, it does not tell us what actually happens in real life when people combine aspirin with other NSAIDs. So no doctor can yet tell you for sure if other NSAIDs will interfere with the heart-protective benefits of taking aspirin. In the meantime, I would advise against taking non-aspirin NSAIDs in large doses for a long period of time on your own if you are also taking aspirin for the heart.

Special medications for RA. There are many medications, other than NSAIDs, that are commonly used to control the inflammation of rheumatoid arthritis. For example, drugs like hydroxychloroquine or methotrexate slow down the immune system attack on joint tissues. Today they are often used early in the course of rheumatoid arthritis to slow its progression. Other disease-slowing drugs less likely to be used today include gold salts and penicillamine. As mentioned above, powerful steroid drugs may be used temporarily during severe flare-ups, but long term use can cause severe side effects, including mood changes, bone weakening, facial swelling, diabetes, and hypertension.

Finally, there are some newer drugs that seem to be even more effective than the others mentioned above. One category is known as TNF (tumor necrosis factor) blockers. Another type actually diminishes the activity of the famous immune system cells known as T cells. These, and other drugs in the pipeline, may be helpful but should be administered only by a physician very skilled in their use—almost always a rheumatologist. So add arthritis to the list of diseases where real expertise can often make a big difference, at least in the more severe cases.

Living with Arthritis: Since it's important to stay as active as you can to improve your muscle strength, it can help to find an exercise companion to motivate you to get out the door. When you're afflicted by a painful flare-up, apply a hot water bottle or heating pad, which can relieve some of the pain and stiffness, or cold applications for unusual swelling.

Some studies have shown that fish oils (omega-3 fatty acids) can reduce arthritis-related inflammation, so it may help to eat fatty fish, like sardines, salmon, tuna, and herring, once or twice a week or to take fish oils in pill supplements. There is also evidence that the popular OTC pills combining glucosamine and chondroitin can be helpful to some arthritis sufferers.

Back Pain

The Basics: Back pain is one of the most common complaints of exercisers and non-exercisers alike. In fact, up to 85 percent of people will have some form of back pain during their lifetime. The highest rate occurs in people between the ages of 45 and 64. Men are slightly more likely to have low back pain than women. There are many other possible causes of back pain but problems with muscles and discs are among the most common.

There are numerous muscles running up and down your back that can get fatigued and tighten when you overuse them or slouch from poor posture. In addition, your spine is made up of 24 individual bones (vertebra), separated by soft discs that provide cushioning. If a disc bulges out from between the vertebra (a condition known as a herniated disc), it can press on the surrounding nerves, causing pain that may travel down your arm or leg.

Prevention & Risk Factors: Certain factors increase your risk of back pain. They include:

- Being overweight.
- Poor posture.
- Osteoporosis (bone thinning).
- Overexercising.
- Weak abdominal muscles.
- Lack of flexibility.
- Lifting improperly.

In fact, the single most important technique to prevent back injury involves proper lifting. When you lift a heavy load, you should bend your knees and squat down to pick up the object instead of bending at your back or waist. That way, your legs, not your back, bear the brunt of the weight as you lift. You should hold the object close to your body to decrease back strain. Also, you should avoid twisting your body to pick up an object. To prevent back pain, it can help to get regular exercise, stretch regularly, and strengthen your back and abdominal muscles. *(See page 46 for tips on stretching.)*

Diagnosis & Screening: Your doctor will want a complete description of your pain, including what it feels like, how severe it is, where you feel

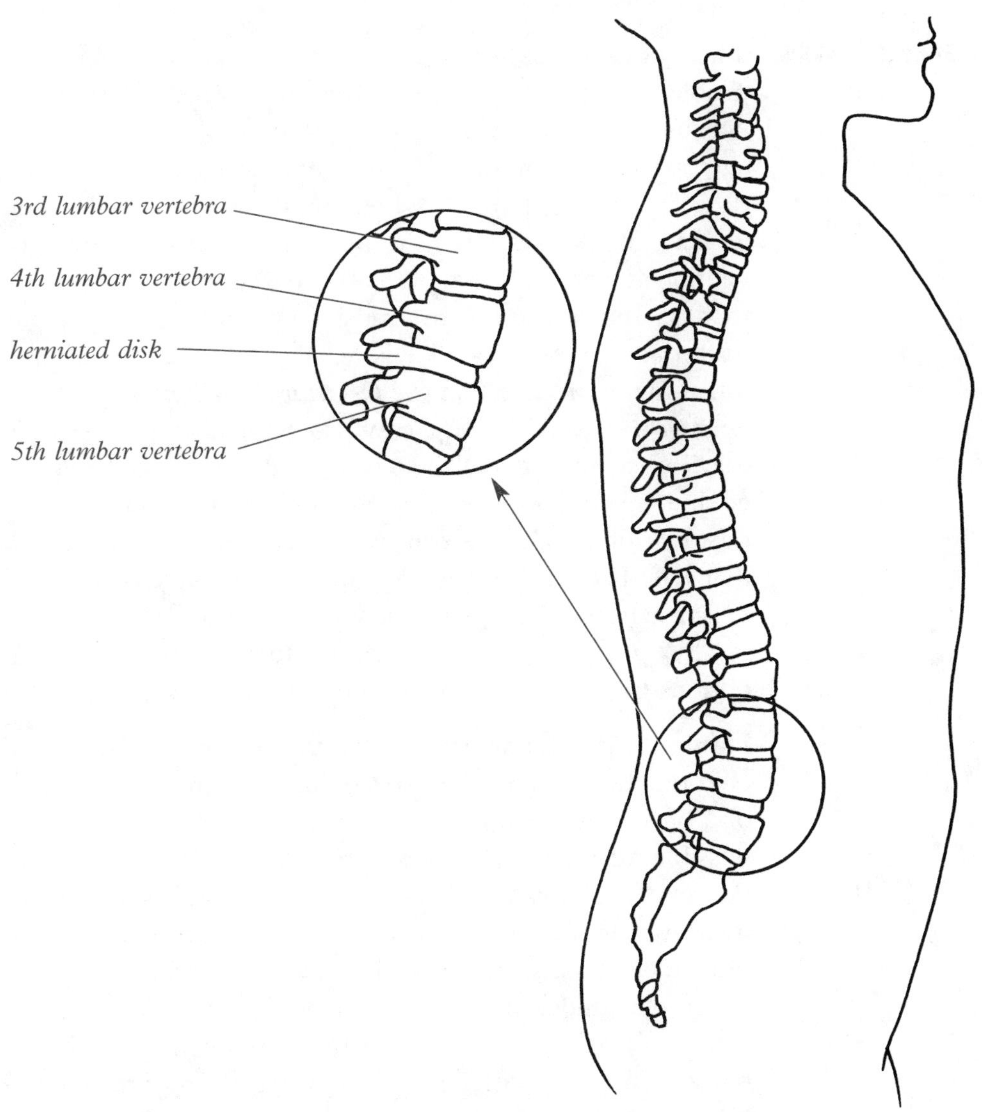

it, when it began, what irritates it, and what makes it feel better. He'll probably also put you through a series of moves to determine if a nerve is involved, and if so, which one. If it is persistent pain lasting longer than two to three weeks, he or she may perform one or several diagnostic tests, including X-rays to examine the bones of the back, or magnetic resonance imaging (MRI), which can provide a view of what discs, nerves, and muscles may be involved.

Treatment Options: The questions of when and how to treat common back problems are complicated and controversial. Partly that's because no matter what you do (as long as you don't keep aggravating the injured area) the vast majority of back problems will get much better on their own within four weeks. That makes it hard to prove that any specific intervention is better than time alone. If the problem appears to be a muscle strain, the most common cause of acute back pain, the usual advice is to take a non-steroidal anti-inflammatory medication *(see the arthritis treatment discussion on page 179)* and "take it easy" for several days. "Take it easy" once meant total bed rest. Today, it usually means getting up and moving around but avoiding positions or postures that make the pain worse. Research has indicated that total bed rest for muscle strains simply delays a return to normal functioning without speeding up recovery.

Beyond these simple measures, there are several other options to consider for acute muscle strain:

Manipulation treatment. There is some evidence that chiropractic treatment can speed healing in the acute phase of a back strain. However, it is important to rule out other possible more serious causes of back pain, such as metastatic cancer, a spinal infection, or a vertebral fracture (as might occur silently in someone with osteoporosis). Chiropractic or massage or physical therapy treatments might be dangerous under those circumstances. There is no good evidence that chiropractic treatment beyond the acute phase makes any difference, so beware of any practitioner who arranges for treatments beyond several weeks! And my own opinion is that good physical therapy and/or massage often accomplishes the same thing as chiropractic.

Acupuncture. Some people swear by this treatment for many forms of pain, including acute back pain. It may be worth a try if the back pain persists beyond a few days.

Percutaneous electrical nerve stimulation (PENS). This technique uses electrical current sent through needles placed into the skin.

Surgery. If the back pain is diagnosed as a herniated disc, the consideration of surgery becomes more rational. However, even with clear-cut evidence of a disc herniation, the typical approach today is that of "watchful waiting," because even when herniated discs are the cause, the pain usually gets better with time alone. There are certain symptoms, such as loss of bladder or bowel control, that are true emergencies and require surgery immediately. And recurrent disc pain in a younger person certainly tips the scale toward surgery as long as there is clear-cut evidence, from symptoms and MRI exams, that the disc is the culprit. Today, disc surgery can often be done through a very small skin incision using various "micro instruments" (so-called percutaneous diskectomy). Other procedures involving injection of dissolving material (so-called chemonucleolysis) are not commonly done in this country because of the slight but real possibility of an allergic reaction to the injected material. Finally, I should point out that bulging discs in the neck (cervical disc herniation) are also very likely to get better with time. Indeed, cervical discs are much more likely to heal on their own than even lumbar (lower back) discs.

Another common cause of low back pain is spinal stenosis. This is a narrowing of the central space in the vertebral column where the spinal cord is located. This problem usually affects people over 65 but can occur at any age. The MRI is the best way to diagnose this problem. Steroid injections into the area affected can often provide temporary relief, but surgery is usually needed for the more severe cases.

Living with Back Pain: As pointed out above, most acute back pain episodes will get better with time, no matter what you do. However, a significant number of people suffer from chronic back pain, often without a certain diagnosis. Such individuals may well benefit from back schools and/or pain clinics where they learn various techniques of daily living to reduce if not eliminate their pain. Preventive back exercises can be particularly helpful in cases of chronic back pain, but these must be taught and learned with care.

Baldness

The Basics: As you age, hair follicles can stop producing new hairs, causing parts of your head to become bald. So-called male pattern baldness is related to a substance called dihydrotestosterone (DHT) which is produced by male hormones called androgens. Too much DHT causes hair follicles to eventually wither away. This typically results in a receding hairline and baldness at the crown of one's head, in the most severe cases creating a horseshoe-shaped fringe around the sides and back of the head. Some men lose virtually all their hair.

Male pattern baldness is responsible for 95 percent of all cases of hair loss and affects about 40 million men. About one-quarter of them begin losing hair by age 30, and two-thirds begin balding by age 60.

Prevention & Risk Factors: Because male pattern baldness is basically genetic, there is really nothing you can do to prevent it. However, reversible hair loss may be caused by any of the following factors.

Illness or major surgery. Physical stress can cause your hair to fall out, but it will probably regrow within a year.

Thyroid or male hormone imbalances. An overactive or underactive thyroid or an imbalance of androgens in your body can cause hair loss, but the loss is usually corrected once the imbalance is corrected.

Medications. Certain drugs, including antidepressants, blood thinners, and especially chemotherapy agents used for cancer treatment, cause temporary hair loss.

Underlying disease. Some severe illnesses, such as lupus, can cause hair loss.

Diagnosis & Screening: If your father or grandfather had a similar pattern, chances are yours is a matter of male pattern baldness. If you don't have a family history of the problem, your doctor will ask you questions about recent events in your life and run diagnostic tests to determine a possible cause of your hair loss.

Treatment Options: There are currently several medical options if you're disturbed by your hair loss.

Minoxidil. This lotion, marketed as Rogaine, works by stimulating your hair follicles to grow new hairs. It's most effective with men who are younger and whose hair loss is recent. If your head is cue-ball bald, you're not a good candidate. It only works while you continue twice daily topical applications. Once you stop, your hair will fall out again rather quickly. Studies show that about 25 percent of men between the ages of 18 and 49 have significant hair regrowth after four months on Rogaine and another 33 percent have minimal hair growth, better known as "fuzz."

Finasteride. This tablet, which is sold as Propecia, slows your rate of hair loss by interfering with the production of DHT. *(This same drug was initially used in larger doses to reduce the size and symptoms of an enlarged prostate gland—see page 294.)* About half of men who take finasteride are able to grow new hair in bald spots if used regularly. Be warned, however: About 2 to 5 percent of people in clinical trials experienced loss of sex drive, impotence, or decreased semen quantity.

Surgery. Using a scalpel to cut small slits in your scalp, surgeons can actually transplant hair from a densely-covered site (usually on the back of your scalp) to a sparsely-covered site. Today this is often done with "micrografts," where the strip of hair-bearing skin is dissected into tiny pieces—some bearing as few as one or two hairs—which are then planted into the bald or thinning area or along a receding hairline. (Years ago, larger grafts were implanted, giving the appearance of "plugs.") If the procedure is well done, many of the grafted hairs will begin to grow in 6 to 12 weeks. Another surgical option is scalp reduction, in which your doctor removes part of your bald scalp and scalp areas with hair are stretched to fill in.

Living with Baldness: Not into the idea of chemical or surgical hair replacement? There's always the good old hairpiece, many of which have improved to look more realistic in recent years. Or, you could simply try a short haircut or a permanent wave, both of which make your hair look fuller. You could also embrace your baldness, which no longer carries the stigma of old age it once did. Modern athletes like Michael Jordan, as well as actors such as Patrick Stewart, have made baldness an attractive look.

Cosmetic Surgery

The Basics: Ten years ago, the thought of cosmetic surgery probably wouldn't have occurred to most men, but surgeons are seeing more and more male patients each year. Men are living longer than ever before, they're in the workplace longer and, often, back in the dating scene in middle or older age. It's natural to want to maintain a somewhat youthful appearance. Moreover, cosmetic surgery has become much more accessible than it used to be. It's not only more affordable, but also less invasive than it once was. Much facial work is now done with lasers—which cut and cauterize (stop bleeding) at the same time—often guided by minimally invasive endoscopes with cameras attached. (Where it used to take two to three weeks to recover from a facelift, now it takes as little as 7 to 10 days.) In liposuction, ultrasound increasingly is used to break up the fat so that it can be sucked out with ever thinner (and purportedly safer) tools. Incisions are smaller, bruising is minimized, and recovery time is faster.

According to the American Society of Plastic Surgeons, the number of plastic surgery procedures performed on men increased by 50 percent between 1992 and 1999. In 1992, the most common surgery requested by men in the United States and Canada was rhinoplasty—a "nose job"—but in 1999, the number one surgery had become liposuction. Plastic surgeons performed nearly 30,000 such operations that year, a 385 percent increase over 1992—and 10,000 more than were done the year before. The next most popular surgery for men was blepharoplasty, a removal of puffy fat in the eyelids. Men also have their noses reshaped, hair transplanted to cover baldness, and prominent ears pinned back.

The following is a brief survey of the more common procedures available.

Liposuction. Contrary to popular belief, the wizardry of liposuction can't turn a fat man into a thin man. Rather, liposuction is body sculpting for patients who are pretty close to their ideal body weight and would like some re-shaping of certain areas. But it's not "weight loss surgery."

In other words, it's for the man who already works out and just can't get rid of that paunch around his middle or those love handles that have sprouted at his waist. There's only so much that can be removed safely, because along with the body fat, the procedure sucks away blood and other body fluids. And it requires a patient with good skin elasticity so that it will shrink to the new, slimmer contour.

The surgeon makes incisions in the groin and/or the navel and along natural skin folds and inserts a straw-like "cannula" (of a variety of lengths and curvatures) attached to a vacuum device. During recovery, which typically takes about two weeks, you may have to wear a girdle-like garment. This surgery can often be done under a form of anesthesia called "tumescent local technique" as an outpatient.

Breast reduction. Gynecomastia is an embarrassing condition in which men appear to have breasts. And like those love handles, breast fat may not respond to exercising and dieting. Less prominent gynecomastias can usually be remedied with liposuction. The more serious cases require gland and tissue removal through an incision along the edge of the areola area, much as in breast reduction for women, but with much less scar production. Doctors send the removed tissue to a pathology lab to check for breast cancer, which is rare in men but can occur. Recovery takes about a month.

Face surgery. Men tend to think of any kind of facial rejuvenation as a face-lift, but in fact there are many separate procedures that can be done in combination or alone, and they all treat a separate part of the face. Often with men, the goal of facial surgery is to remove the hanging tissues and fat deposits associated with aging, but to avoid the wind tunnel look typically associated with face lifts of the past.

Blepharoplasty or eyelid surgery is the most common

facial procedure for men, partly because it's relatively easy to perform and highly effective in making men look younger, since the first signs of aging usually occur around the eyes. Once they hit middle age, many men develop droopy or puffy eyelids, which make them look perpetually tired. In a roughly hour-long operation, the surgeon can remove excess fat and tighten the skin around the eye area, eliminating the "I-didn't-get-enough-sleep-last-night" look.

An actual face-lift raises the loose skin of your neck and cheeks and tightens your face from the eyes down. This is particularly helpful in the neck area where bands of skin and muscle and pockets of fat accumulate. Incisions are typically made in front of and behind the ears, and the skin and the muscles beneath are literally pulled back and up to "tighten" your face.

The third procedure is called a brow lift. As men age their brows tend to get heavy, making them look stern. To counter this, the surgeon literally lifts the skin on the brow and forehead up towards the hairline. Sometimes the surgery requires a long incision across the top of the head (which may not be optimal if you're balding). Other times it's performed endoscopically with three small incisions. Then the muscles are pulled up and anchored with tiny screws that eventually dissolve. The procedure can also be done by simple removal of skin just above the lateral brow. Although it usually achieves a good result, if done improperly it can leave you looking chronically startled.

The Realities of Surgery

Regardless of which part of your body is being operated on, there are surgical problems specific to men. We have thicker, tougher skin than women, which means the surgeon has to work harder to get a natural look. And we have stronger facial features, which means there is more to work with, but also means the work may have to be more subtle. Putting a dainty little nose on a man could leave him just as unhappy as he was with the big hook nose he was born with.

Because hair-bearing skin is rich in blood, men tend to bleed more when they are having facial surgery. And dermabrasion, which is commonly sought by women to smooth their outer skin, isn't done as often on men because it may leave them red in the face.

We also have denser, more fibrous fat, which makes liposuction more difficult. And many surgeons say men don't tolerate pain as well as women, so they have to use more pain medication.

Perhaps the most important issue is expectations. It's important to keep them realistic. You don't have to try very hard to find a surgeon or other doctor claiming to be a cosmetic surgeon to do almost anything you want, whether you need it or not. But keep in mind that how you will look afterwards depends on how you looked before. And you have to be willing to live with the result. "You can't achieve the ideal," is a common refrain among plastic surgeons who are both capable and truthful. The bottom line is they cannot simply reproduce something you've seen in a picture.

Choosing a Cosmetic Surgeon

Even more than many other kinds of surgery, the skill of the surgeon in cosmetic surgery can make a huge difference in outcome. That's because so much of the outcome depends on judgment and "tissue artistry" in addition to standard surgical skills.

Today, the choice of a cosmetic surgeon is very much complicated by the many different kinds of doctors and surgeons who claim that label. Twenty or thirty years ago, a "cosmetic surgeon" was almost always a plastic surgeon—the kind of surgical specialist who trains for at least five years after medical school in both general surgery and plastic surgery and is certified by the American Board of Plastic Surgery. However, today cosmetic surgery may be performed by a dermatologist (skin specialist), ophthalmologist (eye specialist), otolaryngologist (ear, nose, and throat specialist), gynecologist, urologist, or even a nonsurgically trained physician who has (hopefully) taken some special training in the surgery or cosmetic procedures they perform. In short, it can be extremely difficult to find the right surgeon for the procedure you want. And there are some vicious turf battles conducted between various specialists claiming that they are better trained than others for given procedures.

So how do you pick the right "cosmetic surgeon?" If you can get a firm recommendation from your primary care physician, that may be the single best source of good information. Typically, such physicians have learned from many years of referring patients for cosmetic surgery who is good and who is not. Talking with friends who have had good or bad experiences can also be helpful. I would also recommend cosmetic surgeons who are on the staff of reputable hospitals, since that means their credentials and malpractice history have been checked by the hospital. Ask your surgeon to describe his experience with treating your specific problem and ask to see photographs of his work. If this request is not welcomed, you should seek another opinion.

And I am going to tell you that for most procedures involving any actual cutting, I personally would want to choose a cosmetic surgeon who has been trained as a plastic and reconstructive surgeon and is certified by the American Board of Plastic Surgery. (You can call 800-635-0635 for referrals to board certified plastic surgeons in your area.) For liposuction or skin procedures such as dermabrasion or skin peels, dermatologists may be just as good. And for cosmetic surgery of the eye, some ophthalmologists may be fine. Ultimately, experience and skill and honesty about results are just as important as the specific kind of training. But in general, I personally have more confidence in the training of plastic surgeons than I do in the training of other doctors for complicated cosmetic surgery.

Diabetes

The Basics: Insulin, a hormone produced in the pancreas, helps your body utilize blood sugar from the food you eat. People with diabetes have one of two problems: They don't produce enough insulin, or they have a diminished ability to use insulin. As a result, they're not able to modulate their body's blood sugar levels as well as other people, a situation that potentially can adversely affect many parts of the body, including eyes, kidneys, blood vessels, and nerves.

Diabetes affects about 14 million people in the U.S. Most people get it when they're over 40 and have the kind known as Type 2 diabetes (also known as non–insulin-dependent, or adult-onset, diabetes). Type 1 diabetes (insulin-dependent, or juvenile-onset, diabetes) strikes more often during puberty or childhood.

Prevention & Risk Factors: Type 1 diabetes may be inherited, but later life autoimmune diseases or viral infections may put you at increased risk. Type 1 diabetes typically develops suddenly, in a matter of days or weeks, and requires insulin right from the start. Type 2 diabetes, which develops much more gradually, occurs most often in people who are overweight, so if you take steps to keep your weight in check, you're much less likely to fall prey to it.

Diagnosis & Screening: Symptoms of diabetes include increased thirst, increased urination, weight loss, fatigue, nausea, blurred vision, and impotence. In order to diagnose the illness, your doctor will perform a glucose tolerance test, in which you drink a glucose solution to see how your body processes it. Many times a simple blood test that shows a very high blood sugar will be all that's needed to make the initial diagnosis.

Treatment Options: The goal of treatment is to stabilize your blood sugar levels and eliminate the symptoms of high blood sugar. Your doctor will recommend a healthy diet and regular exercise, both of which can help keep your blood sugar under control. Diabetes can be a difficult illness, because it requires a lot of participation on the part of the patient.

If you have Type 1 diabetes, you will have to learn to give yourself a shot of insulin at least once a day to control the amount of sugar in your blood. If you have Type 2 diabetes and it is mild, you may simply need to follow your doctor's lifestyle suggestions by eating a healthy diet, losing weight, and exercising regularly. If these measures don't work, your doctor will recommend that you take one or more oral medications. Various options include:

Sulfonylureas. This class of drugs prompts your pancreas to produce more insulin, but they often stop working after a period of time.

Metformin. This newer diabetes drug prevents your liver from producing glucose and makes body tissue more sensitive to insulin.

Glitazones. This class of medication lowers your glucose levels by making the cells of your body more sensitive to insulin.

Acarbose. This medicine, which you take right after you begin eating, is designed to inhibit the absorption of sugar from your intestine.

Living with Diabetes: Once insulin is required, as it is right from the start in Type 1 diabetes and sometimes down the line in Type 2 diabetes, living with the disease becomes much more difficult because it requires frequent checking for blood sugar levels and the adjusting of insulin injection amounts accordingly. The development of home glucose monitoring (using small devices that provide instant blood sugar readings from finger stick blood samples) have revolutionized the care of insulin-dependent diabetes because it takes the guess work out of knowing what blood sugar levels are at any given moment. However, keeping blood sugar levels within a normal range (80 to 120) is still very tricky and requires a high level of self education and participation.

Some people with insulin-dependent diabetes will choose to use an insulin pump—a device worn to provide constant insulin infusion through a tiny catheter inserted under the skin—rather than multiple insulin injections throughout the day. The device can be used to simulate our body's physiology by providing spurts of additional insulin at mealtimes, just as the pancreas would.

The most important worry for a person taking insulin (and their family and friends) is the possibility of quickly developing hypoglycemia (a very low blood sugar) from taking too much insulin. A person with severe hypoglycemia can quickly become very groggy or even comatose. Therefore, everyone associated with someone with insulin-dependent diabetes (family, friends, coworkers, etc.) should be alert to early warning signs of hypoglycemia (difficulty speaking, thinking, or functioning) and know how to help provide a dose of sugar (fruit juices, glucose tablets, candy, etc.) as quickly as possible. There is no danger in giving sugar to a diabetic because it can always be "controlled" with subsequent insulin. The danger is in withholding sugar when somebody is acting strangely. So when in doubt, give some sugar! If the person has become completely unresponsive, you will have to call for emergency assistance to give sugar intravenously.

The goal of good blood sugar control in a person with diabetes is to help prevent the many possible complications of diabetes. There is excellent evidence from major, large-scale studies that careful control of blood sugar levels in a person with diabetes can make a big difference long term in reducing the risk of complications, especially in Type I but also in Type 2 disease.

Emphysema and Chronic Bronchitis (COPD)

The Basics: When people develop chronic breathing problems as they age, they usually have either chronic bronchitis or emphysema—or both. Indeed, these two conditions so often occur together that they are often lumped together under the label "chronic obstructive pulmonary disease"—or COPD for short. Another reason they are lumped together: Both are almost always caused by a longtime smoking habit. Together, these diseases affect over 15 million Americans; over 80 percent are smokers. Together they are the fourth leading cause of death in this country.

Chronic bronchitis is a chronic state of inflammation in the lining of the breathing tubes leading to the lungs. It is caused by chronic irritation, usually from cigarette smoke, that leads to a thickening and scarring of the lining and causes a chronic phlegm-producing cough. Emphysema refers to the destruction of the lungs' small air sacs—the alveoli—that are crucial for oxygen delivery to our blood. This results in a kind of "merging" of these small air sacs into larger sacs that often trap inhaled air and make it more difficult to breathe. The end result is that there is less surface area for fresh air to come in contact with blood circulating through the lungs. This means that less oxygen gets into our blood from the air we breathe in—and less carbon dioxide gets out of our blood into the air we breathe out. And that leads to the sensation of breathlessness that is the hallmark of this truly awful disease—the sense of having to fight for your breath because you are not getting enough oxygen. Quite frankly, emphysema is one of the most horrific ways to die that I have witnessed as a physician. Many smokers who were dying of emphysema have told me they would rather have had lung cancer, which at least is a quicker death.

Prevention & Risk Factors: Although emphysema is serious, it's actually a largely preventable illness. Don't smoke, and if you do smoke, quit. If you quit, you can at least prevent the progression of the illness, though you can never undo the damage that's already been done to your lung's air sacs.

Other factors can increase the likelihood that you'll develop the disease, especially if you're a smoker. They include:

Exposure to chemical fumes or dust from grain, cotton, wood, or mining. Air pollution and irritating fumes can damage your lungs, making inflammation and emphysema more likely.

An inherited protein deficiency. About 100,000 people in the U.S. are deficient in a type of protein (called alpha-1-antitrypsin) that protects your lungs from being attacked by an enzyme that destroys its elasticity. A blood test can detect the deficiency, which contributes to emphysema in about 20 to 40 percent of people who lack this important protein. Such people must be especially careful to avoid smoking.

Diagnosis & Screening: If you're a smoker and have any of the following symptoms, you should see your doctor:

- Shortness of breath or a feeling that you can't get enough air when you breathe, made worse when you exercise even modestly.
- Coughing and wheezing.
- Excess mucus.

To diagnose the illness, your doctor will observe your breathing to see how hard you have to work to breathe. He'll also listen to your lungs through a stethoscope and will usually perform a number of tests to evaluate your lung function. They include:

Spirometry. For this test, you'll take a deep breath and blow it out as quickly as possible, exhaling through a tube connected to a machine that records airflow and lung capacity.

Chest X-ray. By taking a picture of your lungs, your doctor may be able to diagnose emphysema if it's moderate to severe, but it usually isn't helpful in early stages of the illness.

Arterial blood gas analysis. This blood test checks the levels of carbon dioxide and oxygen in your blood.

Pulse oximetry. In this test, the doctor will attach a small device to your fingertip to measure the amount of oxygen in your blood.

Sputum exam. Looking at your sputum under a microscope can help your doctor check for any infections that may be exacerbating your symptoms.

Treatment Options: Treatment depends on the stage of your illness, but the first thing your doctor will do is tell you to quit smoking, which can slow the progression of the illness. In addition, he or she will probably try one or a combination of the following treatments:

Bronchodilators. These medications, including albuterol, terbutaline, ipratropium bromide, and theophylline, relax the muscles around your airways, helping you breathe more easily. Usually prescribed for people with asthma, your doctor may recommend them for emphysema if you tend to have airway tightness.

Inhaled steroids. Inhaling aerosol corticosteroid drugs can help reduce the inflammation.

Oxygen therapy. If you have severe emphysema, using supplemental oxygen may help you breathe more easily.

Lung reduction surgery. This chest surgery procedure involves cutting out portions of the diseased lung so its remaining section has more room to expand. The surgery can sometimes enhance one's ability to breathe. However, its long-term effectiveness and safety are not proven, and some recent studies suggest that it might actually shorten life in some people.

Lung transplant. If you have severe emphysema and nothing else seems to be working, your doctor may recommend this complicated, risky procedure, in which a surgeon removes one of your lungs and replaces it with one from a donor. The five-year survival rate for people who have a lung transplant is less than 50 percent.

Living with Emphysema:

You'll probably be put on a pulmonary rehabilitation program, which includes education about smoking cessation and medications as well as exercise training to teach you not only good exercises for your body but breathing exercises that can help you feel more in control. You also may find some relief with the following lifestyle changes:

- Avoid airborne irritants, including paint fumes and automobile exhaust, whenever possible.
- Drink at least eight 8-ounce glasses of water a day to keep your lung secretions thin.
- When it's cold outside, wear a scarf around your mouth to prevent the cold air from entering your lungs.
- Avoid the flu by getting a flu shot annually, and get vaccinated against pneumonia every five to seven years. *(See page 72 for more information on adult immunizations.)*

Gallstones

The Basics: Your gallbladder, a small, pear-shaped organ on the right side of your abdomen underneath the liver, stores bile, a greenish fluid that helps in digestion and is produced in your liver. Normally, there is a healthy balance of cholesterol in bile, but when cholesterol concentrations become too high, it forms into deposits, called gallstones, which range in size from as small as a sesame seed to as large as a plum. The concentration of cholesterol in your bile is not related to how much you have in your blood.

Bile reaches your small intestine (where it aids the digestive process) by passing through ducts from the gallbladder, but when gallstones form, they can block these ducts, causing intense abdominal pain.

About 1 in 10 people in the U.S. will have gallstones

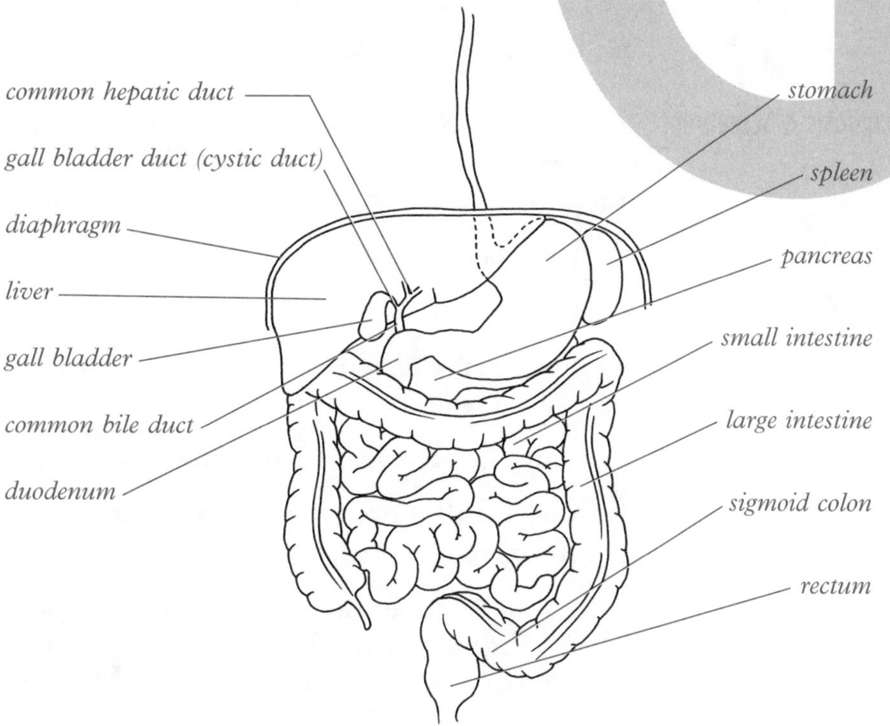

at some point in their lives, though many will never have any symptoms. Men are only about half as likely as women to develop the problem.

Prevention & Risk Factors:

Certain factors make gallstones more likely.

Age. The incidence of gallstones increases as you get older. About 10 to 15 percent of men develop gallstones by the age of 70.

Sedentary lifestyle and being overweight. Even moderately overweight people are at increased risk of gallstones, because extra body weight increases the cholesterol in your bile and causes your gallbladder to empty less frequently. However, obesity is a much greater risk factor for gallstones in women than in men.

Rapid weight loss or a very low–calorie diet. This can disrupt the balance of bile and cholesterol, because it causes your gallbladder to empty less frequently, making bile too rich in cholesterol.

Diagnosis & Screening:

Most gallstones don't produce any symptoms, but when they become large enough to block a duct, they can cause severe pain. There are several trademarks of gallstone pain:

- It's usually sudden and intense.
- It often comes on shortly after you eat something.
- It begins in the upper, right part of your abdomen and may shift to your back or right shoulder blade.
- It may be accompanied by nausea and fever.
- After the pain passes, you may feel a mild ache in the part of your abdomen where the pain started.

If your liver can no longer excrete bilirubin, the yellowish pigment derived from the breakdown of blood cells, your skin and the whites of your eyes may turn yellow (a condition known as jaundice).

It's important to seek treatment immediately if you experience any of the symptoms of gallstones, because in a very small percentage of cases they can lead to fatal complications if untreated. Your doctor will diagnose gallstones based on your medical history and a physical exam, during which he'll check for jaundice and feel your abdomen for tender spots. Other potential diagnostic tests:

Blood test. Your doctor can see if you have an infection by checking your white blood cell count and see if you are jaundiced by looking for excess bilirubin.

Ultrasound. This test uses sound waves to form an image of the organs in your abdomen. The device will be directed to search for gallstones in your gallbladder or bile duct.

Computed tomography (CT or CAT) scan. This test uses computer-generated X-rays to produce an image of the organs in your abdomen.

Endoscopic retrograde cholangiopancreatography (ERCP). If your doctor suspects a gallstone is blocking your common bile duct, he or she may arrange for this test, which can not only identify the gallstones, but, in most instances, treat them. First, the specialist will insert a slender, flexible, lighted viewing instrument down your throat and through your stomach until it reaches the first part of your small intestine (the duodenum). By pumping air to inflate the duodenum, he or she will be able to see the openings for the bile and pancreatic ducts. Next, the doctor will pass a catheter through the endoscope and inject a dye into the bile duct, which helps create a clear visual image of it on an X-ray. If you have a gallstone blocking your bile duct, the doctor will often be able to remove it by using devices that widen the entrance of the bile duct to the duodenum and then gently extracting the stone out of the duct.

Treatment Options: If your gallstones are causing symptoms, your doctor will probably recommend that you have a cholecystectomy, surgery to remove your gallbladder. That's because about

50 percent of people who have had an attack or symptoms caused by gallstones will have another attack within the next year. And when an attack occurs, there is always a chance that it will lead to a serious infection that may require emergency surgery. Therefore, most doctors feel it is better to take the gallbladder out under "elective" conditions—that is, when you're otherwise healthy and no other emergency exists.

Fortunately, today the gallbladder can almost always be removed by laparoscopic surgery. In this approach the doctor makes four small "band aid" incisions in your abdomen, versus the large five-inch (or more) incision required for the old-style gallbladder surgery; traditional "open" surgery is much more painful and requires a much longer recovery period than the laparoscopic approach. Indeed, I would rank the development of laparoscopic surgery as one of the major advances in surgery during the last 20 years. However, if a complication or an unexpected development occurs during laparoscopic surgery, it may be necessary to convert to an "open" large incision to complete the gallbladder removal.

During laparoscopic surgery, the surgeon will pump air into your abdomen and then insert a laparoscope, a thin, lighted instrument equipped with a mini–video camera, into a small incision in your abdomen. With the camera in place, the surgeon can see what's going on inside your body as he or she uses miniature surgical instruments, inserted through other small incisions in the abdomen, to remove the gallbladder

If your doctor doesn't think you're a good candidate for surgery, which is rare, there are several other treatment options available.

Bile salt tablets. If you have very small gallstones, you may be able to dissolve them by taking ursodiol tablets, but you may need to stay on the drug indefinitely, because gallstones tend to recur when people stop taking it.

Sound wave therapy. In this treatment, usually reserved for single stones that are free of calcium and less than 2 centimeters in diameter, high frequency sound waves are used to break up the stone. This is followed by ursodiol tablets.

Living with Gallstones: In some cases, your doctor may find gallstones while performing an X-ray for another reason. If you have gallstones that don't cause any symptoms, most doctors will suggest letting them be. It's good to be aware if you have them, so if you ever develop symptoms, you'll know what's causing them and get treatment quickly. Only about 20 percent of people with "silent" gallstones will develop symptoms from them within 20 years.

Glaucoma

The Basics: Glaucoma, a condition in which there is increased fluid pressure inside your eye, is one of the leading causes of blindness. The increased pressure damages your optic nerve at the back of your eye, which eventually causes vision loss. Trouble is, in its early stages it causes no symptoms, so unless you have regular eye exams, there's virtually no way to know if you have it. About two million people in the U.S. have glaucoma, but only half of them are aware of it.

Prevention & Risk Factors: Although there's no way to prevent glaucoma, if you have regular eye exams you can catch it early and treat it. Some factors may increase the likelihood of developing the disease.

Age. The risk of glaucoma is higher if you're older than 50.

Family history of glaucoma. If your parents or close relatives had the illness, you stand a greater chance of developing it as well.

Steroid medication. Long-term use of this medicine, which many people use for asthma or arthritis, puts you at higher risk for glaucoma.

Diabetes. People with diabetes are more prone to glaucoma.

High blood pressure. This illness can make you more susceptible to glaucoma.

Nearsightedness. This vision problem seems to increase your risk of the illness.

Race. African-Americans are more likely to develop glaucoma. It occurs six to eight times more often and results in blindness more frequently among African-Americans than Caucasians.

Diagnosis & Screening:

Since most people with glaucoma don't notice any symptoms until they begin to lose their eyesight, it's important to get screened for the illness regularly. The American Academy of Ophthalmology recommends that you have an examination every three to five years if you're 39 or older and every one to two years if you're over 50 or have any of the risk factors listed above.

In order to diagnose glaucoma your doctor will take a thorough medical history, then put your eyes through a series of tests.

Measurement of intraocular pressure. This procedure is performed with a tonometer, an instrument designed to measure the pressure within your eye; after some desensitizing eye drops, this test is easily done in an eye doctor's office.

Gonioscopy. In this test, your doctor will place a special lens on your eye to inspect the area between your iris and cornea and see if it's blocked. If it is, the fluid can't drain, which would increase the pressure in your eye.

Ophthalmoscopy. After giving you eye drops to dilate your pupil, your doctor will examine your optic nerve for damage using an instrument called an ophthalmoscope.

Vision perimetry. This test is designed to examine your visual field to see if you've lost any peripheral vision.

Treatment Options:

There isn't a cure for glaucoma, but it can be controlled—and you will need to continue the treatment for the rest of your life. A number of medications have been approved to treat glaucoma. They come in many forms—eye drops, eye inserts, eye ointments, and pills—and contain a number of active ingredients, including epinephrine, which helps remove the fluid from your eye; beta blockers, which reduce the amount of fluid produced by your eye; and prostaglandin analogs, which work by increasing the rate of fluid drainage from your eye. They're all designed to do one thing: lower the pressure in your eye.

If medications don't work or your glaucoma is advanced, your eye doctor may recommend surgery. There are several types, including laser surgery. Your doctor will choose which one you receive based on the severity and type of your illness. Sometimes, preventive laser surgery will be done if you have a "narrow angle" in your eye that increases the risk for developing glaucoma.

Gout

The Basics: Gout is a form of arthritis that affects your joints, usually the big toes, but it also can strike your ankles, heels, knees, hands, fingers, wrists, elbows, or the insteps of your feet. It's caused by a buildup of uric acid, a substance that is produced when waste products from your cells are broken down by your body. When you have too much of it, it can form into sharp, needle-like crystals that settle in your joints and surrounding tissues, causing inflammation and pain. Uric acid usually dissolves in your blood and is excreted in your urine, but people who have gout typically excrete too little of the substance or produce too much of it. More than two million Americans suffer from gout, which affects more men than women.

Prevention & Risk Factors: Although there's no sure way to prevent gout, there are certain circumstances that add to your risk by causing your body to develop high levels of uric acid. They include:

Drinking too much alcohol. If you have more than two drinks a day, you're at increased risk, because alcohol can interfere with the removal of uric acid from your body.

Overeating. Excessive food intake and being overweight may increase your risk of gout because it increases your body's production of uric acid. Purine-rich foods (such as liver or sweetbreads) might be especially troublesome.

Bed rest due to injury or illness. Being incapacitated can somehow trigger an attack of gout.

Diabetes or high levels of fat in your blood. Both of these diseases can interfere with your body's natural uric acid levels.

Family history of gout. Twenty-five percent of people with gout have a family member who suffers from it as well.

Age. The likelihood of developing gout increases as you get older. It most often strikes men for the first time between the ages of 30 and 50.

Diagnosis & Screening:

Symptoms of gout include intense joint pain, inflammation, and redness, typically in the large joint of your big toe. Indeed, sudden joint pain and redness in the big toe is assumed to be gout until proven otherwise. It usually comes on at night, lasts for 5 to 10 days, then subsides gradually over a week or two. Even if the pain goes away, however, it's important to get the condition diagnosed and treated and get on a program to prevent subsequent attacks. Most people will have recurrences after a first attack.

Your doctor will diagnose the illness by taking a medical history and doing a physical examination. He will also perform one or more of the following diagnostic tests:

Blood test. Your doctor will check your blood to assess your uric acid levels.

Synovial fluid examination. If the attack is in a large joint, such as your knee, your doctor may withdraw some synovial fluid, the fluid that lubricates your joint, with a needle to check it for crystals.

X-rays. If gout is well developed, your doctor may take an X-ray picture to see how far it has progressed.

Treatment Options: Your doctor will probably recommend that you take a nonsteroidal anti-inflammatory drug such as ibuprofen or naproxen to relieve your symptoms or a steroidal anti-inflammatory prescription drug such as prednisone. This approach has largely replaced the old standby for treating acute gout—hourly colchicine tablets. Inevitably, colchicine produces too much nausea, vomiting, and diarrhea to warrant its use as first line therapy.

Living with Gout: To prevent future attacks, your doctor may prescribe one of two drugs, probenecid or allopurinol, which lower your uric acid levels. Probenecid, which has fewer side effects, increases kidney excretion of uric acid. Allopurinol blocks the buildup of uric acid in the body.

Headaches

The Basics: Headaches are extremely common. The complaint is the seventh most common one brought to doctors. Although we use the word headache generically, there are actually a number of different types of headaches.

Tension headaches, which feel like you have a tight band around the upper part of your head, are the most common type. They cause mild to moderate aching pain that usually lasts anywhere from two hours to two days. Sometimes they become chronic, however, occurring frequently for a period of six months or more, in which case they can cause intense pain.

Migraines range from moderate to severe and usually have a throbbing or pulsing quality. They can strike one or both sides of your head and typically last 4 to 72 hours. Migraines may be accompanied by nausea and sensitivity to lights or sounds. More than 26 million people in the U.S. suffer from migraines, which are more common in women.

Cluster headaches also tend to occur on one side your head and last for 30 to 90 minutes, during which time you usually have a very intense burning or stabbing pain in your eye or temple. Other symptoms can include eye tearing or redness, a stuffy or runny nose, and sweating on your face. They typically strike every day–even several times a day–over a period of weeks or months. Cluster headaches are unusual in that they tend to occur more frequently in men.

Prevention & Risk Factors: Although scientists are still trying to sort out the biochemical causes of headaches, there are a number of typical triggers for each type. Identifying what triggers headaches in you and then avoiding or minimizing your exposure to those triggers can go a long way toward preventing future episodes.

Tension headaches may be triggered by:

- Emotional stress or depression.

- Eye strain.
- Muscle tension, often caused by poor posture.

Migraines are typically brought on by:

- Diet, particularly red wine; foods prepared with monosodium glutamate (MSG); aged cheeses and other foods that contain tyramine; and preserved meats such as bacon and hot dogs that contain nitrates and nitrites.
- Skipping meals.
- Too little or too much sleep.
- Emotional stress.
- Weather and temperature changes.
- Fluorescent lights.
- High altitude.

Cluster headaches can be precipitated by:

- Alcohol.
- Glare.
- Emotional stress.

Diagnosis & Screening: Your doctor will probably be able to diagnose your type of headache based on your symptoms. In some cases, however, he or she may want to run some tests, such as a CT scan, to be sure there's no underlying problem in your brain.

Treatment Options: Your treatment will depend on the type of headache you have. Tension headaches are typically treated with over-the-counter pain relievers such as aspirin, acetaminophen, ibuprofen, and naproxen or combination products (prescription or over-the-counter) that contain a pain reliever and caffeine or narcotics.

There are a variety of options for migraine treatment, all of which work best when you take them shortly after the headache has begun. Options include aspirin or acetaminophen, both of which may work best when they're taken in combination with an antihistamine, decongestant, or caffeine. In more severe cases, your doctor may prescribe a narcotic or sedative and perhaps an anti-nausea drug. A newer category of drugs known as triptans—which can be given as pills, injections, or nasal sprays—have proven to be very effective for more severe migraine problems.

One of the most interesting new developments in the headache field is the recognition of a phenomenon called "chronic daily headache" that develops in many migraine patients who take OTC pain pills in ever-increasing doses. They become dependent on them to the point where the medications become the cause of headaches rather than a solution. Such patients often need to undergo "withdrawal" from such medications under the direction of a knowledgeable physician.

Because cluster headaches typically last only for a short period of time, they're trickier to treat. Two options that have been shown to be effective, however, are breathing 100 percent oxygen through a face mask and an injection of a triptan drug such as sumatriptan.

Tension headaches often can be prevented with tricyclic antidepressants, anticonvulsants, or beta blockers; migraines can be prevented with beta blockers, antidepressants, calcium channel blockers, and anticonvulsants; and cluster headaches can be prevented with calcium channel blockers, lithium, steroids, and anticonvulsants.

In addition to drug treatments, a number of people find relief from alternative therapies such as biofeedback; relaxation techniques such as yoga, meditation, or guided imagery; or cognitive-behavioral therapy, which is designed to improve your problem-solving and coping skills.

Living with Headaches: Chronic or severe headaches deserve the attention of a physician who specializes in unusual headaches and will therefore take the time to sort out a complicated problem headache. As described on pages 79 and 161, sudden and very severe headaches "unlike anything I have had before" may signal a life-threatening emergency from a burst aneurysm or other source of bleeding in the brain.

Hearing Loss

The Basics: Hearing impairment is one of the most common health problems in the U.S., affecting about 28 million people. Hearing depends on a precise series of events. Sound waves enter your outer ear and travel through your ear canal to your eardrum. The sound waves make your eardrum vibrate, and the vibrations are carried through tiny bones in your middle ear to your inner ear, where the waves are detected by tiny hair cells and turned into electrical impulses. Your auditory nerve sends these electrical impulses to your brain.

There are two main types of hearing loss. *Conductive* hearing loss occurs when sound waves can't get from the outer ear to the inner ear, usually because of some physical impediment to their progress, like wax or fluid, or a problem with the bones of the middle ear. As a result, it's often reversible. Surgery on the bones of the middle ear is quite common today.

Sensorineural hearing loss, on the other hand, which occurs when the hair cells or nerves in your inner ear are damaged, is usually permanent. Some people have a combination of the two.

Prevention & Risk Factors: There are a number of things that can increase the likelihood of hearing impairment.

- Ear wax or fluid, which prevents sounds waves from traveling to the inner ear.
- Punctured eardrum, which can be caused by infection or trauma.
- Sounds louder than 90 decibels—roughly equivalent to

what you hear when you walk within 15 feet of a large truck—can damage your inner ear, causing sensorineural hearing loss. The damage becomes more likely the longer you're exposed to the sound. That's why it's a good idea to wear ear plugs when you're at a rock concert, which typically produces sounds in the range of 100 decibels, or when you're riding a snowmobile or motorcycle, both of which are in the 90-decibel range. As a general rule, if you need to shout to be heard, the noise level is in a range that can damage your hearing.

- Heredity.
- Some head injuries, medications, and certain illnesses can damage your ears, resulting in temporary or permanent hearing loss.

Diagnosis & Screening: If you suspect your hearing is impaired, ask yourself the following questions. If you answer "yes" to three or more, you should have your hearing evaluated.

- Do you often need to ask people to repeat themselves?
- Do you have trouble hearing voices over the phone?
- Is it difficult to follow a conversation when two or more people are talking at once?
- Does it frequently sound to you like people are mumbling?
- Do you find yourself sitting up close to the speaker at a conference or town meeting?
- If you're in a noisy environment, like a ball park or crowded restaurant, is it more difficult for you to hear?
- Do you have more trouble understanding people with high voices, like women and children?

Your doctor can send you to a hearing specialist, known as an audiologist, who will administer an auditory test to determine the extent of your hearing loss. He may also recommend a visit to an otolaryngologist who specializes in ear disorders.

Treatment Options: Your treatment depends on the type and extent of your hearing loss. If your eardrum is punctured or the bones of your middle ear are damaged, your doctor might recommend surgical reconstruction. If wax or fluid buildup is the problem, your doctor should be able to treat this. If your hearing loss is moderate to severe and is the sensorineural type, you may need to be fitted for a hearing aid, which essentially amplifies sounds so you can hear them better, or a cochlear implant, a small electronic device that is surgically implanted under the skin behind your ear. Cochlear implants are used only in people with near-total hearing loss.

Living with Hearing Loss: If you have mild hearing loss, you should be especially vigilant about trying to protect your ears from further damage. Wear ear plugs when you know you're going to be exposed to loud noises or, better yet, try to avoid them altogether.

I would also point out that men are often particularly resistant to the use of hearing aids as a sign of old age or "weakness." However, newer "in-ear" models are difficult to notice, yet can make an enormous difference in quality of life.

Heartburn

The Basics: This extremely common symptom (an estimated 60 million people in the U.S. are affected on a periodic basis, and 15 million people suffer on a daily basis) is known in medical jargon as gastroesophageal reflux disease—or GERD for short. That phrase describes the underlying problem causing "heartburn"—namely, the reflux, or upward flow, of stomach acid into your esophagus, which normally carries food in the other direction from your mouth to your stomach. At the end of the esophagus is a ring of muscular tissue called the lower esophageal sphincter, or LES. Normally, this ring of muscle relaxes usually only when we swallow to allow food to pass into the stomach; it then closes to prevent backflow. But in GERD, this sphincter relaxes often when it shouldn't, allowing backflow. That, in turn, irritates the lining of your esophagus, producing the symptom we call heartburn, because it feels like a burning sensation in your lower chest where your heart is also located. (Your esophagus actually runs behind your heart on its way to the stomach.)

Indeed, one of the problems with heartburn is that it can be confused with angina, which is heart pain that occurs when your heart is not getting enough blood and oxygen *(see page 126)*. Despite our best attempts to educate the public about the differences between heartburn and angina, we doctors still encounter too many people, especially men, who put up with angina for hours thinking it is "just heartburn." And that waiting can sometimes cause extensive damage to your heart or even prove fatal.

In other words, it is important to know the difference between the two. Typically, heartburn occurs after a big meal and/or with lying down or bending over, physical conditions that encourage the backflow of stomach contents. If there is any doubt about the cause of your discomfort, if the sense of burning is brought on by exertion and not eating,

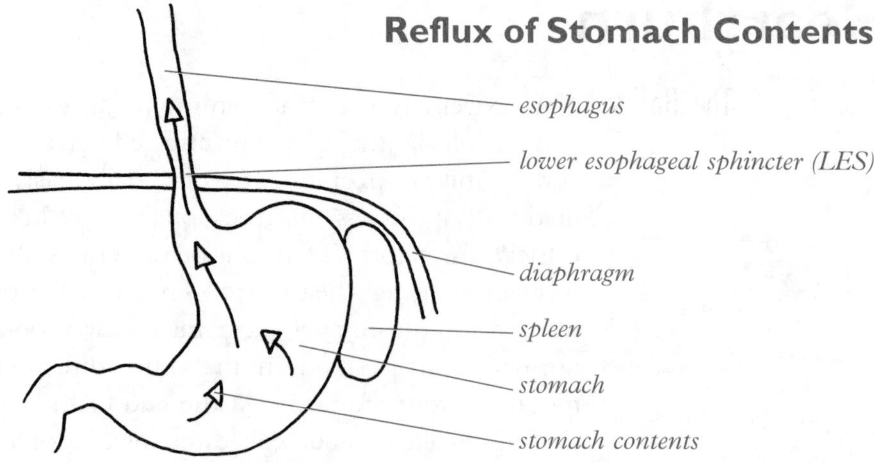

or if it gets worse or is accompanied by other symptoms like sweating and difficulty breathing, you should immediately call your doctor or go to the emergency room.

Gastric reflux can produce other confusing symptoms, such as a chronic sore throat, cough, and wheezing—or even just a persistent feeling of a lump in the throat. Fortunately, there are several tests that can almost always pinpoint gastric reflux as the cause of such symptoms (see below).

Many people are confused about the difference between heartburn and hiatal hernia. A *hiatal hernia* refers to the anatomic condition in which part of your stomach actually pushes up through the opening in your diaphragm through which your esophagus enters the abdomen, where it meets your stomach. In other words, a hiatal hernia means part of your stomach is up in your chest! This anatomic problem may or may not be associated with actual reflux into the foodpipe. The larger the hiatal hernia, the greater the chance of its causing severe heartburn.

Given that heartburn is so common in our society, we tend to minimize its potential seriousness. But if gastric reflux is severe and persistent, it can lead to very real problems in the esophagus, including scar tissue that can block the passage of food and liquids or cellular changes that increase your risk of cancer of the esophagus. Therefore, if

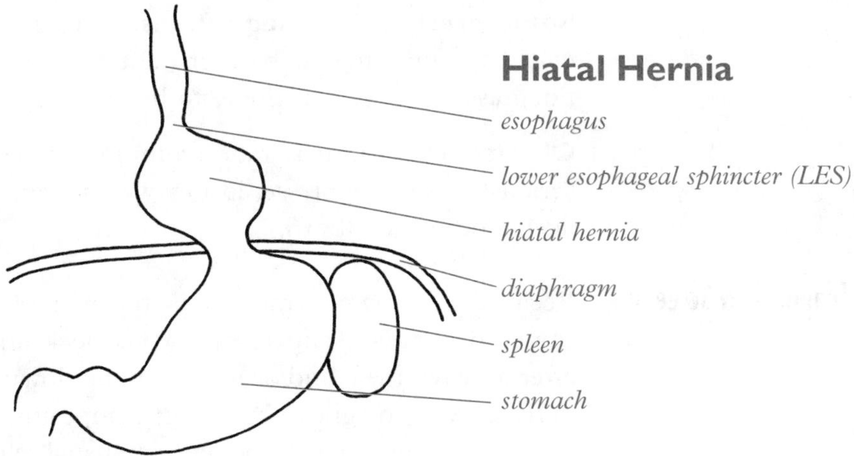

you have recurrent and severe heartburn, you should not constantly gulp antacids. Rather, you should report your problem to your doctor, who can prescribe more potent medications that can actually prevent complications.

Prevention & Risk Factors: There are a number of factors that increase the likelihood of an episode or repeated bouts of heartburn. They include:

Hiatal hernia. As explained above, a hiatal hernia occurs when the upper part of your stomach bulges into your chest cavity through the opening in your diaphragm. It occurs more often in people who are obese and is more common in people over the age of 50.

Diet. Research has implicated a number of possible dietary causes of heartburn, including peppermint, coffee, alcohol, chocolate, citrus fruits and juices, tomato products, spicy foods, carbonated beverages, and anything fried or fatty. So if you're prone to the problem, it may help to systematically try to avoid those foods one by one to see if that alleviates your symptoms.

Smoking. Cigarette smoking causes the lower esophageal muscles to relax and also stimulates excess production of stomach acid. Quitting can reduce the likelihood of heartburn.

Some prescription medications. Certain asthma medicines, calcium channel blockers, and so-called tricyclic antidepressants may contribute to heartburn.

Obesity. Heartburn is more common in people who are seriously overweight, so losing weight can decrease the likelihood of heartburn.

Diagnosis & Screening: Because the main symptom is burning chest pain that sometimes extends up toward your neck and gets worse after a heavy meal and/or when you lie down, heartburn is fairly easy to diagnose based on symptoms alone. A minority of people may experience unusual symptoms such as difficulty swallowing, in which case special tests may be recommended:

Twenty-four-hour esophageal pH study. In this test, your doctor will insert a flexible, narrow tube through your nose and into your esophagus to record levels of acid over a twenty-four-hour period and see if they correlate to your symptoms.

X-rays. Called an upper GI (for gastrointestinal) series, these special X-rays provide doctors with a picture of your esophagus, stomach, and small intestine and can help rule out other possible causes of your pain, including an ulcer *(see page 263).*

Endoscopy. In this exam, the doctor will insert a small lighted tube with a miniature video camera at the end through your mouth and into your esophagus to look for inflamed or precancerous areas. If such areas are found, the doctor will perform biopsies to look at under the microscope for evidence of precancerous changes. This procedure is usually much easier on the patient than it sounds.

Treatment Options: Although heartburn usually isn't considered a serious ailment, it's important to treat it, because over time it can damage the lining of your esophagus, causing inflammation, scarring, bleeding, and ulcers as well as precancerous changes. Most people can find relief through lifestyle changes or medications. Following are some options for those who want to avoid medications:

- Avoid foods that increase your symptoms.
- Don't overeat at any one meal. Heartburn is more likely to come on after a large meal.
- Don't eat within two or three hours of bedtime, because symptoms often get worse when you lie down. If you continue to have nighttime symptoms, elevate the head of your bed six inches or so with blocks under the legs to allow gravity to help keep your stomach

contents where they belong.

- Wear loose-fitting clothing. Clothes that fit tightly around your middle can increase the risk of reflux simply by pushing stomach contents up into your esophagus.
- If you're overweight, try to lose some pounds, and if you smoke, try to quit.

If these lifestyle changes do not solve your problem, or you don't choose to follow them, you will need to turn to medications. There are basically three levels of medication to consider. The most common are the ubiquitous *antacids,* which come in all kinds and shapes and colors. They contain aluminum or magnesium and, today, usually calcium. As their name suggests, they counteract or neutralize stomach acid and can be very effective for mild bouts of heartburn. They typically provide almost immediate relief. I would recommend the cheapest generic brand you can find. If used frequently or in large amounts they can produce diarrhea or constipation and therefore should not be continually used for serious heartburn that requires constant treatment.

There are two newer classes of medications designed to prevent the production of stomach acids in the first place, rather than simply neutralize what the stomach has already made. One class of medicines is known as *histamine (H2) blockers.* These are now widely available (and heavily advertised) as over-the-counter medicines. They are also available in stronger doses by prescription. The other, newer class of medication is known as *PPIs—proton pump inhibitors.* Although they are only available by prescription, they are also widely advertised to consumers and doctors as various drug companies compete for this very lucrative business.

If your heartburn problems are only occasional and predictable—you only get it after eating a big meal, say—you might want to take one of the over-the-counter H2 blockers before you eat. You can talk with your druggist about which one and what dose to choose. However, if your problem is more severe and persistent, the PPI drugs, which are more effective, are the way to go.

In rare cases, medications can't control the problem, and your doctor will recommend a surgical procedure known as fundoplication—a procedure that involves using part of the stomach to wrap around and strengthen the lower esophageal sphincter. Today this procedure can usually be done via the laparoscope, thereby greatly reducing the trauma and recovery time associated with traditional "open" upper abdominal surgery. However, this is a tricky procedure that should be done only by very experienced surgeons and, in my opinion, only as a last resort.

More recently, researchers have been experimenting with ways to strengthen the LES by means of endoscopic procedures—using the same tube-down-the-esophagus approach described above for diagnosis. In one, radiofrequency energy is used. In another, actual suturing is accomplished. And in a third, plexiglass is implanted. All of these must be regarded as experimental until long-term studies on their safety and effectiveness are published.

Hemorrhoids

The Basics: Hemorrhoids are basically varicose veins in your rectum. They occur when normal veins in the area become engorged with blood either because of inherent weakness or due to straining during bowel movements or unusual physical exertion, like lifting something extremely heavy. They can form either inside the anal canal or under the skin around the outside of the anus.

Hemorrhoids will affect more than half of all people in the U.S. at some point in their lives, usually between the ages of 20 and 50.

Prevention & Risk Factors: There are a number of things you can do to prevent hemorrhoids. They include:

- Eat a high-fiber diet. Foods rich in fiber, such as fruits and vegetables, whole wheat bread, and bran, keep your bowel movements soft and regular.
- Drink at least eight 8-ounce glasses of water or its equivalent a day. Adequate fluid intake helps your body produce softer stools.
- Try to get at least 10 to 15 minutes of exercise every day. Staying active will help your body eliminate feces on a regular schedule, making the hard bowel movements associated with constipation less likely.
- Practice healthy bowel habits. Make an effort to empty your bowels when you feel the need to and don't sit on the toilet for more than five minutes, because that position places increased pressure on the veins in your rectum.

Diagnosis & Screening: One sign of hemorrhoids—anal bleeding, or blood in the stool—can be easily confused with other problems, including an anal fissure, colitis, diverticulosis, or colorectal cancer. Doctors tend to be cautious about ascribing rectal bleeding to a hemorrhoid, even if one can be identified. If bleeding is significant and/or occurring for the first time—especially in someone over age 40—I believe a colonoscopy should be performed to rule out cancer in the colon or rectum. Hemorrhoids also can cause itching and pain in the rectum, and you (or someone else) may actually be able to see a lump, much like a small grape, protruding from your anal opening.

In order to diagnose hemorrhoids, your doctor will need to examine your rectal area. He will insert a gloved finger into your anus and may use an instrument such as an anoscope or proctoscope, both of which are hollow lighted tubes that allow him to view the inside of your rectum.

In most cases, your doctor will be able to make a definitive diagnosis quickly and easily using those procedures. If your hemorrhoids are inside your anal canal or aren't readily evident he may want to perform other diagnostic tests to rule out other potential causes of anal bleeding, such as colon cancer *(see page 86)*

Treatment Options: Almost half of all people with hemorrhoids will get a good deal of relief simply by making the lifestyle changes listed in the prevention section. Other things your doctor may recommend:

Sitz baths. Not as complicated as it sounds, this simply entails sitting in several inches of warm (not hot) water for 15 minutes several times a day, especially after bowel movements.

Ice packs. Applying a pack of ice to the area for 10 minutes up to four times a day can reduce the swelling and inflammation.

Over-the-counter hemorrhoid creams or suppositories. These products contain substances like witch hazel, hydrocortisone, or lidocaine that help reduce the itching, swelling, and pain in the area.

Rubber band ligation. If the above first line options aren't effective, your doctor can perform this procedure, in which he ties one or two tiny rubber bands around the base of the hemorrhoid to cut off its circulation. Lacking a blood supply, the hemorrhoid will basically shrivel and die and fall off in a week to 10 days. It's painless and effective about 75 percent of the time.

Infrared coagulation. In this procedure, your doctor uses a beam of infrared light to seal the base of the hemorrhoid, cutting off its circulation. The hemorrhoid will eventually dry up and fall off.

Injection. If your hemorrhoid is inside your anal canal, your doctor may recommend this treatment, in which he injects the hemorrhoid with a substance that causes it to shrink.

Surgery. For hard-to-treat hemorrhoids or large, painful ones, your doctor may refer you to a specialist to perform a hemorrhoidectomy, in which he surgically removes the hemorrhoid and perhaps some surrounding tissue.

Living with Hemorrhoids: Hemorrhoids tend to recur, so it can be helpful to have a stool softening agent or fiber supplements on hand. Take them at the first sign of a flare-up. In addition to following the preventive measures mentioned above, you also should bathe the area daily with warm water (soap can actually irritate hemorrhoids) and dry the area with a hair dryer so you don't have to scrub and irritate it further.

Hepatitis

The Basics: Hepatitis means inflammation of the liver, and it's usually caused by one of three viruses—A, B, or C—that infects your liver. However, certain medications and other substances such as alcohol can cause damage to the liver. When viruses damage your liver cells, the liver may often regenerate, and it can look completely healthy after recovery. This is almost uniformly true of hepatitis A. However, chronic inflammation, as often occurs in hepatitis B and C, may result in permanent loss of cells and replacement with scar tissue.

Hepatitis A, which is excreted in the stool and can thus contaminate food and water, is more common in children than adults and is usually a mild infection. Many times, parents may not even be aware their child is sick. An estimated 50 percent of Americans have been exposed to the hepatitis A virus and have therefore developed immunity to it.

Both the *hepatitis B and C* viruses can exist in body fluids—blood, saliva, semen, tears, and urine—so people are most often infected through sexual activity or sharing needles for injecting drugs. Since rigorous screening of blood donors has been in effect, it's now very rare for someone in this country to contract hepatitis B or C through a blood transfusion, but one can catch either virus if an open cut or sore comes into contact with an infected person's blood. Both hepatitis B and C are more likely to lead to serious, chronic liver disease than hepatitis A.

Because some people recover from hepatitis without ever knowing they were infected, it's difficult to know exactly how common the illness is. Experts estimate that about 200,000 people are newly infected with hepatitis B every year, but about 90 percent eventually clear the virus on their own. About 1.25 million people have a chronic hepatitis B infection, and about 4 million people have a chronic hepatitis C infection (the leading cause of liver transplants). To complicate matters, about half of all chronic carriers don't know they're infected with the illness. Approximately 20 percent of those infected with hepatitis C will, over several decades, develop a severely scarred liver (cirrhosis), and of these about 20 percent will go on to develop liver cancer.

Prevention & Risk Factors: Most children today receive the hepatitis B vaccine as part of their routine immunization program, and it's highly recommended for anyone who engages in high risk sexual or drug behavior or is a health worker. The hepatitis A vaccine isn't routinely given but is available. It's typically recommended for people who are planning to travel in countries with high rates of the illness, including Central and South America, Mexico, and most of Asia, and for men who have sex with for men or use injectable drugs. There is no vaccine for hepatitis C.

There are other steps you can take to prevent exposure to all types of hepatitis.

- Wash your hands after using the bathroom, especially public bathrooms. Since certain types of the virus can be carried in urine and feces, this simple step can be helpful.
- Cover all open cuts and sores. Since the virus can enter your body through an opening in your skin, it's a

good idea to keep cuts and sores covered until they have scabbed over.

- If you are not in a long-term monogamous relationship, use condoms during sex. Although condoms don't provide 100 percent protection, they're the best thing we have to prevent sexual transmission of hepatitis.
- If you are a drug user, don't share needles or syringes. Intravenous drug users are at increased risk of this blood-borne illness primarily because of this unsanitary practice.

Diagnosis & Screening: Hepatitis frequently doesn't cause any symptoms. When it does, they tend to be flu-like—fever, chills, fatigue, nausea, body aches. As the illness begins to attack your liver, you may have other symptoms, including jaundice (a yellowing of the skin and whites of the eyes), and your urine may darken to the color of tea while your stools may become clay colored. Blood tests typically can determine if you're infected with hepatitis.

If you're infected, your doctor also may want to perform periodic blood tests to see how your liver is functioning and perhaps a liver biopsy to help determine the extent of the damage.

Treatment Options: Hepatitis treatments vary depending on the stage of your illness. If you know you've been exposed to hepatitis B recently—for instance, you had unprotected sex with someone who you know is a carrier—your doctor can give you hepatitis B immune globulin within one week of exposure, along with the vaccine. There aren't any good treatments for people with an acute form of the illness.

Chronic hepatitis B infection can be treated with lamivudine (Epivir), an antiviral medication, or interferon, an immune system modulator which is about 40 percent effective in eradicating the virus. For hepatitis C, most doctors opt to use interferon in combination with ribavirin, another antiviral medication. However, chronic liver disease is much easier to prevent than treat—so avoidance of high risk sexual behavior and/or drug abuse (especially alcohol!) is a wise idea.

Hernias (inguinal)

The Basics: A hernia occurs when one body part protrudes through a gap into another body area. Hernias are often, but not always, caused by straining or lifting a heavy object. There are different types of hernias, depending on which body parts are involved. For instance, when tissue from your intestine protrudes through a weak point or tear in your groin, it's called an inguinal hernia. Inguinal hernias are much more common in men than women and account for about 80 percent of all hernias in men. Almost 700,000 men have surgery every year to repair an inguinal hernia. In contrast, a hiatal hernia occurs when part of the stomach protrudes through the diaphragm into your chest cavity *(see page 218)*.

Prevention & Risk Factors: Since many hernias have no apparent cause, it's almost impossible to prevent them. But, anything that puts intense pressure on or in your abdomen can contribute to either an inguinal or hiatal hernia. Common culprits include:

- Violent, persistent coughing.
- Vomiting.
- Straining while going to the bathroom.
- Lifting heavy objects.

Diagnosis & Screening: Some hernias cause no pain or visible symptoms and aren't discovered until your doctor is performing a physical exam. Often with an inguinal hernia, the first sign is a lump or bulge in your groin area. It also may be uncomfortable to bend over, cough, or lift heavy objects. A so-called *indirect* inguinal hernia doesn't cause an evident bulge, because the protruding intestine actually descends into your scrotum, sometimes causing pain and swelling in the scrotum. These are the groin hernias that can become twisted, cutting off the blood supply to the trapped part of the intestine, and causing a surgical emergency.

In order to diagnose an inguinal hernia, your doctor will need to perform a physical exam. He'll look at your groin area, checking carefully for evidence of a bulge or swelling and will palpate your scrotum. He will also insert his finger up through the scrotum into your inguinal canal to check for indirect hernias.

Treatment Options: Most inguinal hernias require surgery, because they often get bigger and may become strangulated. There are two main types of surgery:

Standard herniorrhaphy. In this procedure, your doctor will make a three-inch incision over your hernia and push the protruding tissue back into place, often while stitching a mesh into place to help strengthen the muscle.

Hernioplasty via laparoscope. During this surgery, which is designed to strengthen the muscle wall through which your intestine protrudes, your doctor will make several small incisions in your abdomen, through which he'll insert tiny, tubelike surgical instruments. With them, he'll return your intestine to its proper location and then place a synthetic mesh patch over the weakened tissue.

Living with a Hernia: You can reduce the likelihood that an inguinal hernia will return if you make an effort not to put too much strain on your abdominal muscles.

Intestinal Issues

Many of our emotions seem to reside in our intestinal geography—which is why we often refer to our "gut feelings" about some matter even when our intestines are not officially involved. Nonetheless, our intestines are mysterious organs to most of us. In this section, I am going to briefly highlight some of the common problems that develop in our intestines. First, a brief anatomy and physiology tour is in order.

Structure and Function: The contents of the stomach pass into our intestinal system—first the approximately 21 feet of coiled small intestine and then the approximately 6 feet of large intestine;

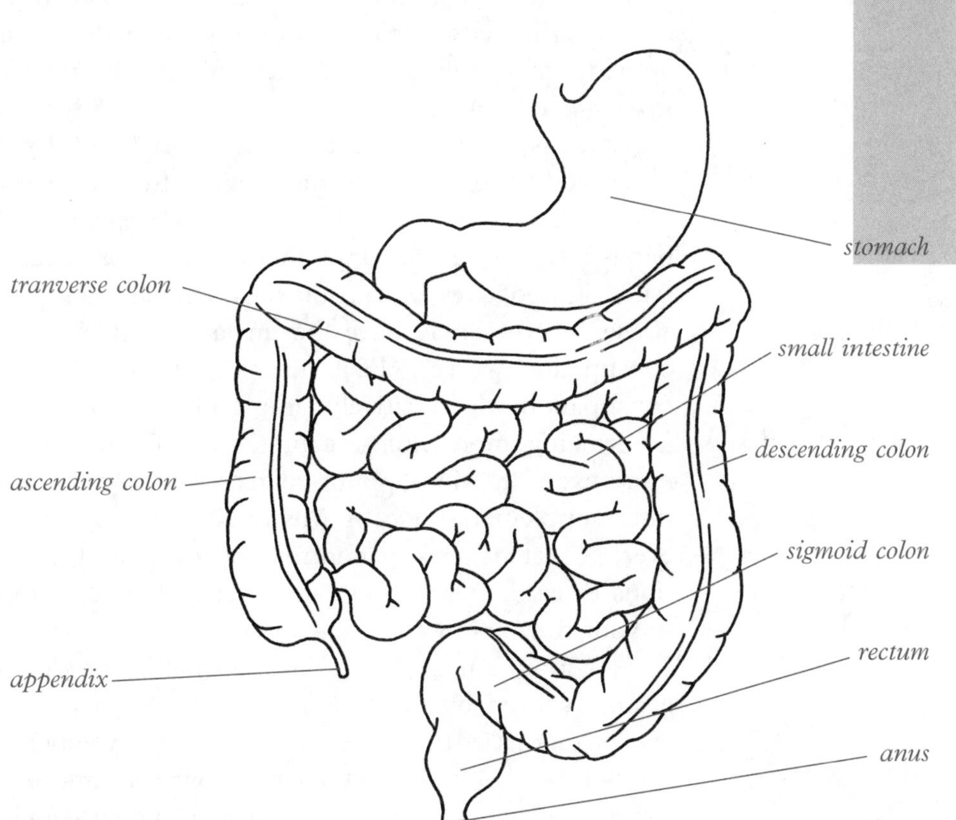

the words "small" and "large" refer to the diameter of each intestine. Much of the digestion of food from the stomach occurs in the first foot or two of the small intestine—the duodenum, which is also where most so-called peptic ulcers occur *(see page 263)*. Most of the absorption of water and nutrients occurs in the remaining two parts of the small intestine, the jejunum and ileum. (I have no idea where these names come from but I have always loved their sound.) The large intestine or colon then absorbs most of the remaining liquid and electrolytes (sodium, potassium, etc.), leaving the solid waste (feces) that eventually passes out through the anus. The last two sections of the large intestine are known as the sigmoid and rectum.

Common Symptoms: The two most common intestinal complaints are constipation and gas. (Vomiting and diarrhea are usually caused by a viral infection or related to foods and therefore "self limited," meaning they get better quickly with time.) *Constipation,* of course, refers to difficulty in having bowel movements, with stools that are often hard and dry. It can be caused by many problems ranging from a diet low in fiber or an unusually sedentary lifestyle to poor "bowel habits" (ignoring the urge to defecate), or medications (such as sedatives or calcium channel blockers), laxative abuse (overuse may have the unwanted effect of making constipation worse). That means you can often reduce constipation with relatively simple lifestyle changes, such as drinking more fluids, eating more fiber, and getting more exercise. Many senior citizens find a psyllium-based fiber supplement such as Metamucil very helpful. However, persistent constipation may be a signal of a more serious disease, even colon cancer, and should be reported to your doctor.

A certain amount of *gas* is a normal by-product of digestion caused by the action of intestinal bacteria on digested food. (In this case, "normal" is very much in the ear—or nose—of the beholder.) However, intestinal gas can also be greatly increased by swallowing air (often associated with anxiety) or consuming carbonated drinks. People with milk (lactose) intolerance usually have gas problems. Certain foods, such as beans, cabbage, and cauliflower, are notorious gas producers. Various home remedies can be helpful (peppermint, anise, or chamomile teas), and over-the-counter medications containing simethicone are occasionally useful.

Diagnostic Tests: There are many ways that doctors can view the insides of the gastrointestinal (GI) tract, including the intestines, and I am going to briefly describe them here.

Endoscopes. In this procedure, the doctor inserts an endoscope, a flexible tube with fiber-optic lights at the end, either through the mouth or the anus to look at the upper or lower parts of the digestive tract. Endoscopes can be inserted through the mouth to examine the esophagus, the stomach, and the duodenum (the first part of the small intestine). They can also be inserted through the anus to examine either the last one-third of the colon (using a type of endoscope called a sigmoidoscope) or the entire colon (using a colonoscope). Biopsies and other procedures can often be performed with instruments that can be threaded through the endoscope. Endoscopy has revolutionized the diagnosis of many digestive conditions and has increasingly replaced barium X-rays for that purpose.

Barium X-ray exams. With these procedures, you first swallow a substance called barium (in the case of upper GI exams) or your doctor inserts it via a tube through the anus (in the case of lower GI exams). Barium then shows up as a white chalk on X-rays and therefore outlines the various structures of the digestive tract. As mentioned above, these exams have been increasingly replaced by procedures like endoscopy, which allows direct visual examination of the linings of the various organs, and biopsies which remove tissue samples for further examination.

Small intestinal exams. Unfortunately, the small intestine often exists in a sort of "no-man's land" between the places endoscopes can reach from above (by mouth) or below (through the anus). One way to visualize the small intestine is by a so-called small bowel X-ray. In this procedure, you swallow barium, then X-rays are taken when the barium swallowed by mouth is passing through the small intestine. However, this techique is not as good as direct visual examination would be. Recently, scientists have developed a tiny camera that takes pictures of the small intestinal lining as it passes through the digestive tract. This disposable camera takes two pictures per second, which are then transmitted to a receiver worn on your belt; the device is then inserted into a special computer set-up for rapid viewing and screening of the over 50,000 pictures that have been taken during the camera's eight-hour passage through the digestive system! In experimental use to date, this camera has proven very valuable in uncovering problems in the small intestine that cannot be detected in any other way. And researchers are hopeful that it can be perfected to take useful pictures of other areas of the digestive tract that are currently best seen with endoscopes.

Diverticulosis/Diverticulitis

Diverticulosis occurs when small balloon-like pouches push out from the inner lining into the wall of the colon. Such out-pouchings are very common, occurring in up to half of all Americans over age 60. If the mouth of an out-pouching (a diverticulum) gets blocked, perhaps by a piece of hard stool, it can get infected, a condition known as diverticulitis. Sometimes the infected diverticulum can burst into the abdominal cavity and cause life-threatening peritonitis (infection of the lining of the abdominal cavity). A diverticulum can also bleed and produce bloody bowel movements. The cause of diverticulosis is unknown, though the most prevalent theory is that a lack of fiber in the diet can lead to constipation, which in turn leads to increased pressure in the colon that produces the out-pouchings. In the most serious cases of diverticulitis, surgery may be required to remove the affected area of the colon.

Inflammatory Bowel Disease (IBD)

We use this term to describe two conditions—Crohn's disease and ulcerative colitis—in which the wall of the intestine becomes significantly inflamed. *Crohn's disease* can involve the small or large intestine, though it most commonly occurs in the last part of the small intestine. *Ulcerative colitis* occurs only in the large intestine. Both can produce a wide range of serious symptoms, including abdominal pain, diarrhea, blood and pus in the stool, anemia, and weight loss. There are many medications that can be used to control symptoms, but if they do not work, surgery may be required either to remove affected areas of the intestine or to clean out abscesses that can form. Ulcerative colitis that affects the entire colon for more than eight years increases the risk for colon cancer and mandates periodic colonoscopy exams to look for early cancerous changes. Because of the wide range of medications used to treat these conditions today, the expertise of a gastroenterologist (a doctor who specializes in digestive diseases) can often make a big difference.

Irritable Bowel Syndrome (IBS)

This very common problem (estimated to affect one out of every six Americans at some point in their lives) has many other names, including spastic colon, mucous colitis, and functional bowel disease. As that last name suggests, the hallmark of the condition is that no visible inflammatory changes can be found when the colon is examined (unlike ulcerative colitis), but there are very real (functional) symptoms, including cramping, bloating, and diarrhea. The cause of this disorder is a great mystery, but many physicians believe that stress and diet (including high-fat foods, gas-producing vegetables, sorbitol-containing gums and drinks, caffeine, and alcohol) play a role in most cases. Getting more fiber in the diet can sometimes be helpful. Medications designed to slow down the activity and spasms of the bowel can be helpful, as can antidepressants in low doses.

Kidney Stones

The Basics: The kidneys, two bean-shaped organs located in the middle of your back below your ribs, are the most essential part of your urinary tract. Their job is to remove waste from your blood and convert it into urine, which is then sent to your bladder via narrow tubes called ureters. Kidney stones develop when certain chemicals in your urine crystallize into solid specks that can grow into stones. About 10 percent of people in the U.S.—80 percent of them men—will develop a kidney stone at some point in their lives. Men between the ages of 20 and 40 are particularly susceptible.

Prevention & Risk Factors: There are certain factors that may increase your risk of developing kidney stones. They include:

- Living in warm climates that promote dehydration, which lead to amore concentrated urine.
- A family history of kidney stones.
- Urinary tract infections *(see page 264)*.
- Kidney disorders.
- Gout *(see page 209)*.
- Too much vitamin D in your diet, which increases your blood calcium levels.

- Taking diuretics (drugs to help you eliminate excess water from your system), calcium-containing antacids, or protease inhibitors (drugs that treat HIV and AIDS).

Diagnosis & Screening: Sometimes, very small kidney stones don't cause any symptoms and pass out silently in your urine. However, when larger stones move through your urinary tract, symptoms can include an intensely sharp, cramp-like pain in the area of your back near your kidneys (or in your lower abdomen) as well as nausea, vomiting, and blood in your urine. If the stones get stuck and block the flow of urine from the kidneys, they can cause severe damage to the kidneys. If you have any of these symptoms, your doctor will probably perform a CT scan of the abdomen or a special X-ray of the urinary system, which will provide him or her with an image of your urinary tract, including any possible obstructions.

Treatment Options: Often, treatment is fairly simple. After the pain has been effectively treated, your doctor will have you drink two to three quarts of water a day to encourage your body to pass the stone. In 90 percent of cases, a kidney stone will pass out in the urine on its own. If you don't pass the stone or

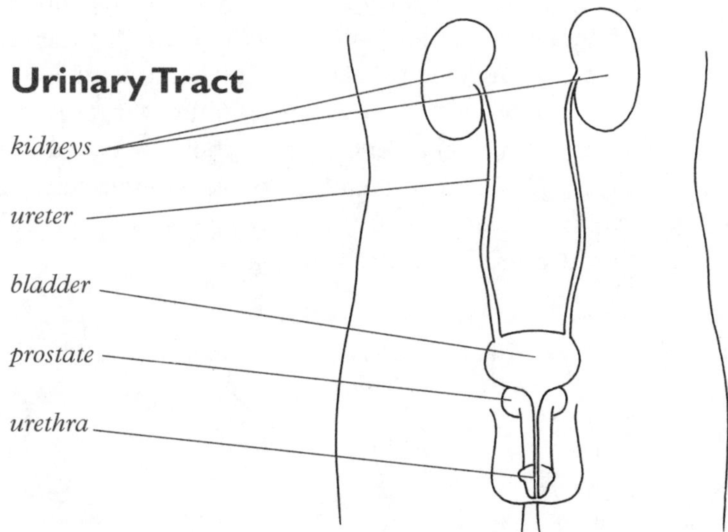

it's blocking the flow of urine, various procedures may be necessary. They include:

Extracorporeal shockwave lithotripsy. This procedure uses shock waves delivered by a special machine to break up the stones. Your body eventually excretes the fragments in your urine.

Percutaneous nephrolithotomy. For larger stones, surgical removal through an incision in your back may be required.

Ureteroscopic stone removal. This technique is most often used if your kidney stones are located in your lower ureter, the tube that connects your kidneys with your bladder. In this procedure, the doctor passes a ureteroscope, a small instrument, through your urethra and bladder into your ureter. Once the ureteroscope gets to the stone, the doctor either removes it or breaks it up using shock waves or electrical energy.

Living with Kidney Stones: Once you've had a kidney stone, you are at increased risk for having another. Your doctor will encourage you to increase your intake of fluids and may suggest modifications in your diet if an analysis of your stone indicates that it contains specific components that may be reduced by dietary changes. A recent study demonstrated that a low-salt, low-protein diet was much more effective in preventing recurrences than the low-calcium diet often recommended. If analysis of your stone reveals that it contains uric acid, your doctor may prescribe medications to reduce uric acid levels in your body.

Macular Degeneration
(Age-Related)

The Basics: In the back layer of your eye (the retina) is an area called the macula, which is important for sharp vision and helps you perform detail-oriented work like reading. The macula is especially important for central vision (allowing you to see things right in front of you). In people with age-related macular degeneration, the macula begins to malfunction, causing a number of vision problems, including blurred or fuzzy central vision, and an actual "hole" in the center of their field of vision. Since it doesn't affect peripheral vision, it usually doesn't cause complete blindness. If only one eye is affected, the normal eye may compensate and "cover" the loss of vision.

Age-related macular degeneration is the leading cause of vision loss worldwide. It can affect people as young as 40, but it strikes more often in the 55- or 60-plus age range and affects from 15 to 30 percent of people 75 and older.

Prevention & Risk Factors: Although scientists still aren't certain what causes age-related macular degeneration, they say there are steps you can take to ward off this vision-impairing illness.

Don't smoke. Researchers have found that tobacco interferes with your body's ability to absorb lutein, a nutritional antioxidant found in some fruits and vegetables. Lutein is important because it protects your retina from the harmful effects of ultraviolet light—a potential contributor to macular degeneration.

Keep your blood pressure and cholesterol in check. Studies have shown a correlation between high blood pressure and high cholesterol and the incidence of macular degeneration.

Wear sunglasses when you're outside. Protecting your eyes from the sun's ultraviolet rays can help keep the structures within your eyes, including your retina and macula, healthy and free from damage. Choose sunglasses that provide 99 to 100 percent protection from both ultraviolet A (UVA) and B (UVB) rays. Ones with side panels and a shield at the top offer the best protection.

Eat a well-balanced diet rich in fruits and vegetables. A diet rich in antioxidants, protective substances found in fruits and vegetables, can help keep your eyes functioning optimally in general and may help prevent macular degeneration in particular.

Diagnosis & Screening: After the age of 65, you should have an annual vision test, during which your doctor can check the health of your retina and macula. And at any time, if you have any of the symptoms of macular degeneration, including blurred or distorted vision (straight lines can appear wavy), or a "hole" in your central vision, you should see an eye doctor who will perform a number of tests to determine if you have the disease.

Treatment Options: Experts recently reported a breakthrough in the treatment of this often debilitating disease. In a study sponsored by the National Eye Institute, researchers found that in people who already have some level of macular degeneration, high levels of antioxidants and zinc can significantly reduce the risk of developing advanced stages of the disease. In fact, the risk of developing more severe problems was 25 percent lower in people who took a high-dosage combination of vitamin C (500 milligrams), vitamin E (400 IU), beta-carotene (15 milligrams), and zinc oxide (80 milligrams) every day. Although the nutritional therapy isn't a cure, it may help prevent the progression of the disease in people with the most common form of the illness, known as "dry" macular degeneration.

People with so-called "wet" macular degeneration, in which the capillaries of the eye are affected, may benefit from laser therapy or photodynamic therapy, in which doctors use a combination of light and a light-sensitive drug to slow the progression of the illness.

Living with Macular Degeneration: Since there is no known cure for the illness, most people who develop it will need to cope with some degree of vision impairment. Fortunately, there are a number of low-vision aids, from magnifying glasses to bright lights, that can help you see more clearly. Your doctor may also suggest that you monitor your vision at home using an Amsler chart which detects blurred vision.

Male Menopause

The Basics: Confusion abounds about this controversial subject, partly because of its name. "Male menopause" makes this condition sound like the male equivalent of female menopause, a definitive, well-accepted, universal change in women's hormonal status as they reach middle age. But unlike the rather sudden and dramatic drop in hormones that occurs in women, male menopause, which is sometimes called "andropause" or "viropause," refers to the slow, gradual waning of male hormones, including testosterone, that begins when a man is in his 30s and can be exacerbated by psychological symptoms that occur during mid-life. Starting at about age 40, most men experience a drop in male hormone (testosterone) levels of about 10 percent per decade. The rate of decline in testosterone varies greatly among men.

Prevention & Risk Factors: Since a decreasing level of testosterone is a normal part of the aging process, there's no easy way to prevent it, and in many men it causes no problems. Certain factors may increase the likelihood that a drop in testosterone will cause other common symptoms of andropause. They include:

- Drinking too much.
- Smoking.

- High blood pressure.
- Poor diet.
- Lack of exercise.

Diagnosis & Screening: Since male menopause is still very controversial within the medical community, your doctor may not have the interest or expertise to analyze your concerns. Your best bet, if you think you might be having a problem, is to seek the help of an endocrinologist, a doctor who specializes in treating hormonal disorders. After a careful exam, he or she may want to do a blood test to check the level of your total testosterone and may check what's called your "free active testosterone" level as well.

Treatment Options: Doctors remain unclear about the benefits of testosterone supplements in men whose levels have dropped as a result of normal aging, but that is currently the only treatment. Methods of delivery include injections, given about every two weeks; patches, which deliver a dose of the hormone through your skin; and gels, which you rub onto the skin of your lower abdomen, upper arm, or shoulder. However, testosterone replacement therapy carries considerable risk and in my opinion should only be done under the guidance of an expert physician. The risks include cardiovascular disease, benign and malignant prostate disease, and sleep apnea.

Living with Male Menopause: Whether you choose to try testosterone replacement therapy or not, it might be worthwhile to address some of the symptoms of "middle age" separately. If you've gained weight, start exercising. If you're struggling with depression or mood swings, seek the help of a psychologist or psychiatrist, who can suggest a number of treatment options for those problems. *(See Minding the Mind on page 315 for more information.)*

Memory Loss

The Basics: Most people start having trouble remembering things as they age. That's because our brains lose cells as we get older and our bodies produce less of the chemicals that our brain cells need to work. There's another factor possibly at work as well: brain overload. Some experts speculate that the older you are, the more memories you have stored in your brain, so you may simply have trouble accessing a specific name or incident because you've accumulated so many memories. *(See also Alzheimer's Disease on page 173.)*

Prevention & Risk Factors: There are a number of things you can do to help keep your mind sharp.

Learn new things. Just as your muscles atrophy if you sit on the couch all day, your brain starts to slow down if you don't push it to learn. No matter how old you are, if your brain is active, it makes new connections between nerve cells, which usually helps your mental functioning. Here are a few brain "workouts" that can keep your mind fit: Do crossword puzzles; take an unfamiliar route to work; take up a new hobby, like model airplane building, painting, or playing the piano; read the newspaper and discuss current events with other people.

Exercise. Even 30 minutes of aerobic exercise can boost blood flow to your brain, which feeds the cells and keeps them working properly. Researchers have also found that it may prompt your brain to create new cells.

Find what helps you relax—and do it. The hormone cortisol, which is released when you're under stress, can interfere with the proper functioning of your brain, especially concentration. Whether it's yoga or biofeedback, find a stress reliever that works for you. *(See page 337 for a discussion of stress.)*

Eat a healthy diet. Many researchers believe that antioxidants found in fruits and vegetables boost brain functioning, and research is ongoing to find which ones are the most beneficial. For example, a recent study conducted by the National Institute on Aging found that when animals were fed extracts of blueberries, strawberries, and spinach, their memories improved. Likewise, a grossly inadequate intake of B vitamins (found in low-fat milk and yogurt, bananas, seafood, whole grains, green peas, and other foods) can impair your memory.

Get plenty of rest. Although short-term sleep deprivation isn't likely to do any long-term damage, it can make you feel like your brain is on loan.

Consider depression. Depression inhibits short-term memory and concentration. *(For more information on depression, see page 320.)*

Stay away from Ecstasy. This recreational drug, also known as methylenedioxymethamphetamine or MDMA, affects your hippocampus, the part of your brain associated with learning and the consolidation of new memories. Researchers have found that people who take the drug as infrequently as twice a month for a year show a marked drop in their ability to remember things.

Check your medications. Certain medications, such as Valium and Elavil, can cause memory problems, as can illnesses like hypothyroidism, diabetes, and vitamin deficiencies. If you're having noticeable problems, it's a good idea to seek the help of a professional to get to the bottom of it. Make sure to tell him or her about all the medications you are taking.

Diagnosis & Screening: If you are concerned about memory loss, your doctor will perform a physical exam as well as ask you a number of questions about the types of things you can't remember. He or she will probably do some diagnostic tests to check your short-term and long-term memory and may want to do a CT scan of your head, which provides a detailed picture of your brain. Blood tests may also be done if your doctor suspects you have an underlying illness like hypothyroidism or diabetes.

Treatment Options: If a medical problem appears to be at the root of your memory problems, your doctor will treat its underlying cause. If it's thought to be simply a part of the normal aging process, he or she will likely recommend that you take some of the above steps to help keep your memory sharp.

Living with Memory Loss: If you feel like you've lost a bit of your mental edge, there are ways you can compensate for it. For instance, you can develop a system for helping you remember things—writing appointments down on a calendar, putting your keys and sunglasses in the same place every time you walk in the door, or repeating new information you hear several times to implant it more firmly in your brain.

O

Osteoporosis

The Basics: Osteoporosis, which literally means porous bones, is a disorder that is characterized by decreased bone strength. The bones of people with osteoporosis are less dense and less structurally sound than those without the illness, putting them at increased risk of fractures. Although osteoporosis has traditionally been considered a women's disease, researchers now know that it strikes both sexes, but in somewhat different ways. While women tend to lose bone mass after menopause, men lose it later in life and are more likely to suffer from secondary osteoporosis, or osteoporosis that is caused by taking certain medications or other illnesses. In fact, 30 to 60 percent of men with osteoporosis fall into this category.

Osteoporosis affects two million men, but another three million are at risk for the disease, according to the

National Osteoporosis Foundation. One in eight men will suffer an osteoporosis-related fracture during his lifetime, although the risk is slightly lower for African-American males than white males.

Prevention & Risk Factors: Osteoporosis is, in large part, a preventable illness. Make sure you get adequate amounts of calcium and vitamin D. Bones contain lots of calcium, and the mineral is critical for their strength and integrity. If you're under 65, many experts recommend 1,000 milligrams every day, and if you're over 65, some say 1,500 milligrams a day. Vitamin D helps your body absorb calcium, so the two go hand in hand. Ordinarily, as little as 10 minutes of sunlight each day is enough to facilitate calcium absorption, but if you live in an area where you receive little natural light, you should talk to your doctor about taking vitamin D supplements. Indeed, there is growing evidence that people who live in northern climes without much sun exposure during a large part of the year are at considerable risk for vitamin D deficiency—another reason to take a daily multivitamin containing vitamin D. *(See the vitamin chart on page 22.)* And I will again point out that a very high protein diet can leech calcium out of bones in potentially dangerous amounts.

The big question is how you should get the calcium and vitamin D you need. If you listen to the dairy industry, you would think the only honorable way is to drink lots of milk. In fact, milk is an excellent source of calcium and vitamin D, but unfortunately it is also an excellent source of saturated fat. Therefore, I believe adults should consume only low-fat or skim dairy products as a source of calcium and vitamin D.

Finally, I will point out that there are some data to suggest that men who consume more than 2,000 mg of calcium a day might be at increased risk for prostate cancer. (One theory: Too much calcium slows the production of active vitamin D, which is known to retard the production of cancer cells.) However, there is also some evidence to suggest calcium might lower the risk for colon cancer.

At this point, the evidence for either one of these effects is not solid enough to offer any precise recommendation. Therefore until and if more evidence becomes available I would limit my intake of calcium to no more than 1,500 mg of calcium a day (that's from both food and supplements combined) and instead rely on a good exercise program to help strengthen bones. (I will also urge you to read the section on calcium in Dr. Willett's book, *Eat, Drink, and Be Healthy,* in which he discusses the pros and cons of calcium and his concern about too much calcium in the diet.)

Other ways of reducing your risk of osteoporosis include:

Make weight-bearing exercise a part of your daily routine. Although strength training can help increase bone strength as well as muscle strength, you don't need to lift weights to do weight-bearing exercise. Any activity that requires you to support your entire body weight, including walking, running, racquet sports, and team sports, will place extra stress on your skeleton, prompting it to build more bone. At the same time, these activities increase your strength, agility, and balance, all of which make falling down less likely.

Don't overindulge in alcohol, and don't smoke. Although there's no specific osteoporosis-related recommendation regarding the amount of alcohol it's safe to consume, studies show that alcoholics are at increased risk for the disorder, and smoking can have a deleterious effect on bone health.

Be especially careful to adhere to a bone-preserving lifestyle if you have any of the following risk factors:

Increased age. The risk of osteoporosis increases beginning in middle age. Bone mass peaks at about age 30, at which point the rate of bone deterioration often begins to outpace the rate of bone building in your body.

Low weight and body mass index. Thin people are more likely to suffer bone loss than normal-weight or overweight people.

Family history of osteoporosis. If one or both of your parents had the illness, you're at increased risk for developing brittle bones. The amount of bone mass you build early in life is genetically predetermined. Also, Caucasians and Asians are at higher risk than African-Americans.

Personal history of bone fractures. If you've broken a bone, it could be an indication that your bones are weak and predisposed to osteoporosis.

Use of steroid drugs, such as prednisone, often used to treat asthma or arthritis. This is the most common form of drug-induced osteoporosis. In one study, people who took 10 milligrams of prednisone for 20 weeks lost 8 percent of the bone mineral density in their spines.

Other medications. If you take anticonvulsants, certain cancer treatments, or aluminum-containing antacids on a regular basis, you could compromise your bone health.

Hypogonadism. Male hormones secreted by your testicles influence your skeletal health. As a result, the loss of testicular function or the loss of the hormone testosterone increases the risk of osteoporosis.

Diagnosis & Screening: It's important to know that doctors often forget to look for osteoporosis in men, so ingrained is our attitude that it affects women almost exclusively. As a result, it makes sense to raise the subject with your doctor, especially if you've had any symptoms of the illness, including a loss of height, change in posture, sudden back pain, or a fracture.

Your doctor will diagnose osteoporosis by asking you about your medical history, assessing your risk factors, conducting a physical exam (including blood and urine tests, which can help identify secondary causes of osteoporosis), and performing a bone density test of your spine, hip, or other sites. Bone mineral density accounts for about 70 percent of bone strength. There are several different types of tests that can measure bone density. Some independent clinics may push screening for osteoporosis that is unnecessary or inaccurate.

Treatment Options: Your course of treatment depends on the specific cause of your illness. If you developed osteoporosis as a result of hypogonadism, for instance, you may be given male hormone replacement therapy. Your doctor will almost certainly recommend that you make dietary and lifestyle changes that can contribute to bone health and may also recommend that you take one of the following medications:

Bisphosphonates. There are several newer drugs that fall into this category, and they are often prescribed for people who have steroid-induced osteoporosis.

Calcitonin. This medication can slow or stop bone loss. It is given by injection or as a nasal spray.

Living with Osteoporosis: If you have osteoporosis, you should take extra care not to fall down. Make sure any rugs in your home are firmly secured to the floor, the hallways and stairwells are well lit, and floors aren't slippery. In addition, you should avoid medications that make you drowsy or dull your senses since they make a slip or trip more likely.

Sinusitis

The Basics: You might think it strange to include sinusitis on a list of diseases every man should know about, but I do so because I have learned over the years that it is one of the most misdiagnosed and misunderstood of all common medical problems. One recent medical study suggests that chronic sinusitis can cause more disability than congestive heart failure, lung disease, and back pain combined. I don't know for sure if that is true, but it does suggest that chronic sinusitis causes far more suffering than most people—and many doctors—realize.

We humans have four pairs of air-filled spaces that are located basically above, behind, and below the eyes—in the bones of our forehead, nose, and upper jaw. These spaces, or sinuses (frontal, maxillary, ethmoid, and sphenoid), contribute significantly to the quality of the sound of our voice (which is why our voice sounds so nasal when they are plugged up) and they help to clean and warm the air we breathe in through our nose. However, their main activity too often seems to be causing a pain in the head when they become inflamed and infected. That can result from anything that plugs up the pinpoint openings that drain from the sinuses into the nose. When that happens, mucus builds up in the sinuses, providing a breeding ground for infection. The combination of blockage and infection produces the typical symptoms of acute sinusitis—feelings of pressure and congestion in the affected areas, headaches, fever, and, in the very worst cases, a body wide blood infection that can produce shaking chills. Many cases of acute infection are misdiagnosed simply as "headcolds" or even as "the flu." And many cases of chronic sinusitis—an infection that lasts more than three weeks—can produce confusing body wide symptoms that can occasionally be misdiagnosed as all sorts of other problems, including chronic fatigue syndrome or arthritis.

Prevention & Risk Factors: Nasal allergies, nasal polyps, serious colds—anything that can block the openings into the sinuses—can lead to sinusitis. Therefore, preventing or treating such problems quickly can reduce the risk for actual sinusitis. Other practices designed to keep the nasal passages clear include frequent gentle blowing of the nose, lots of fluid consumption to keep nasal and sinus mucus flowing, warm facial packs, and periodic steam inhalation.

Diagnosis & Screening: As I indicated above, one of the reasons sinusitis so often turns into a troublesome chronic problem is that it is so often misdiagnosed as something else. Therefore I would recommend that anyone who has unexplained facial or head symptoms see an ENT (ear, nose, and throat) doctor who specializes in sinus problems. One tool that has revolutionized the diagnosis of sinus problems is the nasal endoscope, a very thin fiber-optic tube that can be inserted into the nose for a direct visual examination of the openings into the sinuses. The other tool that can be extremely helpful in diagnosis is a CT scan of the sinuses which can show very clearly which ones are blocked.

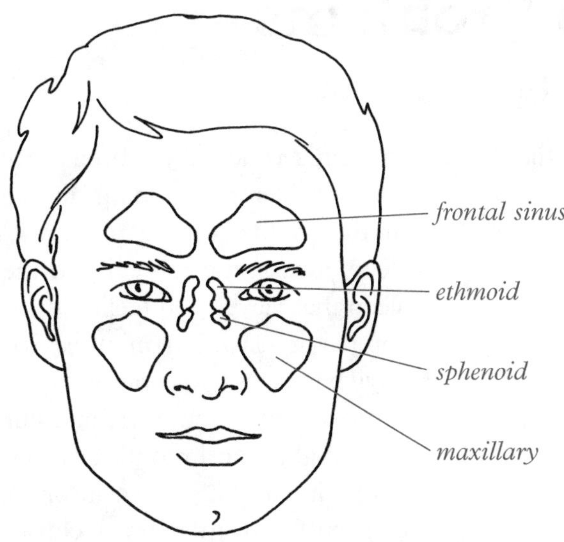

Treatment Options: There are many medications (antibiotics, decongestants, nasal steroid sprays, antihistamines) and procedures (suction through the endoscope, flushing, etc.) that can be used to treat acute sinusitis. However, when infections are recurrent and/or do not respond to other treatments, surgery to enlarge the openings that drain the sinuses should be considered. Old style sinus surgery involved incisions in the face or mouth and was very traumatic and potentially dangerous. Modern sinus surgery involves the use of an infrared guidance system that allows the surgeon to insert an endoscope through the nose and remove bone and enlarge openings in a very precise and safe manner. However, this surgery requires experience and skill and should be done only by physicians who truly specialize in this kind of procedure. There are now approximately 300 image guidance systems for sinus surgery in the U.S., so this surgery is becoming more available. It should be done only when non-surgical measures are inadequate, but in the right hands it can provide huge relief to people who suffer severe chronic sinusitis.

Sleep Problems

Insomnia

The Basics: Insomnia is actually a broad term for a number of sleep-related problems, including difficulty falling asleep, waking up in the middle of the night with difficulty getting back to sleep, awakening too early in the morning, and poor quality sleep that leaves you feeling un-refreshed in the morning. Insomnia is classified in three ways: transient insomnia lasts anywhere from one night to several weeks; intermittent insomnia comes and goes; and chronic insomnia hits sufferers most nights for a month or more. About 30 to 40 percent of adults in the U.S. have insomnia occasionally, and 10 percent suffer from it on a chronic basis. Women are about twice as likely to experience sleep problems as men, but people of both sexes complain of difficulty sleeping as they age.

Prevention & Risk Factors: You're better off trying to prevent a bout of insomnia than trying to cure it once you have it, because the condition can snowball quickly. Often labeled as "learned insomnia," it happens this way: After a few nights of insomnia, you start worrying about getting enough sleep when you get into bed, which can make it more difficult to nod off. To prevent insomnia, or to break a "learned" cycle, you should maintain a "sleep-friendly" lifestyle. Here are some useful and time-honored tips:

Try to go to bed only when you're sleepy, so you don't lie there tossing and turning, a situation that can actually cause subsequent nights of insomnia.

Don't use your bedroom for anything other than sleep or sex. If you work in your bedroom, you may begin to associate the room with work and stress, neither of which are conducive to sleep. The idea is to set up a "sleep association" in your mind, much as Pavlov did with his dogs, so you'll automatically feel ready to sleep when you go in your bedroom.

Maintain a regular schedule. Go to bed and get up at the same time every day.

Get some exercise every day, but not within three hours of bedtime, because it can rev your body up, making it difficult to fall asleep.

Avoid alcohol within three hours of bedtime. It's been shown to cause middle-of-the-night awakenings.

Avoid caffeine, which is a stimulant, within six hours of bedtime. Some people are so sensitive to caffeine that any consumption after the morning is problematic.

Start winding down about an hour or so before bed. Don't watch disturbing television programs, pay bills or do anything that's likely to cause you to worry. Instead, do something relaxing, like taking a bath or reading a book, especially a dull one.

Make sure you create a sleep-friendly environment in your bedroom. Both excessive heat and excessive cold can make it difficult to get to sleep and stay asleep, as can too much light or noise. Try to make your room as dark and quiet as possible. If you live in a noisy area, try using a white noise machine to block the sounds of the environment; I personally have found such machines very useful, especially when traveling.

Diagnosis & Screening: Your doctor can often diagnose insomnia based on your report of your sleep habits as well as common symptoms, which include fatigue, low energy, difficulty concentrating, and irritability.

However, sleep experts are increasingly turning to so-called sleep studies to sort out less obvious sleep problems such as sleep apnea and restless legs syndrome. Such studies involve an overnight stay in a special sleep lab hooked up to various recording devices that help diagnose specific sleep problems more precisely. While such studies are sometimes performed too readily, many primary care doctors sometimes wait too long to order sleep studies in people with chronic sleep problems that do not respond to usual lifestyle changes or other treatment measures.

Treatment Options: Your doctor may recommend that you try over-the-counter sleep aids, if your insomnia hasn't gone on long. But you should only take such medication for several weeks, because beyond this time, it is apt to lose its effectiveness. If your insomnia recurs after stopping a short course of medication, your doctor may refer you to a sleep specialist or recommend one of the following approaches:

Relaxation therapy. In this treatment, you can learn techniques to relax your body and decrease stress so you'll feel more able to fall asleep.

Sleep restriction therapy. Ironically, forcing yourself to get less sleep for several nights can make you so tired that you konk out the second your head hits the pillow. Sleep specialists have devised specific programs that can help thwart a case of insomnia.

Cognitive behavioral therapy. In this approach, your doctor will provide you with a variety of information about habits that are conducive to a good night's sleep and put you on a schedule that includes spending less time in bed.

Prescription medications. There are a number of drugs that doctors may try to help you beat a bout of insomnia. They include benzodiazepines, which were originally developed to treat anxiety; hypnotics such as zolpidem (Ambien) and zaleplon (Sonata), which make you feel sleepy; and tricyclic antidepressants, which often have a sedating effect. (The newer SSRI antidepressants often make insomnia worse.) All prescription medications for insomnia have potential side effects—and the potential for developing psychological habituation if not actual physiological dependence. Therefore they must be used carefully for short periods of time under the direction of a physician.

Melatonin. Although frequently touted as a sleep-enhancer, studies of the hormone melatonin have shown spotty results. At this point, most experts say it's probably most helpful for preventing or relieving sleep problems related to jet lag or shift work.

Herbal remedies. A number of herbal solutions are sold as sleep potions, including valerian root, hops, kava, chamomile, passionflower, and lemon balm, but since most of them haven't been tested with rigorous scientific studies, their true effectiveness is unknown. If you plan to try an herbal remedy, be sure to let your doctor know. Some (such as valerian) can cause side effects or may interfere with the effectiveness of other medications.

Restless Legs Syndrome

One of the most common but least recognized causes of sleep disturbance is the condition known as restless legs syndrome—or RLS for short. Some experts suggest that 5 to 10 percent of adults suffer from this, though most of them don't know it. The problem tends to run in families. As the name suggests, the main symptom is a vague feeling of restlessness or aching in the legs, particularly at rest; the problem often disappears with activity or movement. People afflicted with RLS often have a hard time sitting through concerts or other events that require their legs to be at rest for long periods. Sometimes the problem is obvious during sleep because jerky leg movements wake the person and partner. In others the problem is much more subtle and is diagnosed only during a sleep study. Since it is so common, the problem should be suspected in anyone with a sleep problem that has no obvious explanation. Fortunately, there are several medications that very effectively treat this condition, and many people afflicted describe these medications as a "miracle" when they first start taking them.

Sleep Apnea

The Basics: Sleep apnea refers to a condition in which a person temporarily stops breathing many times during the night, in some cases hundreds of times. The typical sequence is that breathing stops, followed by a sudden snort and awakening, followed by quickly falling asleep again. The person afflicted often does not realize what is happening but a sleeping partner may be alerted by the sudden snorts. Often this problem is not diagnosed until an actual overnight sleep study is done.

The most common type is known as obstructive sleep apnea, caused by the actual blockage of the airway at the back of the throat when throat muscles relax. The likelihood of obstruction is increased by extra weight, which increases the amount of tissue in the back of the throat; an enlarged tongue, tonsils, or uvula (the soft tissue that hangs down at the back of the roof of the mouth) can also contribute. Much less common is so-called central apnea, which is caused by a problem in brain control over the muscles that cause breathing.

Obstructive sleep apnea is most common in overweight men with large necks, though it certainly can occur in normal-weight men and women. It is estimated that 18 million Americans suffer from some degree of sleep apnea. In its most serious form, sleep apnea can significantly increase the risk for heart attacks and strokes.

Prevention & Risk Factors: Although there's no easy way to prevent sleep apnea, there are some things that can increase your risk for the problem. They include:

- Being overweight. The condition has been shown to be more common in people who weigh too much, probably because they have more flesh at the back of their throats, making an obstruction more likely.
- A physical abnormality in your throat or nose.
- High blood pressure.
- Drinking alcohol and taking sleeping pills or tranquilizers, all of which can cause your throat muscles to relax.

Diagnosis & Screening: If you have any of the following symptoms of sleep apnea, you should discuss the problem with your doctor.

Excessive daytime fatigue or sleepiness. People with sleep apnea often fall asleep at inappropriate times, like at work or in the middle of a phone conversation, because they're so tired from all the mini-awakenings in the night. Sleepiness may manifest itself in a number of other ways, including difficulty concentrating or paying attention, irritability, and poor judgment.

Periods of not breathing during sleep. Although you may not be aware of anything amiss, your partner is likely to notice that you stop breathing for periods in the night.

Snoring. Because apnea causes a rebound snort once you start to breathe again, your partner may tell you that you snore very loudly.

Frequent nighttime waking. If you feel like you wake up a lot over the course of the night, and you do so with a jolt, you may be suffering from sleep apnea.

If your doctor suspects you have sleep apnea, he or she will perform a physical exam of your mouth and throat. Your doctor will confirm the diagnosis by doing one or more of the following tests:

Polysomnography. In this test, your doctor will hook you up to a machine to record a variety of body functions, including eye movement, heart rate and muscle activity, while you sleep.

Multiple sleep latency test (MSLT). This test measures how quickly you fall asleep during the day. If you fall asleep within 5 to 10 minutes, it could mean you have a problem.

Blood gases check. Your doctor may also want to measure the amount of oxygen in your blood when you sleep.

Treatment Options: A simple first step is trying to sleep on your side; a variety of devices may help you do this—even sewing a ball in the back of your pajamas. Sleep apnea is much more common when you're lying on your back, a position that makes the muscles in the throat collapse into your airway. If you're overweight, weight loss is a good idea as well. If these interventions don't work, your doctor will likely try one of the following treatments:

Continuous positive airflow pressure (CPAP). This treatment is administered via a machine that you place on your bedside table. When you go to sleep, you place a plastic mask over your nose. The mask is connected to a tube that comes from the machine, which supplies a steady flow of air through your nose, thereby keeping your airway open.

Dental devices. Your doctor may recommend that you wear a mouth-guard–like device when you sleep to keep your tongue away from your airway. This treatment is best for people with mild apnea.

Rapid maxillary expansion. This orthodontic treatment actually expands your upper jaw in about three weeks, helping reduce the pressure in your nose and improve your breathing.

Surgery. Typically used only for very severe cases of sleep apnea, there are a couple of options your doctor may use:

- Tracheostomy, in which your doctor inserts a tube through your neck into your windpipe, is disfiguring but almost always successful.
- Uvulopalatopharyngoplasty, in which your doctor removes soft tissue from the back of your throat, has only about a 50 percent success rate, though it usually reduces any associated snoring.
- Radio frequency ablation. This technique, which is still considered experimental, uses radio waves to destroy a small amount of tissue at the base of your tongue.

Snoring

The Basics: Snoring happens when air flowing through the back of your throat causes the tissues there, including your soft palate and uvula (the pink flap that hangs down at the back of your throat), to vibrate. Men are 10 times as likely to snore as women, although researchers aren't able to explain why. Snoring itself usually isn't medically serious, though it can certainly raise havoc with your sleeping partner. However, about 5 percent of people who snore have sleep apnea (see above), a condition that can be life threatening.

Prevention & Risk Factors: There are a number of things that can increase the likelihood of snoring. They include:

Being overweight. Extra weight can compress the tissue at the back of your throat, making snoring more likely.

Alcohol, sleeping pills, and tranquilizers. Because they relax your body's natural breathing mechanism, they increase the amount you snore.

Sleeping on your back. Snoring is more common in this position, because the tissues of your throat tend to cave in.

Smoking. The smoke from cigarettes irritates the membranes in your nose and throat, causing them to swell and secrete more mucus, both of which increase the chance that you'll snore.

Diagnosis & Screening: Your doctor will ask you or your partner to provide a detailed description of your snoring, including how loud it is, when it typically occurs, and if you have any other symptoms, like excessive daytime sleepiness.

Treatment Options: Your doctor will recommend weight loss, if you're overweight, a strategy that is typically quite effective. He'll also recommend that you sleep on your side instead of your back; there are many devices designed to force you to do this—even pajamas with a ball sewn in the back. If your problem doesn't seem to be getting any better, continuous positive airflow pressure and the various surgical procedures for sleep apnea (see above) can also be useful in treating serious snoring. Laser destruction of excess tissue at the back of the mouth has become popular for treating snoring, but it is very important to have this done by a throat specialist who is very experienced. Knowing how much tissue to destroy is a fine art. Doctors need to destroy enough to decrease the snoring but not destroy so much that they cause an unwanted change in speaking quality.

Thyroid Disease

The Basics: The thyroid is a butterfly-shaped gland located in the front of your neck just below your Adam's apple. Your thyroid makes and stores hormones that help regulate your heart rate, blood pressure, metabolism, and body temperature, among other things.

There are two main problems that can affect your thyroid. *Hypothyroidism* means your gland is underactive. It's the most common thyroid disorder. *Hyperthyroidism,* on the other hand, occurs when your gland makes too much thyroid hormone, or is overactive.

Thyroid disease, which affects about 12 million people in the U.S., is eight times more common in women than in men.

Prevention & Risk Factors: There's no way to prevent a thyroid disorder, but you may be at increased risk if you have one of the following illnesses or conditions:

Thyroiditis (also known as Hashimoto's disease). This illness, in which your immune system mistakes your thyroid for a harmful invader, is the most common cause of hypothyroidism.

Low-iodine diet. If you don't get enough iodine in your diet, a rare occurrence in the U.S. thanks to our heavy use of iodized salt, you're at increased risk of developing hypothyroidism.

Graves' disease. This illness, which affects primarily women, is the main cause of hyperthyroidism.

Diagnosis & Screening: A simple blood test can detect a thyroid disorder. You can have hypothyroidism for years without knowing it, because symptoms are often slow to develop. When they do appear, you're likely to have fatigue, weight gain, decreased appetite, constipation, and decreased sex drive—all evidence of your thyroid slowing down.

If you have hyperthyroidism, you may be tired, too, but most of the symptoms will be the opposite: weight loss, nervousness, rapid heart beat, increased sweating, and more frequent bowel movements.

Treatment Options: If you have an underactive thyroid, your doctor will put you on medication that contains thyroid hormone. You will have to slowly increase the dose until you have a normal amount in your blood. You'll have to take the medication for the rest of your life and have your blood thyroid level checked on a regular basis.

If you have an overactive thyroid, your doctor will probably prescribe anti-thyroid medication to reduce the amount of thyroid hormone in your blood. In addition, he or she may recommend that you take beta blockers to prevent your heart from beating too fast. In some instances, this approach doesn't work. Plan B is usually treatment with radioactive iodine, which destroys part of your thyroid gland, or, as a last resort, surgery to remove part of the gland. People who have these treatments for hyperthyroidism may eventually become hypothyroid so they need periodic blood testing to check their thyroid status.

Ulcers

The Basics: Our understanding of the cause and treatment of ulcers not caused by medications such as NSAIDs and steroids has undergone a true revolution during my lifetime as a physician. When I was in medical school in the 1960s, we were taught that ulcers were caused by stress and spicy foods leading to excess stomach acid, so the treatment was to change your life and diet and take plenty of antacids. Today we know that most peptic ulcers—those open sores that develop in the inner lining of the stomach (gastric ulcers) or the first part of the small intestine called the duodenum (duodenal ulcers)—are caused by a bacterium called Helicobacter pylori—or H. pylori for short. In other words, most ulcers are an infectious disease that should be treated with antibiotics!

The story behind this revolutionary change in our thinking really revolves around one man—Dr. Barry Marshall, a physician from Australia who slowly but surely proved the hypothesis that most ulcers were, at root, caused by a bacterium and then courageously convinced the medical establishment that ulcers were an infectious disease. He was often laughed off the stage at medical meetings but finally proved his case to a skeptical medical establishment that still believed stomach acid was the basic cause. And the ultimate proof was in the pudding of treatment: If people with ulcers known to be H. pylori positive are given an effective program of antibiotics as part of their treatment, only about 3 percent will have a recurrence within one year. If they are not given antibiotics, 90 percent will have a recurrence!

Unfortunately, the H. pylori bacteria are very common in our world, especially in poor countries with bad sanitation. In this country, about 60 percent of people over age 60 carry the H. pylori bacteria but only about 10 percent of people under age 30 (who presumably have grown up with better sanitation) are infected. Therefore, even though ulcers are still quite common—about one in ten American men will develop an ulcer during his lifetime—we might expect to see a significant drop in the incidence of ulcers in the future, at least in developed countries.

The H. pylori bacteria cause ulcers because unlike most germs, they can thrive in stomach acid. Duodenal ulcers are the most common and usually occur in men between age 30 and 50; stomach ulcers tend to occur later in life and more often affect women.

Prevention & Risk Factors: One radical strategy would be to give antibiotics to everyone to prevent ulcers from ever developing. And given that H. pylori infection also increases the risk for stomach cancer, this possibility of giving prophylactic antibiotics is being tested in some areas of the world where both H. pylori infection and stomach cancer are a major problem. However, in the U.S., where stomach cancer is much less common, this approach would almost certainly cause more problems (side effects and resistance to antibiotics) than it would solve.

There is another fairly common cause of ulcers that we can sometimes prevent—namely ulcers that develop in people taking larger than usual amounts of aspirin or other nonsteroidal anti-inflammatory drugs like ibuprofen. *(For more information on NSAIDs, see page 181.)* Smoking can also increase the risk of ulcers, especially in association with these other bad health practices. Older people are especially susceptible to the ulcer-causing effects of anti-inflammatory medicine and can rather easily develop life-threatening bleeding from such ulcers, even sometimes with relatively moderate use of these drugs.

Diagnosis & Screening: The main symptom of an ulcer is pain in the upper part of your abdomen, in the area between your navel and the lower end of your breast bone. The pain gets worse when your stomach is empty and at night. You may also vomit blood or have black, tarry stools from ulcer bleeding. Sometimes an unexplained anemia from slow bleeding will be the first signal of an ulcer.

To diagnose an ulcer, your doctor will ask you about your symptoms, including when you feel pain and if it gets worse or better after eating. He also may perform one or several of the following diagnostic tests:

Blood test. In this test, your doctor looks for the presence of H. pylori in your blood. Today blood tests are replacing older breath tests since they are easier and cheaper.

Upper gastrointestinal X-ray. For this test, commonly called an upper GI series, you'll have to drink barium, a white, metallic liquid that coats your digestive tract, making it easier to see an ulcer on the X-ray.

Endoscopy. This procedure is much more accurate than an upper GI series. It provides an up-close look at your stomach and duodenum. The doctor will insert a long, narrow tube with a small camera attached to it down your throat and into your stomach and small intestine.

Biopsy. If your doctor sees an ulcer during an endoscopy, he may remove a small amount of tissue from it to check it for the presence of H. pylori. This is more likely if the ulcer is in the stomach.

Treatment Options: Today, ulcers caused by H. pylori are very effectively treated with antibiotics to kill the bacteria plus acid-reducing drugs to promote healing. The acid-reducing drugs are the same ones used in the treatment of heartburn *(see page 221)*. There are several different combinations of antibiotics and acid-reducing drugs that can be used. They differ somewhat in cost, convenience, and the risk for side effects, but the good news is that they all seem to be effective. And because they are so effective, surgery for ulcers is almost never necessary today.

Urinary Tract Infections (UTIs)

The Basics: As blood circulates through your kidneys, various "waste products" are removed and urine is produced. From the kidneys, your urine is transported to your bladder via thin tubes called ureters, and your bladder stores the urine until you find time to go to the bathroom, when it's eliminated from your body through your urethra when you urinate. Adults typically produce about a quart and a half of urine every day.

More than nine million people contract urinary tract infections every year. Although they affect women much more frequently than men (partly because women's urethras are shorter and closer to the rectum, so bacteria don't have to travel as far to set up an infection), these infections become more common as men age, striking as many as 15 percent of men over age 65.

Prevention & Risk Factors: In men, urinary tract infections typically are caused by an obstruction to the flow of urine. When urine pools, it becomes a good breeding ground for bacteria. Two typical

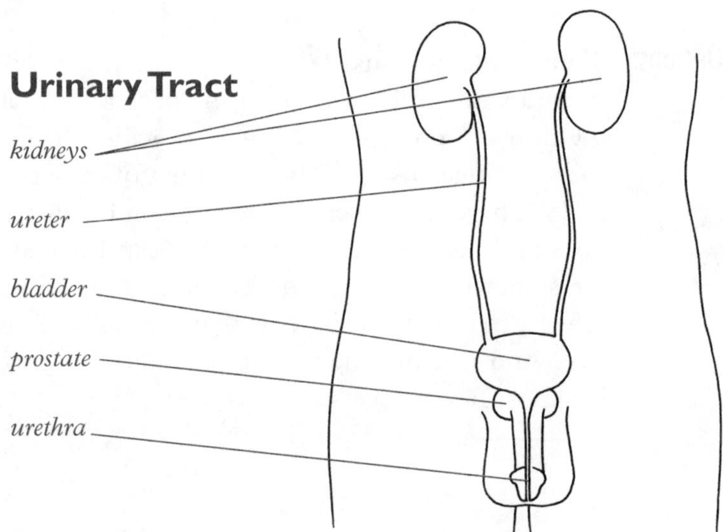

causes of obstruction in men are kidney stones and an enlarged prostate gland. Both of these increase your risk for developing a UTI. Other factors that can increase your risk include having a catheter, or tube in your bladder that helps you void urine, or having diabetes, which causes an increased risk for infection generally. Unprotected sex with a risky partner increases the risk of sexually transmitted diseases that can cause UTIs *(For more information on STDs, see page 296).*

There are several preventive measures you can take to reduce your risk of developing a UTI. They include:

- Drink at least eight 8-ounce glasses of water a day (or its equivalent). If you're physically active or live in a warm environment that causes you to sweat a lot, you may need to drink even more.
- If you have an underlying condition that predisposes you to UTIs, drink a glass of cranberry juice every day. Because it's very acidic, it seems to inhibit the growth of bacteria in your urinary tract.
- Urinate when you feel the need. Urinating frequently will wash bacteria from your urethra.
- Wear a condom during sex to prevent bacteria from entering your urethra.

Diagnosis & Screening: Your doctor may suspect that you have a UTI based on your symptoms, which typically include a frequent urge to urinate, even when little urine is present; pain and burning during urination; pain in the lower abdomen or on one side of your back (flank); and cloudy or reddish urine. The diagnosis is confirmed with a urinalysis, in which a sample of your urine is tested for the presence of pus and bacteria. Your doctor may inspect the prostate and bladder through a fiberoptic tube inserted through the penis. He or she may also perform an intravenous pyelogram, a special X-ray of your urinary tract that is done after an opaque dye is injected into your bloodstream. This can reveal structural abnormalities that may be causing the problem.

Treatment Options: UTIs can be treated with a number of different antibiotics. The one your doctor chooses will depend on the underlying cause of your infection and the type of bacteria that is causing it. Because UTIs can be quite painful, you may also receive medication to relieve the discomfort. Drink plenty of water and reduce caffeine and alcohol, both of which can be dehydrating and exacerbate the problem.

Varicose Veins

The Basics: The arteries in your body carry blood from your heart to the rest of your tissues and organs. Veins do the opposite—they carry blood from your organs and tissues back to your heart, often working against gravity and pushing the blood "uphill" to do so. Your veins keep blood from flowing backwards thanks in large part to a series of tiny one-way valves, which allow blood to flow toward your heart but not backward. When these valves malfunction, blood pools in your veins, leading to varicose, or bulging, veins.

Although they can strike any veins in your body (even in your testicles, a condition known as a varicocele), varicose veins are most likely to crop up in your lower legs, where the valves have to work especially hard to maintain blood flow toward your heart. About 40 million people in the U.S. have varicose veins, a condition that's about twice as likely to strike women as men.

Varicose veins should not be confused with blood clots in the deeper veins of the legs, a condition known as DVT (for deep vein thrombosis). Such clots are potentially dangerous when they break loose and travel through the veins to the heart and into the lungs, where they can cause a sudden and dangerous blockage known as a pulmonary embolism. There is little or no correlation between varicose veins and deep vein thrombosis, though sometimes before performing a varicose vein stripping (see below) the physician will want to study the deeper veins to make sure there is no blockage to alternative blood flow once the superficial varicose veins have been removed. Deep vein blood clots can cause generalized pain and swelling in your leg even though the superficial veins look normal. Such symptoms should be reported to your doctor right away because of the potential danger of "traveling" blood clots.

Prevention & Risk Factors: There are a number of factors that increase the likelihood of developing varicose veins. They include:

Family history of varicose veins. If your parents or close family members had varicose veins, you're more likely to develop them as well.

Being overweight. The more you weigh, the more pressure there is on the valves in your veins, making leakage more likely.

Having a career in which you're required to stand for long periods of time. When you stand in the same position, your blood doesn't move around your body as well, so valves may malfunction.

Being sedentary. Muscles help the blood to pump through your veins, so when muscles are not used, your blood doesn't pump as efficiently as it should.

Age. Varicose veins first appear in many people around age 30, but the chance of developing them increases the older you get, because your veins often lose elasticity and stretch out, making valves looser so they don't seal properly.

Diagnosis & Screening: Symptoms of varicose veins include an achy or heavy feeling in the area; enlarged, blue veins that are visible through your skin; an itchy vein; leg swelling; or skin ulcers or brown-looking skin near your ankle. To diagnose varicose veins, your doctor will ask you about your symptoms and examine the area in question. He may also perform an ultrasound test to check for the presence of a blood clot.

Treatment Options: Typically, you can ease the symptoms of varicose veins by making a few lifestyle changes—losing weight; exercising; keeping your legs elevated to encourage blood flow back to your heart; avoiding long periods of standing; wearing elastic support stockings, which help the muscles of your legs push blood upward toward your heart; and, if you have swelling and pain, taking an over-the-counter anti-inflammatory.

If your condition doesn't improve with those simple measures, your doctor may recommend one of the following treatments:

Sclerotherapy. In this outpatient treatment, your doctor injects a chemical called a sclerosing agent into your vein to scar the vein and collapse its walls, rendering it useless. Since blood can re-route itself to healthier veins, it's not dangerous to do this, and it often solves the problem in smaller, more superficial varicose veins.

Laser surgery. This newer strategy, in which doctors use a laser to shut down small varicose veins, is becoming more common.

Vein stripping. In this technique, also performed on an outpatient basis, your doctor actually removes the malfunctioning vein through small incisions in your ankle and groin, literally pulling out or "stripping" the vein.

CHAPTER 7

Your Sexual and Reproductive Health

The male sex organs produce sperm cells (or spermatozoa) and male sex hormones and direct them to their appropriate targets. The health of your reproductive system is affected by many of the same things that affect the health of the rest of your body—diet, exercise, sleep, stress. If you maintain good physical and emotional health, you should be able to maintain sexual potency well into your senior years, barring direct injury or diseases that affect the reproductive system.

Eating a low-fat diet, maintaining an ideal body weight, and staying physically active can help prevent hardening of the arteries, or atherosclerosis, and adult-onset diabetes, both of which can diminish your sexual functioning. *(See pages 124 and 196 for more information on atherosclerosis and diabetes.)* Drinking too much alcohol and smoking can take a toll on your sexual health as well.

The principal male sex hormone, testosterone, is present in very low levels in boys prior to puberty. At puberty, the pituitary gland produces two hormones—luteinizing hormone and follicle-stimulating hormone—that trigger special cells in your testicles to produce testosterone.

Under the influence of testosterone, a young boy begins to develop secondary male sexual characteristics. His shoulders broaden and muscles enlarge. He gets facial hair, pubic hair, and hair in his armpits and on his chest and legs. His genitals change, too. His penis grows longer and wider, and his body becomes capable of producing sperm.

Testosterone has a psychological influence as well. Boys become more aggressive and they begin to take an interest in sex. Male reproductive hormones are essential for the normal growth, development, and maintenance of the prostate. Although men continue to produce sex hormones after middle age, the levels of testosterone begin to fall gradually, much more gradually than the drop in female hormones during menopause. *(See page 241 for a discussion of "male menopause.")*

Here's a look at how each part of this elaborate system looks and functions—and what can go wrong.

The Penis

About 90 percent of all erect adult penises are between five and seven inches long. There is actually very little correlation between the length of a flaccid penis and its length when it's erect.

The **foreskin,** which is actually two layers of skin, covers the head of the penis (called the *glans*) in an uncircumcised male.

The extremely sensitive **glans** (or *glans penis)* is the smooth, shiny head of the penis.

The **urinary meatus** is the opening at the tip of the penis where urine and semen exit the body. (The **urethra** is the tube inside the penis that carries urine and semen out of the body.)

The **corpora cavernosa** are large areas that run the length of the penis and fill with blood during erections.

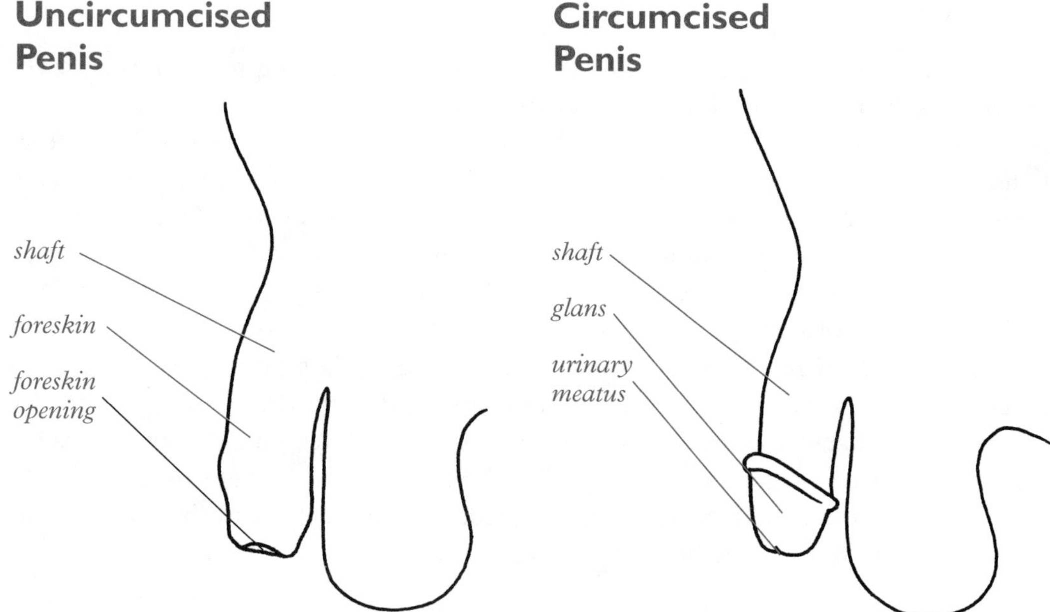

Keeping the Penis Healthy

The way your penis works is fairly straightforward. When sexually aroused, the nervous system signals the circulatory system to send blood to the genitals. As the corpora cavernosa in the penis become engorged, an erection results.

Every part of the penis, including the foreskin (if present), shaft, and glans, is sensitive to touch, though the glans, which contains hundreds of nerve endings, is by far the most sensitive. It plays a significant role in sexual arousal and may trigger orgasm.

Your mother was right: It's important to keep your genitals clean. The best way to do it: Gently wash the surface of your penis with mild, non-deodorant soap every day. If you're not circumcised, you'll need to clean under your foreskin, where bacteria can build up, as well.

Wearing a condom during sex is the best way to avoid contracting a sexually transmitted disease (STD) such as AIDS or herpes. Choose a latex condom, and check it for holes or signs of wear before you put it on. Roll it on carefully, according to the package instructions, so it doesn't tear. Don't use oil-based lubricants (such as petroleum jelly) when you're wearing a condom, because they dissolve the latex. Condoms should fit snugly. If yours doesn't, it's more likely to break. Breakage isn't very likely, but it happens about 2 percent of the time.

Circumcision

About 60 percent of boys in America are circumcised, meaning their foreskin is removed shortly after birth. This once almost standard procedure has become much more controversial in recent years. Those who are against circumcision argue that it diminishes erotic pleasure by exposing the sensitive tip of your penis to daily abrasion and other nerve-damaging stimulation; that it leaves an infant's glans unprotected from feces and ammonia in diapers; and that it can diminish sexual performance, because some people believe the foreskin is supposed to enhance the gliding action of your penis during sex.

On the other hand, those who believe circumcision is a good idea say that an intact foreskin provides a favorable environment for the growth of bacteria, thereby increasing the likelihood of penile and urinary tract infections. There is also a slightly increased risk for penile cancer in an uncircumcised male. In its most recent statement, the American Academy of Pediatrics basically said that either decision made by parents is medically acceptable.

Penile Fracture

The Basics: When your penis becomes erect, the erectile chambers (corpora cavernosa) inside your penis fill with blood and your penis becomes more rigid. If your erect penis suffers some trauma—if, for example, you bump it against your partner's pubic bone or even the mattress of your bed—there's a small chance it could bend sharply and suffer a fracture, in which the blood-filled erectile chamber actually ruptures.

Prevention & Risk Factors: Fractures tend to occur more frequently in men who have longer-than-average penises. Scenarios in which this is more likely to occur include:

- When you are having intercourse, especially with your partner on top. The majority of penile fractures occur during sexual activity with a partner, but it can happen when you masturbate, though this is very rare.

- During rough sports or strenuous physical activity—particularly if you're not wearing a cup for protection.

Diagnosis & Screening: When your penis fractures, you may hear a loud snap, which will be followed by intense pain. Within an hour, you'll be able to see a bruise and your penis will be swollen. About 20 percent of the time, the urethra (the tube in your penis that carries urine from your bladder) is injured as well.

Diagnosis is usually fairly simple and is based on the symptoms of bruising and swelling. Your doctor will perform a physical examination, paying special attention to your penis and the surrounding area. If it cannot be determined whether your penis sustained a fracture, your doctor may recommend a penile ultrasound, an imaging test that provides a view of the structures within your penis and that can check for areas of leakage.

If your doctor suspects your urethra has been injured as well, he'll perform a urine test to check for the presence of blood in your urine.

Treatment Options: Surgery to repair the rupture is the most effective treatment. The sooner you have it repaired, the better your prognosis for a complete recovery.

Penile Swelling or Inflammation

(Balanitis)

The Basics: Swelling or inflammation of any part of the penis could be the sign of a number of disorders. Balanitis or inflammation of the head of the penis (the glans penis) is most common in uncircumcised men. Symptoms of balanitis may include redness, itching, soreness, and a foul-smelling discharge. White or red blotches or lumps may appear on the glans, which may also look shiny or waxy. In severe cases there is swelling.

Balanitis may be caused by poor personal hygiene. Allergic reactions—to substances both natural and store bought—can also lead to balanitis. Some men are allergic to thrush (a yeast infection caused by the fungus candida) in a woman's vagina or to rubber, spermicides, deodorants, or the perfumes in soaps and detergents. In addition, streptococcal bacteria in a woman's vagina transmitted during sexual intercourse can cause a problem. Strenuous sexual activity and certain medications may also be responsible for the condition.

A yeast infection is not common in men but is extremely common in women and can be transmitted to a man (particularly if uncircumcised) during sexual intercourse. Symptoms include pain and redness of the penis.

Herpes and syphilis also cause sores on the penis. *(For more information on these sexually transmitted diseases, see pages 298 and 300.)*

Prevention & Risk Factors: Balanitis is usually caused by poor personal hygiene. Men at risk of developing balanitis are those who are uncircumcised and who do not clean their penis regularly. It is especially important for uncircumcised men to wash their genitals every day using mild soap without added perfume. Underwear should also be washed regularly.

Diagnosis & Screening: Balanitis is usually detected during a physical examination to rule out other conditions that produce similar symptoms, such as STDs. If balanitis is severe you may also have to undergo a test for diabetes because severe balanitis can be a sign of diabetes.

Yeast infections are usually diagnosed by examining any discharge or by taking a swab of the area and sending it to a lab for a culture.

Treatment Options: If balanitis is caused by thrush (candida) you will probably be given an antifungal drug. If it is caused by a bacterial infection, you will receive an antibiotic. If your doctor suspects that it was triggered by an allergic reaction, he or she may recommend allergy testing. If the problem recurs often and is caused by a tight foreskin, your doctor may recommend circumcision.

Penile Warts

The Basics: A virus called human papilloma virus (HPV) causes penile warts, which are usually transmitted sexually in adults through intercourse *(see also STDs, page 296)*. Penile warts can also occur in children without sexual contact, particularly children who are in diapers.

Penile warts, which are soft, wart-like or cauliflower-like growths on the penis, are relatively common. You may see just one or a cluster of these flesh-colored growths. They often appear two to three weeks after exposure to the virus but can appear up to 18 months after sexual transmission.

There are more than 60 different types of human papilloma viruses, some of which are associated with an increased risk of cancer of the penis.

Prevention & Risk Factors: Condoms offer some protection against penile warts, though the virus may "shed" beyond the area covered by the condom. As with all STDs, your risk increases with the number of partners and amount of sexual activity you have. You are also prone to penile warts if you're suffering from another viral infection such as the flu, HIV, Epstein-Barr, or herpes. Since warts thrive in a moist environment, it's important to keep the area as dry as possible.

Diagnosis & Screening: A physician usually makes a diagnosis during a physical examination and by taking a tissue sample, which is examined under a microscope.

Treatment Options: Your doctor may recommend any of the following treatments:

- Application of the medicine podophyllin to remove the wart.
- Standard surgery.
- Laser surgery, in which the wart is removed using a beam of high-powered light.
- Cryosurgery, in which the wart is frozen with liquid nitrogen applied to the area.
- Injection of the drug interferon.

Living with Genital Warts: There is no cure for HPV infection, which frequently recurs. However, there are a number of simple and effective treatment options. Left untreated, the warts can enlarge and become quite uncomfortable, so it's best to deal with them early on. Even though the warts may disappear after treatment, you can still transmit the virus to a sexual partner so you should always wear a condom to help prevent this from happening.

Peyronie's Disease

The Basics: If your penis is injured when you're playing sports, say, or having sex, it can develop scar tissue, which restricts blood flow to the area. A similar condition known as Peyronie's disease, named after Francois de la Peyronie, a French physician who first reported the illness in the mid-1700s, can develop spontaneously without injury. Depending on how extensive it is, the scar tissue can cause a number of problems, from erectile dysfunction (because it impedes the blood flow to your penis) to a noticeable bend in your penis where the scar tissue is located. In some men, the bend is so dramatic that they can't have intercourse.

Peyronie's disease can go away on its own, without any treatment. In about half of affected men, it gets worse over time. It occurs in about 4 percent of men, most of whom are older than 40.

Prevention & Risk Factors: Although there's no way to prevent the condition, there are certain things that increase your risk. They include:

Damage to your penis. In most acute (sudden-onset) cases, an injury sets off the problem. If the area is damaged repeatedly, it increases your chance of having long-term problems.

Family history of Peyronie's. Although there's not a lot of good data, it appears that the illness is more likely to strike if you have a relative who had it.

Medications. Drugs such as beta blockers, used to treat high blood pressure, may boost the likelihood of developing Peyronie's.

Other scarring diseases. An illness called Dupuytren's contracture, which causes scarring on the palms of your hands or the soles of your feet, may increase your risk for the illness.

Diagnosis & Screening: In order to diagnose the illness, your doctor will perform a physical exam of your penis. Penile ultrasound can also be helpful.

Treatment Options: Your doctor may try medications first, although none has been proven to be effective. Some that may work include topical or oral vitamin E; vitamin A; injections of steroids into the scar tissue; or oral colchicine, an anti-inflammatory drug used to treat gout.

Surgery is an option as well, and although it's quite successful, your doctor may recommend waiting as much as a year or more before trying surgery to give the illness a chance to go away on its own. Surgical options include:

Scar excision. In this technique, the doctor removes the scar tissue from your penis and patches it with skin from your hip area.

Nesbit plication. This surgery attempts to straighten your penis by removing normal tissue on the opposite side of your penis from the scar tissue.

Saphenous vein graft. In this method, your doctor cuts the scar tissue to straighten the penis, then covers the cut with a vein graft.

Penile prosthesis. In some cases, your doctor may suggest inserting a prosthesis into your penis to straighten it out.

Phimosis

(Tightening of the Foreskin)

The Basics: When the foreskin becomes so tight that it cannot be drawn back from the head of the penis, the condition is called phimosis. This disorder can develop anytime from early childhood on. In small children, the foreskin is stuck to the glans, but as boys get older, it normally retracts to expose the glans. In some cases, however, the foreskin remains attached to the glans until after puberty.

Phimosis can also develop when the foreskin becomes scarred from frequent thrush (yeast) infections. Men with phimosis frequently have painful erections. In severe cases, the condition can interfere with urination.

Prevention & Risk Factors: Obviously, phimosis only affects uncircumcised men. If you cannot retract your foreskin enough to wash it properly, this may lead to infection. Trying to force back the foreskin will only cause painful cracks on its inside, which will scar as they heal and make the condition worse.

Diagnosis and Screening: Usually the physician conducts a physical examination to determine the severity of the condition and choose the best treatment plan.

Treatment Options: Your doctor will probably recommend circumcision. *(For more information on circumcision, see page 274.)* In some cases, you may first be asked to use steroid creams to relieve the condition, but circumcision will probably still be required.

Priapism

The Basics: Usually, your penis becomes erect when blood flows into it in response to sexual stimulation. But in men with priapism, the penis becomes erect without any stimulation, and the erection won't go away—in other words, the blood won't drain—even if you ejaculate. The condition, which is rare, is considered a medical emergency when it occurs. It typically strikes one of two age groups: children between the ages of 5 and 10, and men between the ages of 20 and 50. In about half of men it causes erectile dysfunction.

Prevention & Risk Factors: Certain men are more likely to have a bout of priapism than others. Factors that increase your risk:

Medications. Drugs that you inject into your penis to treat impotence are a common cause of priapism. It also can be caused by drugs used to treat psychotic illness, including thorazine and chlorpromazine.

Sickle-cell disease. This illness accounts for about one-third of all cases of priapism. About 40 percent of men with sickle-cell disease will have the problem at some point.

Marijuana use. Smoking this drug may cause priapism in rare cases.

Diagnosis & Screening: If you've had an erection that has lasted more than four hours, it's important to see your doctor immediately. Left untreated for as little as 12 hours, priapism can lead to impotence or to the development of scar tissue.

Your doctor will diagnose priapism based on your report

of how long you've had an erection. Let your doctor know any medications you've been taking and if you smoked marijuana recently. It may also be necessary to draw some blood from your penis for a blood gas measurement.

Treatment Options: Your doctor's approach will depend on how long you've had the problem. Some options:

Decongestants. If you've had the erection for less than four hours, your doctor may start with decongestants, like pseudoephedrine and terbutaline, to decrease blood flow to your penis.

Aspiration. In this method, your doctor places a small needle into your penis to remove some of the blood.

Other medications. Although aspiration usually works, priapism can recur. If it does, your doctor may give you epinephrine, a drug that causes your blood vessels to constrict.

Inserting a shunt. If you're still having problems, your doctor may need to implant a shunt into your penis to drain the blood into the surrounding tissues.

Other Causes of Penile Pain

Penile disorders are usually at the root of pain or discomfort in that area, but sometimes, problems in other reproductive organs can lead to penile pain. Conditions that may cause your penis to hurt include:

- Inflammation of the prostate gland *(see Prostatitis on page 290)*
- An infection or inflammation of the urethra (called nonspecific urethritis), which is usually caused by the sexually transmitted disease chlamydia *(see also STDs on page 297)*
- An autoimmune syndrome of the joints called Reiter's syndrome, which can cause pain and discharge from the penis. (Other symptoms of Reiter's syndrome include low-grade fever, aching joints, and redness in the eyes.)

The Testicles and Scrotum

Just to make sure we are all on the same anatomical page, I will remind you that most of us men have two testicles, one on each side of the skin sac, called the scrotum, that hangs under the penis. The testicles inside the scrotum are "connected" to the lower pelvic area of the abdomen by a cord of blood vessels (both artery and veins), nerves, and the vas deferens, a thin tube that transports the millions of sperm produced by the testicles. (That's the basis for the terrible joke I first heard in medical school, that there is a "vas deferens" between the male and female.)

Testicular Cancer

The Basics: Unlike many cancers, testicular cancer tends to strike young men. Although testicular cancer accounts for just 1 percent of all cancers in men, it's the most common form of cancer in men between the ages of 15 and 35. It's more common in white men than in African-American men. In 2002, there will be an estimated 7,500 new cases of testicular cancer, and 400 deaths from the disease.

Cancer of a testicle occurs when its cells begin to divide uncontrollably, forming a tumor, or mass of abnormal cells. Depending on the type of cancer it is, it may spread, or metastasize, to other parts of the body. There are two general types of testicular cancer: seminomas, which account for about 30 percent of all testicular cancers, and nonseminomas, which have a variety of subtypes.

Prevention & Risk Factors: Researchers have yet to unravel the exact cause of testicular cancer, but studies show that several factors increase your chance of developing the disease. They include:

Undescended testicle. Usually, the testicles drop from inside the pelvic area down into the scrotum before birth, but in some boys, the testicle doesn't move down, a condition that places them at 10 times greater risk of testicular cancer—even if they underwent surgery to move the testicle into the scrotum.

Abnormal testicle development. Rarely, testicles don't develop fully or there's some problem with development, both of which increase the risk of testicular cancer.

Klinefelter's syndrome. This chromosome disorder, which causes low levels of male hormones, breast enlargement, and sterility also increases the risk of testicular cancer.

History of testicular cancer. If you've had the disease in the past, you're at greater risk of developing it in the other testicle.

Diagnosis & Screening: Doctors sometimes examine the testicles during routine physical exams, but there are no standardized screening regimens for this illness. As a result, it's a good idea to make sure you know the general shape, size, and feel of your testicles so you'll be aware of changes if they appear. Since most testicular cancers are found by men themselves, I believe that men between the ages of 15 and 40 should "self-examine" their testicles on a regular basis—every two to three months.

Here's how to do a testicular self-exam: After you get out of the bath or shower, when your scrotum is relaxed, put your foot up on the side of a bathtub or toilet and gently feel each testicle. Roll the testicle between your thumb and forefingers. The testes are oval shaped and should feel smooth, firm, and fairly equal in size, although it's normal for one testicle to be slightly larger than the other. Check for lumps or anything that feels different, such as sore spots or a change in skin texture. Most lumps are found on the side of the testicle, but they can show up on the front, so it's important to check the entire area with care. Don't worry about the small tube slightly to the back of each testicle. This stringy structure is the epididymis, a network of tubules through which sperm cells pass as they mature. By becoming familiar with the way your testicles feel, you'll be able to tell when something is different. If you find something unusual, see your physician right away. Not all lumps are cancerous, but it's important to make sure.

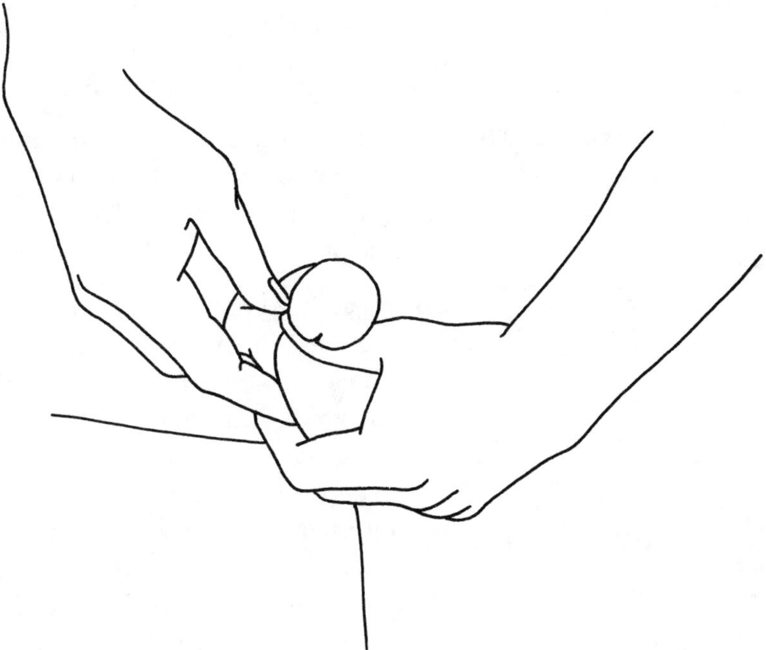

In addition to self-examination, you should be on the lookout for the following symptoms and see your doctor immediately should any of them appear:

- Swelling or lumpiness.
- A feeling of heaviness, pain, or discomfort in the scrotum.
- A dull ache in the groin or lower abdomen.
- Fluid collecting in the scrotum.

If testicular cancer is suspected, your doctor will examine your testicles for lumps and, if it doesn't feel normal, order an ultrasound examination, which uses sound waves to form an image of the inside of the testes. If an ultrasound is inconclusive, your doctor may order a blood test to measure your level of tumor markers, substances that your body produces in greater-than-normal amounts when you have cancer. Or, your doctor may feel it's best to biopsy or even remove the testicle, a procedure called inguinal orchiectomy, so a pathologist can look at the cells under a microscope.

Treatment Options: The most effective treatment approach depends on the type of cancer, the extent of the cancer, and your age and general health. Following are the most common approaches:

Surgery. Inguinal orchiectomy, the same procedure that may be used for biopsy, is the surgery of choice for testicular cancer. In this approach, the doctor makes an incision in your groin and removes the affected testicle. As long as you have one remaining healthy testicle, you can still have an erection and produce sperm, but 90 percent of men will be infertile because of abnormal sperm production. If you have lymph nodes removed, it may interfere with your ability to ejaculate. If you would like to have children, you must talk to your doctor about banking some of your sperm before surgery.

Radiation. In this approach, high-energy X-rays are used to kill cancer cells in the lymph nodes in the abdomen. Although seminomas are highly sensitive to radiation, non-seminomas are not.

Chemotherapy. After surgery, your doctor may recommend that you take a round of cancer-killing drugs to target cancerous cells that may have spread to another part of your body. One commonly used combination of drugs is cisplatin (Platinol), bleomycin (Blenoxane), and vinblastine (Velban). The use of chemotherapy has dramatically increased the survival rate, even when testicular cancer has spread widely throughout the body, as in the case of bicyclist Lance Armstrong.

Bone marrow or stem cell transplant. In a bone marrow transplant your doctor will remove your bone marrow, treat it with drugs that kill cancer cells, and then freeze it while you have high-dose chemotherapy (and perhaps radiation) to destroy any cancer cells that remain in your body. When you're finished with chemotherapy, your doctor thaws your treated bone marrow cells and puts them back into your body through a needle in a vein. Today, so-called "stem cells" from the blood are more likely to be used instead of bone marrow.

Living with Testicular Cancer:

After orchiectomy, the side of the scrotum where the testicle was removed may look and feel empty. To restore a more natural look, you have the option of having an artificial testicle, or prosthesis, that has the same heft and texture as a normal testicle surgically implanted in the scrotum. The prosthesis is filled with silicone gel and it comes in a number of sizes to match your remaining testicle.

Common side effects of chemotherapy include hair loss, nausea, vomiting, diarrhea, fatigue, and mouth sores. It may permanently reduce your sperm count.

Recent data suggests that men treated for testicular cancer may be at higher risk for heart and kidney disease later in life.

Other Testicular and Scrotal Problems

In addition to testiculer cancer (see above), here are several other more common problems that can arise in the testicles or scrotum.

Inflammation/Infection

Usually, only one testicle is affected, although both can be.

The resulting symptoms are usually obvious: swelling of and significant pain in the affected testicle. This is a condition that should be treated as quickly as possible since prolonged infection can result in infertility, especially if both testicles are affected. One of the more common causes of testicular infection is the mumps virus, which is one of the reasons why it's so important to get vaccinated with the MMR vaccine—against mumps, measles, and rubella (German measles)—in childhood. Sometimes the pain and inflammation are caused by epididymitis, an infection in the collection of tubules on the surface of the testicle that collect sperm and feed them into the vas deferens.

Torsion

This is a condition in which the testicle gets twisted, thereby twisting the artery and vein and cutting off blood supply to and drainage from the testicle. It is most common during adolescence but can occur at any age. *It is a true emergency.* If the testicle cannot be "untwisted" by hand, immediate surgery is required. Fortunately, the pain and swelling from this problem are usually so severe that it drives the afflicted male to seek quick medical attention.

Scrotal Swellings

Sometimes the scrotum will enlarge because of swelling of structures other than the testicles. In these cases, there may be some pain but is it not usually severe, unlike problems with the testicles. The structures most commonly affected are the veins (varicocele), but other structures such as the membranes around the testicles (hydrocele) or the epididymis (spermatocele) can also develop painless swelling.

Obviously any abnormality of the scrotal sac—painful or not—should be taken seriously. In any complicated or uncertain case, a urologist, the specialist for such problems, should be consulted quickly.

Male Reproductive System

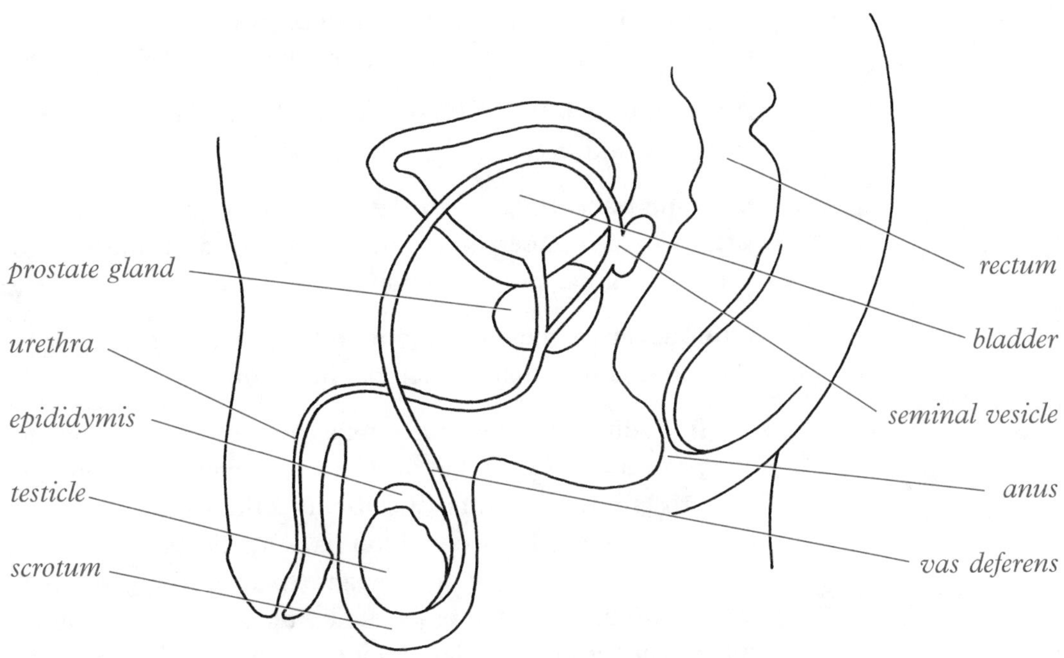

The Prostate

Your prostate is a walnut-size gland located just below your bladder that produces the fluid necessary for ejaculation. Your prostate actually wraps around your urethra, the tube through which you urinate. The prostate gland begins to grow during adolescence, reaching its full size in your 20s. In some men, the prostrate grows again in old age. In fact, about two out of every three men who reach the age of 70 have an enlarged prostate, which can cause difficulty urinating.

Prostate enlargement can be caused by cancer, but more frequently, such enlargement is benign (called benign prostatic hypertrophy, or BPH). Though benign, you shouldn't ignore the condition, because enlargement of the prostate often results in urinary retention caused by the obstruction of the urethra.

Prostate cancer was covered in Chapter 4 *(page 103)*. Here I'll address prostatitis and BPH, the two most common conditions affecting the prostate.

Prostatitis

The Basics: Any condition in which the prostate becomes inflamed is known as prostatitis. There are three basic kinds of prostatitis:

Acute bacterial, which comes on very suddenly and dramatically and is caused by a bacterial infection.

Chronic bacterial, which develops slowly and often persists over a number of months or even years and is also caused by a bacterial infection.

Nonbacterial, the most common type, which is caused by something other than a bacterial infection.

In addition to these infections, men often complain of a very vague but very real problem with pain in the area of the prostate for which no specific infectious or other cause can be found. This condition is sometimes labeled as *prostatodynia* which literally means "pain in the prostate." This condition is often associated with some of the symptoms of infection or enlargement—such as difficulty starting or maintaining urination—but the prostate feels normal during an examination and a urine test doesn't show any signs of infection such as bacteria or pus cells. Not surprisingly, men with this problem often end up with other psychological symptoms, including depression and sexual dysfunction. There is no predictably effective treatment other than sympathy and support, but doctors usually try so-called alpha-blocker drugs, which can relax the muscles at the neck of your bladder, making the flow of urine easier.

Sexually active men between the ages of 20 and 35 are the most susceptible to acute prostatitis. About 35 percent of men over the age of 50 have chronic prostatitis at some point. Among young and middle-aged men who visit the doctor with genital and urinary problems, prostatitis is the cause one-quarter of the time.

Prevention & Risk Factors: Although there's no surefire prevention strategy, there are some things you can do to decrease the likelihood of prostatitis. They include:

Wash your hands after bowel movements. Because prostatitis is often caused by infection with a bacterium known as E. coli, which typically makes its home in your colon, you can reduce the transfer of the bacteria by being religious about washing your hands after using the restroom.

Drink lots of fluids every day to flush any bacteria out of your bladder.

Wear a condom when you have sex with a new partner or with anyone whose sexually transmitted disease (STD) status is uncertain. Certain common STDs, such as gonorrhea, chlamydia, and trichomonas, can cause acute prostatitis.

Diagnosis & Screening: In order to determine whether you have prostatitis, your doctor will perform a physical exam of your groin area and ask you if you've had any of the following symptoms:

- Fever.
- Chills.
- Pain in the low back, abdomen, and/or pelvic floor.
- Pain during urination, ejaculation, and/or bowel movements.
- Inability to completely empty your bladder.

You'll also need to provide a urine sample, which may reveal the presence of bacteria or white blood cells, which indicates the presence of infection. Your doctor may also massage the prostate to provide fluid for analysis.

Treatment Options: Treatment varies depending on the cause of the problem, assuming your doctor is able to determine the cause. If it's thought to be caused by a bacterial infection, you'll be put on antibiotics, sometimes for as long as six to eight weeks. Doctors often prescribe trimethoprim-sulfamethoxazole or the newer fluoroquinolone antibiotics, such as Cipro. If antibiotics don't work, your doctor may recommend surgery to remove all or part of your prostate, but the treatment is typically performed only on older men, because it can cause sterility or impotence.

BPH
(Benign Prostatic Hypertrophy)

The Basics: Past the age of 50, most men's prostate glands start to enlarge to some degree and will eventually cause some problems with urination. This general type of prostate enlargement is called benign prostatic hypertrophy, more commonly referred to as BPH.

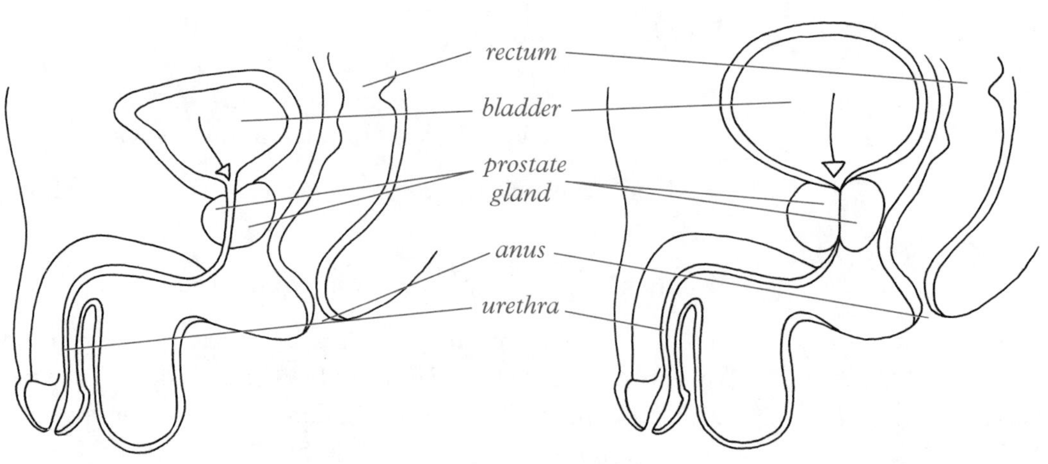

A normal prostate gland

The enlarged prostate gland blocks the flow of urine

The usual, rather annoying symptoms of BPH, which range from mild to severe, include:

- Frequent need to urinate, especially at night.
- A feeling of urgency when you need to urinate.
- Difficulty starting or stopping the flow of urine.
- Less urine output with each attempt.
- Diminished force of the urinary stream.

Prevention & Risk Factors: Enlargement of the prostate seems to be associated with aging and its accompanying hormonal changes. Since virtually all men can expect their prostate to enlarge to some degree as they age, many men are now taking a growing interest in alternative treatments, herbal remedies, vitamin supplements, and dietary changes to address the issue. None of these have been subjected to rigorous scientific scrutiny, and I suggest you talk to your doctor before trying them. I have been particularly impressed by the many men who report improvement with saw palmetto even though scientific studies haven't found measurable changes in urine flow from its use.

Diagnosis and Screening: A doctor can often diagnose BPH simply based on your description of the relevant symptoms. In order to do a physical examination of your prostate, your doctor will need to insert a gloved finger into your rectum to feel for an enlargement of the prostate gland. To rule out cancer your doctor may ask you to take a blood test for PSA, or prostate specific antigen. *(See Prostate Cancer on page 103 to learn more about this test.)* Imaging studies of the pelvis or bladder may also be performed to help diagnose BPH or rule out other possible causes of your urinary symptoms.

Treatment Options: This is one of the most difficult areas in which to give advice, because so much depends on the subjective feelings and needs of the individual. There is nothing dangerous about benign enlargement of the prostate unless it reaches a point where it causes complications, such as urinary tract infections or bladder stones, because of urine backup and pooling. However, the symptoms of BPH as described above can definitely be annoying and, for some men, even embarrassing—such as standing at a public urinal and whistling an entire Mozart sonata while waiting for your stream to start.

Studies suggest that the majority of men with mild enlargement will either improve or stay the same and that only 10 to 20 percent will get progressively worse. Therefore those of you with mild symptoms may choose to "wait and see." However, if even mild symptoms bother you, talk with your doctor about taking medication, which might help. There are two kinds of drugs currently approved for treating the symptoms of mild to moderate enlargement:

Finasteride (trade name, Proscar) is a drug that shrinks the prostate by reducing androgen (male hormone) levels. However, it often takes three to six months to produce changes. And it may reduce levels of PSA, thereby reducing the accuracy of the test in detecting cancer. *(For more on PSA levels, see page 107.)*

Alpha blockers, such as terazosin (Hytrin) and doxazosin (Cardura), act much more quickly than finasteride by relaxing the muscles in the prostate and bladder. However, they can cause side effects such as dizziness, fatigue, and dangerously low blood pressure. Most physicians believe they are somewhat more effective than finasteride, though results can certainly vary.

If enlargement and/or symptoms are more severe, you may want to consider one of the many surgical procedures now available for removing or destroying part of the enlarged prostate gland. They include:

Transurethral resection of the prostate (TURP). This is still the most common surgical procedure for benign enlargement. It involves inserting a probe through the urethra in the penis (under anesthesia, of course) and burning away some of the excess prostate tissue. Many men will experience minor side effects such as bleeding and temporary incontinence. About 1 percent will experience more serious long-term incontinence, and 2 to 5 percent will experience impotence. Another common side effect is so-called retrograde ejaculation, meaning that during male orgasm (ejaculation) the semen goes backward into the bladder rather than out the penis. A man can still experience full sexual pleasure—though obviously he will be infertile—but some men find the condition "unnerving."

Transurethral incision of the prostate (TUIP). This is a variation on TURP in which small incisions are made in the prostate to allow the urethra to expand. The complication rate is lower than with TURP, but it is usually only effective for minimally enlarged glands.

Transurethral microwave therapy (TUMT). This variation uses microwaves to destroy excess tissue. Studies show it has fewer complications than TURP but about half of men who have it will require a repeat treatment within one to two years.

There are other techniques being studied, but all are designed to cut out or destroy excess prostate tissue. If you are having severe symptoms, one of these surgical procedures is probably the way to go, though you'll lose little (except some time and money) by trying medications first.

Living with BPH: There are a couple of myths surrounding the prevention of prostate enlargement. One is that sexual activity (either too much or too little) makes a difference. There's no proof of that. Another is that periodic massage of the prostate gland (by the doctor's finger inserted in the rectum) can help. There's no proof of that either. What can help is decreasing your intake of caffeine and alcohol, both of which are diuretics that increase urine production. If nighttime urination is a problem, it also can help to drink less fluid before you go to bed. You might also check with your doctor to see if any medications you are taking (such as antihistamines or decongestants) could be making your symptoms worse.

Sexually Transmitted Diseases (STDs)

One in five people in the U.S. has or has had an STD, according to the American Social Health Association, a group that tracks such information. Nearly 70 percent of STDs strike people younger than 26, but fewer than half of people between the ages of 18 and 44 have ever been tested for an STD other than AIDS (HIV). One important point that must be directed especially at men: A recent study in France suggests that men are seven times more likely than women to hide the fact that they have an STD. That's not only morally wrong, but medically dangerous! Knowing about STDs—how they're transmitted and what to do about them—is one way to protect yourself and your partner. Use this chart as another tool in your safe-sex arsenal.

Safe Sex

Abstinence is the only way to truly prevent STDs, so what follows are some "safer" sex tips—precautions you should take every time you have sex:

- Use a new, sealed latex condom every time you have vaginal or anal sex.
- During oral sex, a non-lubricated latex condom should be used on a man. On a woman, a condom can be cut open to cover the genital area.
- If at all possible, be monogamous (and insist that your partner is as well).
- Use a spermicide containing nonoxynol-9 which is effective against some STDs. If you use any other lubricants, be sure that they're water-based: Petroleum jelly and other lubricants containing oil can damage latex condoms.

STDs

CHLAMYDIA

The Basics: Chlamydia is caused by a bacterium called Chlamydia trachomatis. About three million people are infected annually, and, although statistics show that the majority of them are women, men are rarely tested for the illness so they probably have the infection more than is realized. Untreated chlamydia can cause an infection in your urethra, inflammation of the prostate, and swollen, painful testicles.

Symptoms: About half of infected men have no symptoms, but it may cause painful urination, a discharge from your penis, or an inflamed rectum.

How It's Transmitted: Through sexual intercourse or contact with an infected partner's bodily fluids.

Prevention: There's no guaranteed prevention method, but you can decrease your risk by wearing a latex condom during all sexual contact with any partner who hasn't been tested for the illness. (Women are even more likely than men to have no symptoms when infected.)

Treatment: Oral antibiotics such as doxycycline, azithromycin, erythromycin, and ofloxacin.

PUBIC LICE (CRABS)

The Basics: Pubic lice, known in the vernacular as "crabs," infect the hair and skin around the genitals. They're actually small, wingless insects, which use their crab-like claws to attach. They need blood to survive. Every year, there are about three million cases of crabs in the U.S.

Symptoms: Itching in your pubic area, which usually starts within five days of the infestation, and blue spots or bites. You may also see small, whitish gray or rust-colored crab-like parasites or tiny, shiny, oval-shaped eggs.

How It's Transmitted: Through skin-to-skin contact with an infected person. You also can catch crabs from infested towels, bedding, or clothing.

Prevention: Aside from abstinence or having sex only with uninfected partners, there's no way to prevent it.

Treatment: A cream rinse called permethrin, or a shampoo called lindane. You also need to wash all clothing and bedding in water that's at least 140 degrees Fahrenheit.

GENITAL HERPES

The Basics: Genital herpes is usually caused by the herpes simplex virus, HSV-Type 2, although we now know that HSV-Type 1, which typically causes cold sores around the mouth, can also infect the genital area. About 45 million people ages 12 and older—and one in five men—are infected.

Symptoms: Most of the time, there are no symptoms, so many people who are infected don't know it. The initial infection often causes genital blisters and flu-like symptoms within two weeks. Symptoms recur an average of four or five times a year, but they typically become less noticeable.

How It's Transmitted: Through direct contact, including kissing; sexual contact with an infected partner's vagina, mouth, or anus; or skin-to-skin contact. It can be transmitted even if your partner isn't having a skin outbreak.

Prevention: There's no surefire prevention, but it can help to use latex condoms during all sexual contact with a partner whose status is unknown. If you know your partner is infected, avoid sex during active outbreaks and use latex condoms in between.

Treatment: There's no cure, but antiviral medications can shorten outbreaks.

GENITAL WARTS

The Basics: Genital warts are caused by the human papilloma virus (HPV), but not all of the more than 60 strains of the virus cause warts. There aren't good statistics on how many men are infected, but it's known to be very common. *(See page 277 for more details.)*

Symptoms: Often there are no symptoms. Sometimes, warts may appear on your penis, scrotum, anal area, and/or groin within several weeks of exposure.

How It's Transmitted: Through skin-to-skin contact during vaginal, anal, or oral sex. It's most contagious when warts are present but may be spread even in the absence of warts.

Prevention: Having sex only with uninfected partners. Wearing a condom provides only partial protection, because it doesn't cover the entire genital area.

Treatment: Although there's no cure for the virus, your immune system may clear it on its own. Doctors can treat warts by freezing them with liquid nitrogen; applying chemicals such as podophyllin or trichloracetic acid; cutting them off; or burning them off with an electrical current or laser.

GONORRHEA

The Basics: Gonorrhea, sometimes called "the clap," is caused by a bacterium called Neisseria gonorrhoeae. The Centers for Disease Control and Prevention receives about 400,000 reports of cases of gonorrhea every year, but the disease is undoubtedly much more widespread. If untreated, the bacteria can spread in your blood to your joints.
Symptoms: Only about half of infected men have symptoms, which can include burning during urination, a yellowish white discharge from your penis, and painful, swollen testicles. Rectal infection causes discharge, anal itching, soreness, bleeding, and painful bowel movements. Symptoms appear within 2 to 30 days.
How It's Transmitted: Through sexual contact with an infected partner's vagina, mouth, or anus. There's a 20 percent chance you'll catch the illness after one episode of vaginal intercourse with an infected woman.
Prevention: Condoms don't provide complete protection, since they don't cover the whole genital area, but they can decrease your risk of contracting the illness.
Treatment: Antibiotics, such as ceftriaxone, ciprofloxacin, and erythromycin.

HIV and AIDS

The Basics: Human immunodeficiency virus (HIV) is a virus that gradually weakens your immune system and causes acquired immunodeficiency syndrome, or AIDS. As many as 900,000 people in the U.S. are infected with the virus, and about 775,000 people have actual AIDS.
Symptoms: Many people don't have any symptoms for years, but about half of people infected with HIV develop AIDS within 10 years. Early symptoms may include weight loss; dry cough; night sweats; recurrent fever; fatigue; swollen lymph nodes in the armpits, neck or groin; diarrhea that lasts more than a week; white spots on your tongue or throat; and red, brown, pink, or purple blotches on the skin of your mouth, nose, or eyelids.
How It's Transmitted: Through contact with the blood, semen, or vaginal secretions of an infected partner. Transmission from blood transfusions today is extemely rare.
Prevention: Wear a latex condom during all sexual contact, and don't perform oral sex without protection unless you're sure of your partner's status. Don't have sex with someone who has any other STD or open sore, because it increases your risk of contracting HIV.
Treatment: Although there's no cure for HIV or AIDS, there are a number of antiviral medications that can slow the rate at which HIV weakens your immune system.

SYPHILIS

The Basics: Syphilis is caused by the bacterium Treponema pallidum. There are about 70,000 cases in the U.S. every year, and the illness is slightly more common in men than women. Untreated, it can damage your brain, nerves, eyes, heart, blood vessels, liver, bones, and joints.

Symptoms: Symptoms can appear between 10 and 90 days after contact with an infected partner, but the average is 21. They begin with a single sore that is firm, round, small, and painless and typically appears on the penis, scrotum, or anus or in the rectum. Other symptoms that may develop later include a rash that looks like copper pennies on your hands and feet; fever; mouth and throat sores; swollen lymph nodes; patchy hair loss; weight loss; muscle aches; and fatigue.

How It's Transmitted: Through direct contact with a syphilis sore or with a symptomatic person.

Prevention: Although it's not 100 percent effective, wearing a condom during all sexual contact can reduce your risk.

Treatment: The antibiotic penicillin.

TRICHOMONIASIS

The Basics: This common STD is caused by the bacterium Trichomonas vaginalis. Despite the name, it infects both men and women but is much less likely to cause symptoms in men. It can hide out in the urinary tract or the prostate. You can infect your sexual partner even if you have no symptoms.

Symptoms: Trichomoniasis (sometimes called "trich" for short) can cause frothy and/or painful urination, especially in the morning. The testicles are more rarely infected and can become painful.

How It's Transmitted: Like so many STDs, trichomoniasis is easily spread through sexual intercourse.

Prevention: Again, like most STDs, the best method of preventing spread is the appropriate use of condoms.

Treatment: Because this is a bacterial infection, appropriate antibiotics will usually quickly cure the disease.

Special Health Concerns for Homosexuals and Bisexuals

Because many sexually transmitted diseases are more common in the gay community, it's especially important for men who have sex with men to be cautious about their choice of partners and be diligent about using latex condoms during sexual encounters. Here are some things you may not be aware of that can help you stay safe:

- HIV can be transmitted through oral sex with another man. One study found that nearly 8 percent of recently infected men in San Francisco were probably infected through oral sex.
- Your risk of catching any STD is higher if you regularly have anal sex. The reason: There's more friction during anal sex, so it's more likely to cause mini-tears in your rectum through which bacteria and viruses can easily pass. Using a water-based lubricant can decrease your risk of tears by decreasing friction.
- Although correctly and consistently using condoms can prevent HIV transmission about 85 percent of the time, the method doesn't work as well for a number of other STDs, including genital herpes, human papilloma virus, and syphilis.
- Condoms break about 2 percent of the time.
- Although spermicides such as nonoxynol-9 kill many of the viruses and bacteria that cause STDs, they're not 100 percent effective.

Sexual Function Problems

Problems with sexual functioning are among the most common, but least talked about, conditions men experience.

Delayed Ejaculation

The Basics: Ejaculation happens when the muscles in your genitals contract and expel seminal fluid, including sperm, from your penis. Ejaculation is caused by a combination of physical stimulation and emotional input, and it's typically the latter that becomes a problem if you're having trouble ejaculating during sexual contact. Although there's no specific time limit that defines the term "delayed," if you take more than a half hour to ejaculate (without trying to hold back), you may fall into this category.

Delayed ejaculation isn't a common problem. In fact, there aren't good statistics on how often it occurs, but it becomes more common as you age, occurring more frequently in men over the age of 50.

Prevention & Risk Factors: There are a number of factors that increase your chances of delayed ejaculation. They include:

Emotional issues, like fear or guilt. Typically, men with delayed ejaculation are trying to cope with some sort of emotional issue about the sexual encounter. Perhaps you're fearful that your partner will get pregnant, or you feel guilty about having sex because of your religious upbringing. If you're able to ejaculate quickly when you masturbate, it could be an indication that the problem during partner sex is emotional rather than physical.

Alcohol consumption. Drinking too much dulls your senses, which means that your ability to feel the sensations in your penis—a critical element in ejaculation—will be diminished as well.

Health problems. Although rarely the culprit, it's worth discussing whether a health problem like diabetes could be contributing to your problem.

Medications. In some men, medications like antidepressants or anti-inflammatory drugs can interfere with the ability to ejaculate.

Diagnosis & Screening: If you feel you take too long to ejaculate, describe the problem to your doctor. You will undergo a physical exam, and your doctor will ask you a number of questions about the problem. It's important that you convey not only physical details, but emotional ones as well, because they often are the underlying cause of delayed ejaculation. Depending on the likely cause, your doctor may refer you to a sex therapist, a psychotherapist, or a urologist.

Treatment Options: The course of treatment will depend on what's at the root of your problem. A sex therapist will give you tools to explore your feelings about sex as well as offer suggestions for alternatives, including hand or mouth stimulation, that may help you ejaculate more quickly. A psychotherapist may want to treat you individually or include your partner in the process to clear away any emotional roadblocks. And a urologist will treat physical problems that could be interfering with your ability to ejaculate.

Premature Ejaculation

The Basics: In contrast to delayed ejaculation, the cause of premature ejaculation is usually unknown. Most men feel the desire to ejaculate within two or three minutes of initiating sexual contact that involves stimulation of the penis. So the definition of "premature" is very much influenced by the desires of a given couple.

There aren't good statistics on premature ejaculation, but it's thought to be the most common sexual complaint among men, and it probably affects all men at least occasionally in their sexual lives. It's more common in young or sexually inexperienced men.

Prevention & Risk Factors: Certain factors may increase the likelihood of premature ejaculation. They include:

Age and inexperience. Young men are more likely to ejaculate sooner than they'd like, because they haven't yet learned to control their sexual responses.

Emotional issues, like fear or guilt. If you're afraid of getting your partner pregnant, say, or catching a sexually transmitted disease, it may cause you to ejaculate too early. Likewise, if you feel that sex is bad or shameful, it can interfere with your ability to prevent quick ejaculation.

Diagnosis & Screening: Although the timing of ejaculation is somewhat arbitrary, if it happens before you actually engage in intercourse or within seconds of insertion, or if your partner is routinely dissatisfied, you should talk to your doctor about what you can do to combat the problem. You'll be asked a number of questions about how and when ejaculation typically occurs, and your doctor may refer you to a sex therapist or psychologist for treatment.

Treatment Options: If underlying relationship issues are the root of the problem, a couples therapist can help you sort them out by talking about what's happening between you and your partner. Likewise, a therapist trained to treat sexual problems may recommend a variety of strategies to help delay ejaculation. They are successful about 95 percent of the time.

Stop-and-start method. In this treatment, you engage in sexual activity until you feel like you're about to ejaculate. To prevent ejaculation, you need to stop the stimulation for about 30 seconds, then start again. You continue in this vein until both you and your partner are ready for you to ejaculate.

Squeeze method. With this method, you have a normal

sexual encounter until you feel like you're about to ejaculate, at which point you or your partner gently squeezes the tip or base of your penis for a few seconds. Wait about 30 seconds before resuming sexual contact and repeat the procedure until both you and your partner are ready for you to ejaculate.

Biofeedback. This therapy helps you become aware of the muscles that control ejaculation and learn to relax them at will in order to control the timing of ejaculation.

Different sexual positions. The traditional man-on-top position is probably the most difficult in which to control ejaculation because it's more likely to stimulate the delicate nerve endings at the tip of your penis. Try instead the side-lying position or have your partner be on top.

Antidepressants. Some studies have found that low doses of antidepressant medications such as Prozac and Zoloft can slow down ejaculation, in many cases with dramatic effect.

Impotence (Erectile Dysfunction)

The Basics: One definition of impotence is the inability to sustain an erection that's sufficiently firm for intercourse more than 25 percent of the time. Your penis has two chambers filled with muscles, veins and arteries that run from its base to its tip. When you get an erection, physical and mental stimulation cause the muscles in these chambers to relax, making extra space for blood to flow into them. As the chambers fill with blood, your penis expands and stiffens.

There are a number of problems that can interfere with the process of getting and maintaining an erection, including diseases that damage the arteries, muscles, and tissues of the penis; pelvic surgery that injures nerves and arteries near the penis; many medications; and psychological issues. Whereas it was once believed that most impotence was psychological, it is now thought that more than 80 percent of cases of erectile dysfunction are caused by physical problems.

Impotence is a common problem, affecting as many as 30 million men in the U.S. Although it can strike at any age, it's most common in men over the age of 50. The problem occurs in about 5 percent of 40-year-olds and as many as 25 percent of 65-year-olds. That said, it's not a necessary consequence of aging.

Prevention & Risk Factors: A wide variety of problems can interfere with your ability to sustain an erection. They include:

Diseases. Diabetes, kidney disease, alcoholism, atherosclerosis, vascular disease, and multiple sclerosis all can prevent normal erections, making physical illnesses the number one cause of the problem. Between 35 and 50 percent of men with diabetes struggle with impotence.

Medications. Certain drugs, including hypertension drugs, antihistamines, antidepressants, appetite suppressants, and tranquilizers, can interfere with the impulses from the brain and nerves that tell the muscles in your penis to relax.

Prostate surgery. If you suffer nerve or artery damage during prostate surgery, you may be left with erectile dysfunction.

Smoking. Because it affects blood flow, smoking can interfere with sexual functioning.

Recreational drug use. Alcohol, cocaine, and marijuana all can compromise your ability to get an erection.

Low testosterone. Adequate levels of this male hormone are necessary to maintain an erection. Overall testosterone deficiency is an uncommon cause of impotence.

Emotional issues, like stress, guilt, and fear of sexual failure. Although it's not usually the primary cause of impotence, emotional issues often play a contributing role in many cases.

Long-term bicycle riding. Although doctors are uncertain of the connection, some believe that spending hours on a hard bicycle seat can injure the nerves and blood vessels that are crucial to getting an erection. They recommend standing up on your pedals occasionally to relieve the pressure in the area, avoiding bumpy roads, and wearing padded shorts and using bike seats that are specially designed to provide a gentler ride.

Diagnosis & Screening: Your doctor will diagnose erectile dysfunction based on a wide variety of information, including your medical history and medication use; your sexual history; and a complete physical exam. Your doctor also may perform one or several of the following diagnostic tests:

Blood tests. Analysis of your blood may be able to reveal underlying diseases that could be contributing to erectile dysfunction.

Hormone measurements. If low testosterone is playing a role, you can pinpoint it by checking your hormone levels.

Nocturnal penile erection test. Since healthy men typically have two to five erections while they sleep, this test, in which a pressure-sensitive strap is placed over your penis during sleep to detect any nighttime erections, can help your doctor find out whether there's some underlying physical problem that's interfering with your ability to attain an erection. If you have erections during sleep, it is likely that psychological issues are the cause of your problem.

Ultrasound. This test can measure blood flow into and out of your penis.

Psychosocial examination. This evaluation may highlight psychological factors that may be contributing to the problem.

Treatment Options: Once your doctor has diagnosed impotence, a course of treatment may include one or a combination of the following options:

Viagra (sildenafil). I begin the list of treatment options with this medication because it is usually the first choice today in both self and physician directed treatment for impotence. It is also being widely used by men who obtain it through the internet and black market sources without a physician's direction. Therefore it is important to know the pros and cons of Viagra use.

Viagra acts by boosting levels of a natural chemical called guanosine monophosphate that causes blood vessels in the penis to enlarge, increasing blood flow into the penis. (It actually acts indirectly by blocking the enzyme that normally inactivates guanosine monophosphate.) It is important to understand certain facts about Viagra, including:

- The drug by itself does not increase sexual desire and will only act if a man is sexually aroused.
- Various reports indicate that anywhere from 10 to 30 percent of men using Viagra will have minor side effects ranging from headaches, facial flushing, and stomach upset to temporary visual changes that distort colors and brightness. However, potentially fatal drops in blood pressure can occur in men who also take nitrate medicines for heart disease. Nitrate drugs should therefore not be used in combination with Viagra. Indeed, any man with heart disease should be cleared by his cardiologist before using Viagra.
- There is no good evidence that the drug will improve erections in young, perfectly health men. However, since most men as they age have at least some degree of blockage in their arterial system, including the arteries carrying blood to the penis, it can often enhance sexual performance in such men.
- It works well in the majority of men with impotence, although it is less likely to work when severe diabetes or spinal cord injury is the cause of impotence.
- The drug is not effective in all men, and it is not effec-

tive in all attempts in a given man. Some experts report that it will not work in anywhere from 20 to 40 percent of men who try it.

Other medications. Alprostadil is another medication that can increase blood flow into the penis. It can be injected into the base of the penis (a procedure that most men find less distasteful in actual use than it sounds) or placed inside the tip of the penis in pellet form. Because it is not absorbed into the bloodstream, it does not produce side effects elsewhere in the body, although it can produce pain at the injection or insertion site. Unlike Viagra, it produces an erection in the absence of mental sexual excitement. Experts report about a 90 percent success rate with injection. There are several other medications now in the research pipeline but not yet approved by the Food and Drug Administration.

Testosterone. Given in shots or skin patches, this male hormone can be helpful for the approximately 5 percent of men with hormone deficiency.

Vacuum devices. To use this device, you place your penis in a plastic tube, then pump air out of the tube to create a vacuum around your penis. This action pulls blood into your penis, and, in order to maintain the erection, you place a plastic band around the base of your penis to keep the blood in your penis. You can leave it on safely for about a half hour.

Surgery. There are several procedures that a surgeon can do to help you get erections, including implanting an erection-causing device into your penis; reconstructing your arteries to increase blood flow to your penis; or repairing any veins that allow blood to leak from the tissues of your penis.

Yohimbine hydrochloride. This substance found in tree bark has been used for ages as an aphrodisiac, but controlled clinical trials have yet to prove that it's effective. Even so, some men say they benefit from it.

Infertility

The Basics: The ability to impregnate a woman depends on a number of factors, including the timing of intercourse, hormonal factors, and the quality and quantity of your sperm. Probably the most important component of male fertility is your sperm's ability to swim quickly and in a straight line — qualities referred to as "motility." When you ejaculate, you release between 100 and 600 million sperm, but even in the best of circumstances only about 15 percent are healthy enough to fertilize a woman's egg. Because a woman's vagina is a fairly hostile environment for sperm, only about 100 or so are able to survive long enough to make it to a woman's fallopian tubes, where the egg is usually waiting, and typically, only one is likely to actually penetrate the outer coating of the egg and achieve fertilization.

Sixty percent of couples conceive a child within six months of having unprotected intercourse, and 85 percent of couples conceive within the first year. Infertility is usually defined as the inability to conceive after one year of regular, unprotected intercourse. If, after a year, your partner hasn't become pregnant, one or both of you could have a problem with fertility. About one in 10 couples in the U.S. are infertile, and in about a third of those cases, the cause is male infertility, and in another third, it is female. In the remainder, both partners may have difficulty conceiving or the cause is unknown. Although experts long believed that male sperm quality started declining at about age 40, newer information seems to show that is doesn't change significantly until your mid-60s.

Prevention & Risk Factors: Certain factors can have an impact on either the quality or quantity of your sperm, or both. They include:

- Testicle problems, including a physical injury, varicose veins in the scrotum (known as a varicocele), sperm duct blockages, or testicular damage from infections like mumps.

- Use of alcohol; cigarettes; illegal drugs, including anabolic steroids and cocaine; and medications, including cimetidine (Tagamet), sulfasalazine (Azulfidine), corticosteroids, and phenytoin (Dilantin).
- Retrograde ejaculation. Men with this problem ejaculate into their bladders instead of through their penises.
- Sexually transmitted diseases.
- Hormonal abnormalities.
- Radiation treatment to the groin area.
- Temporary low sperm counts can be caused by high fever, stress, overheating (from baths or even tight underwear), excessive exercise, obesity, and low levels of dietary selenium and zinc.

Diagnosis & Screening: If you and your partner are having trouble getting pregnant, your doctor will perform a number of tests as well as take an extensive medical history. Since more than 90 percent of male infertility is caused by low sperm counts, poor sperm quality, or both, the most important screening test your doctor will perform is to analyze a sample of your sperm. There are several categories of abnormal sperm production.

- Oligospermia means you have fewer than 20 million sperm per cubic centimeter of semen.
- Azoospermia means you have no sperm at all.
- Dysspermia means you have low quality sperm. If at least 50 percent of your sperm swim normally, you have average quality sperm, but if less than 40 percent are able to move in a straight line, your sperm motility is considered "low quality."

Treatment Options: The treatment approach your doctor takes depends in large part on what is causing the problem. You may be put on medication if you have a hormone deficiency or infection, or your doctor may recommend surgery if a sperm duct is blocked or you have a scrotal varicose vein that seems to be causing the problem. If you have retrograde ejaculation, poor sperm quality, or a low sperm count, your doctor may try to place your sperm in your partner's uterus when she is ovulating (artificial insemination) to try to achieve a pregnancy.

More recently, researchers have developed a technique whereby a single sperm can be directly inserted into the female egg. Known as intracytoplasmic sperm injection (ICSI), this technique is used as part of the process of in-vitro fertilization (IVF) in which the egg is fertilized in the lab and any resulting embryo is then implanted in the woman's uterus. Obviously such advanced techniques require real expertise and it is important to do your homework in finding a competent fertility specialist and clinic, especially since the fertility industry is still largely unregulated. I think that two questions are especially important to ask of any fertility clinic:

What is the live birth rate? Clinics often report their pregnancy rates, which can be much higher than the rate of actual successful "take-home" results. In interpreting these results it is also important to know the kind of problems being treated. Some clinics can stack their results with easier cases.

What is the rate of multiple births? Some clinics try to achieve better success rates by implanting more embryos in the uterus than is ideal, and that practice should be reflected in a higher than average multiple birth rate.

Finally, I cannot resist pointing out that adoption may be a wonderful alternative to fertility treatment for couples who cannot achieve pregnancy. I know many couples (including my wife and I) who have been so blessed.

Family Planning

Most men spend years trying to avoid making their partners pregnant. It can be the focus of much of our reproductive lives. Choosing a birth control method requires thought and discussion with your partner, since the majority of commonly used birth control options are made for women. The ideal contraceptive fits your lifestyle, is easy to use, and is reliable. For instance, if you're in a monogamous relationship, the type you use may be different than if you're single and dating. Following are the most widely used methods of birth control:

Abstinence and natural family planning (the "rhythm method"). Natural family planning involves abstaining from sexual intercourse during the times of the month when your partner is fertile, which is slightly before and during ovulation. There are several ways your partner can track ovulation, including taking her temperature every morning. The rhythm method works if you're religious about tracking ovulation, but that can be a tall order. About 25 percent of people who use this method get pregnant during the first year.

Barrier methods. The condom is the barrier method of choice for men. In addition, your partner has a number of barrier options, including the female condom, the diaphragm, the cervical cap, or the contraceptive sponge. Used correctly and consistently, the male condom is an effective method of contraception, with about a 3 percent accidental pregnancy rate in the first year of use. Couples who don't use it consistently have a 14 percent pregnancy rate, however. The cervical cap has anywhere from a 9 to 40 percent accidental pregnancy rate, and the diaphragm has a 6 to 20 percent accidental pregnancy rate.

Withdrawal. Withdrawing your penis from your partner's vagina prior to ejaculation has roughly a 4 percent accidental pregnancy rate in couples that have been using the method consistently and correctly for about a year. That rate jumps to 19 percent in couples who aren't as conscientious.

Other female contraceptive measures. Such measures include the birth control pill, an implanted intrauterine device, and hormones by injection.

For women: the morning-after or missed-period pills. If you think you might have had sex at a time when your partner was fertile, you can still prevent pregnancy if she takes the so-called morning-after pill for five days after unprotected intercourse.

Sterilization. During vasectomy, a doctor cuts or ties off the tubes (called vas deferens) that carry sperm out of your testicles. The procedure takes less than a half hour, is very safe, and is usually done under local anesthesia. The failure rate for vasectomy is very low and any potential complications (such as bleeding, scrotal swelling, or infection) are usually minor.

Reversal of vasectomy is quite possible today and depends upon the length of time since the surgery, the skill of the surgeon, and the extent of the original procedure. Subsequent pregnancy rates range from 20 to 60 percent. If a large amount of the vas deferens has been removed, reversal is less likely.

Your partner could also have a tubal ligation. This female sterilization procedure interrupts the continuity of the fallopian tubes, which transport the eggs to the uterus.

Making Sperm (Spermatogenesis)

Males begin making sperm at about age 12, thanks to the influence of male hormones, which trigger special cells in your testicles. Your body stores sperm cells in the ductus deferens until they're used for ejaculation.

The sperm-making process is sensitive to heat. So wearing tight clothes, which increases the temperature in your testicles, or taking hot baths can reduce your sperm count dramatically. Although it's not reliable enough to use as a form of contraception, heat can interfere with your attempts to conceive if you and your partner are trying to get pregnant.

PART THREE

Minding the Mind

Let's say, for the sake of argument, that you're a paragon of physical health. You actually go to the doctor for checkups and screenings. You're careful about what you eat, and, when you do indulge in the occasional hot-dog-and-chips meal, you're conscientious about following it with one that contains an extra helping or two of good things that come directly from the earth (think: broccoli, carrots, apples). You're a regular at the gym or in your home basement, where you do both strength training for your skeletal muscles and aerobic exercise for your heart. You even routinely use sunscreen! So, you've got your bases covered, right?

Not so fast. If you're not paying attention to the mass of nerve cells and chemicals that makes up your "gray matter," you're still missing a big component of overall health and well-being—with a surprisingly strong emphasis on the former. Study after study has found that what's going on in your brain can affect more than just your mood. Depression, stress, and hostility—and the lack of sleep that often accompanies those problems—might suppress your immune system, making you more susceptible to everyday illnesses like the common cold and maybe even potentially life-threatening diseases. Depression can also lead men especially to self-medicate, typically with addictive substances such as drugs or alcohol, which—in addition to exacerbating depression—can also take a terrible toll on the body.

On the flip side, understanding a little about what makes your mind tick, and taking the time to keep your "mental muscles" as fit as your physical ones, can help you function more efficiently at work, get more joy out of play, have more satisfying interpersonal relationships, and feel more fulfilled about your life in general. In the next few chapters, you'll find a guide to the most important health issues that originate in the often-overlooked recesses of the mind, with some emphasis on issues often especially difficult for men.

Are Emotional Problems Really Illnesses?

As a young physician many years ago, I shared the then general attitude that "emotional" problems could and should be solved by "willpower" and "tincture of time." However, the dramatic discoveries about brain chemistry of the past several decades—and several dramatic personal encounters with effective drug treatment of emotional/psychological upheavals in close friends—have convinced me that many if not most of these problems are caused in large part by biochemical changes in our brain. I admit that our understanding of these changes is still far from precise and that our medical treatments are still often lacking in pinpoint application to a very specific biochemical target. But even the imprecise understandings and resulting treatment we now use is so often dramatically effective that it reinforces the concept of "chemical imbalance" as the major cause of many of these problems. Therefore I believe the word "illness" is the correct one. And the analogy so often used today—that treating mental illness with medication is like treating diabetes with insulin—is, I think, largely correct even though I would admit that our understanding of the biochemistry of diabetes is more advanced and precise.

At this point I also want to raise a very sensitive and complicated issue—namely whether our society and our health care system is encouraging the overuse of medications as an "easy answer" to life's problems—and a way to save money for the health care system by avoiding costly psychotherapy. Indeed, some of the newer medications for depression and anxiety (see below) are usually so safe and effective that many primary care physicians are prescribing them for their patients without ever referring them to a mental health professional for evaluation and treatment. That in turn has some in the mental health field crying foul—saying that such a quick fix approach is denying people with emotional illnesses the benefit of a combination approach, namely medications to quickly help relieve symptoms and psychotherapy to explore possible underlying personal, social, and family dynamics that might be contributing to the problem. Obviously this is a debate that is not going to be quickly settled but it is an important one because we should not let professional or economic bias prevent our using what is truly best for the person who is suffering.

How Do You Know If You Need Help?

Before proceeding to specific problems, I think it is important to address two generic questions: How do I decide when I should seek professional help for emotional or mental problems? And what kind of professional should I go to for these kinds of problems? The first question is often difficult to answer because it involves trying to separate the normal ups and downs of life from those situations that are potentially more serious. One study conducted by the American Psychological Association found that nearly half of all people in the U.S. don't know when it's appropriate to see a mental health professional. I am going to offer one very simple way of deciding: If the question "Do I need help?" even enters your mind, it is probably time to seek help.

But now comes an even more difficult question—where do I go for help? If you have a good relationship with a primary care physician, that is usually a very good place to begin. *(See page 68 for information on finding a primary care physician.)* Such physicians have a lot of experience in referring their patients to mental health professionals since these problems are so common, and they have had a chance to learn which ones work best for different kinds of problems. But even with such guidance, it is helpful to know something about the different kinds of professionals available so I will list them with a brief description of each:

Psychiatrist. A physician who has specialized in mental health with at least four years of training after medical school. Like all licensed physicians, psychiatrists can prescribe medications and admit people to the hospital when necessary.

Psychologist. A non-physician who has postgraduate training in mental health, often a Ph.D. in clinical psychology. Psychologists cannot prescribe medications but they often work closely with psychiatrists who will do so for their patients when necessary.

Psychiatric social worker. As the name suggests, a person trained in social work with further special training, usually a master's degree, in areas of mental health such as drug abuse or family counseling. Such professionals often work in an agency setting or with psychiatrists and/or psychologists.

Psychoanalyst. A person who has had special training in the form of therapy known as psychoanalysis, a form of therapy that explores past relationships and experiences and how they impact our behaviors and relationships in the present. Psychoanalysts receive three to five years of postgraduate training at what are called psychoanalytic institutes. Many psychologists and social workers are also trained in psychoanalysis.

Therapist. A person who wants to call himself a therapist can do so regardless of any specific training. Usually "therapists" have one of the kinds of degrees described above, but it is always worth asking about the specifics. Therapists who work in hospitals or recognized mental health agencies are almost certain to have legitimate training and credentials.

Again, if you are being guided in your choice by your primary care physician, you will probably not have to worry about these choices. I will point out that most primary care physicians, because they are physicians themselves, will tend to have a bias toward psychiatrists, who are also physicians. And there is often a "turf battle" between psychiatrists and psychologists as to which can provide the "best" help for people suffering from mental and/or emotional problems. Psychiatrists argue that because they are also trained as physicians, they can provide the "complete" diagnostic and treatment package, including medications when necessary. This complete package comes at a price: Psychiatrists' fees are typically much higher than those of psychologists or social workers. Psychologists argue that they have often spent more time in actual psychological testing and psychotherapy (often described as "talking therapy") and are therefore less likely to quickly and unnecessarily prescribe medications. My own opinion is that it is much more important to find the personality right for you rather than deciding which kind of professional is best.

So if you are faced with an emotional problem, what should you do? Again, if you have a good relationship with your primary care physician, I would trust him or her to make the right recommendation. But ultimately, you are the one who has to feel comfortable with the person you are seeing and you shouldn't hesitate to ask for a change if you are not satisfied with your care or progress.

Finally, I will tend to use the words "mental" and "emotional" and "psychological" interchangeably. Experts like to make distinctions but for our purposes, they all refer to the same arena of concerns.

CHAPTER 8

Depression and Other Mood Disorders

Let's face it: The area north of our neck is *terra incognita* for lots of men. We tend to ignore psychological problems, and, even in the new millennium, there's still enough of the leather-hide cowboy in many of us to feel uneasy when it comes to acknowledging and dealing with our emotions.

Unfortunately, such attitudes can be life threatening. Although almost twice as many women as men suffer from serious depression (2 to 4 percent of men as opposed to 4 to 8 percent of women in any given year), depressed men are much more likely to take their own lives, a fact that experts blame in part on many men's reluctance to acknowledge their illness and seek treatment. In other words, neglecting the mental component in your overall stay-healthy approach could leave you not just unhappy, but dead. Enough said.

Forms and Faces of Depression

Approximately 19 million adults in the U.S. suffer from some form of depression, and a recent study sponsored by the World Health Organization and the World Bank found that major depression is the leading cause of disability not only in the U.S. but worldwide.

Given its prevalence and its undeniable economic impact, you'd think we'd all be as familiar with this illness as we are with the flu—that we'd easily be able to recognize its symptoms and readily see a doctor when we feel we're sick. But the truth is, there's still a stigma attached to emotional problems, especially depression, perhaps because it doesn't jibe with the typical "pull-yourself-up-by-your-bootstraps" American mentality so often still embraced by men as the "ideal."

Although effective treatments have been available for years, many people—again, especially men—still believe that they can talk themselves out of even serious depression, much like they'd talk themselves out of a passing bad mood. Another common myth is that depression is somehow your own fault, that it's a sign of a weak character—a characterization that goes deeply against the grain of most men. As a result, as many as two-thirds of people suffering from this illness never receive treatment (again, men are more likely to suffer in silence than women), despite the fact that scientific studies have consistently shown that about 80 percent of people who are treated will get much better.

The most important first step in overcoming the shame attached to seeking treatment for depression is to truly accept that depression is a disease with proven physiological components. In fact, the most recent brain imaging technologies have shown that the brains of depressed people often function differently than those of people who are not depressed. Many experts now believe that depression is usually caused by an imbalance in the brain's neurotransmitters, the chemicals that help nerve cells communicate with one another.

There are three main types of depression. Here's a rundown of their signs and symptoms.

Clinical depression

Clinical depression is sometimes called major depressive disorder or unipolar major depression. It is the type most of us think of when we hear the word depression. Symptoms typically include:

- A persistent feeling of sadness.
- Loss of interest or pleasure in activities that you once enjoyed, including sex.
- A significant change in appetite or body weight (some people lose weight, others gain it).
- Trouble sleeping or excessive sleepiness.
- Feeling physically slowed down, or, conversely, feeling anxious and agitated.
- Loss of energy.
- Feelings of worthlessness or guilt.
- Problems thinking, concentrating, remembering, or making decisions.
- Recurrent thoughts of death or suicide.

Your doctor will usually make a diagnosis of clinical depression if you have five or more of these symptoms over the course of two or more weeks. Clinical depression can range from mild, which typically means that you have a handful of symptoms and feel somewhat affected by it in your everyday activities, to severe, which means you have a majority of the symptoms and it almost always prevents you from participating in your normal daily activities.

No matter how severe it is, depression tends to be recurrent. Studies have shown that the relapse rate after having one bout of depression is about 50 percent, and after two bouts about 70 percent. University of Washington researchers recently found that certain personalities may be more prone to recurrences. In their study, the people at the highest risk for recurrent bouts of major depression were more likely to be hostile and aggressive, have low levels of dependency on other people, and report lower levels of satisfaction from recreational activities.

Bipolar disorder

The second main type of depression, bipolar disorder (also known as manic-depressive illness), affects about 1 in 100 people and is characterized by bouts of major depression alternating with periods of abnormally elevated mood, or mania. People who suffer from this illness go beyond the normal mood swings we all experience now and then. The manic phase of the disease is typically characterized by at least three of the following additional symptoms:

- A grandiose sense of self esteem.

- A decreased need for sleep.
- Increased talkativeness.
- Racing thoughts.
- Distractability; physical agitation or increased goal-directed activity.
- Participating in pleasurable activities that carry a high risk of painful consequences, such as wild spending sprees leading to significant debt.

The "high" and "low" episodes that characterize bipolar disorder are unpredictable. They can last anywhere from several days to several months, and in between, sufferers often feel completely normal.

Dysthymia

Also called dysthymic disorder, dysthymia is a less severe but more chronic form of depression. In fact, one of the criteria for a diagnosis of dysthymia is feeling sad and blue for at least two years. Sufferers typically have at least two of the other symptoms of major depression (see above) as well. People who suffer from dysthymia are more likely to have a bout of full clinical depression at some point in their lives, so even though it's less serious than the other forms of the illness, treatment is still critical.

Recognizing Depression

Depression goes beyond the normal blues or sadness that most of us experience during the typical upheavals of everyday life. It's a true medical disorder. How do you distinguish depression from run-of-the-mill melancholy? In order to receive a medical diagnosis of depression, you usually have one of two key symptoms—loss of interest in things you used to enjoy, whether it's golfing, work, food, or sex; and feeling sad, blue, or down in the dumps—for most of the day every day for at least two weeks. In addition, you usually have at least three of the other symptoms of clinical depression listed above. If you don't meet all the criteria for true depression but have some of the symptoms, you may have dysthymia or a very mild form of the illness, both of which should be brought to your doctor's attention.

Depressed people often have a number of other physical or psychological symptoms, including headaches, other physical aches and pains, digestive problems, sexual problems, excessive pessimism and anxiety, or excessive worry. If you feel you might be suffering from depression, it's worth mentioning your symptoms to your doctor, who may refer you to a mental health specialist.

Causes of Depression

Because depression seems to run in families, leading researchers believe that there's a significant genetic component to the illness. It also can be caused by a variety of other factors, from physical illness or medications to alcohol or drug abuse. Traumatic experiences, like the loss of a loved one or a career crisis, can trigger a bout, especially in someone who is genetically predisposed to the illness. Depression may also be caused by the emotional environment in which you grew up. But keep in mind that it also can occur out of the blue, with no discernible cause, and can come on gradually, so that your withdrawal from activities and people is barely noticeable as it is happening. Bipolar disorder has a genetic component as well, but it also can be precipitated by another medical health problem, like a head injury or certain neurologic conditions.

In recent years experts have also identified lack of sunlight during the winter, and especially in more northern or southern regions of the earth with longer nights, as a major cause of depression. (It is usually labeled as SAD, for seasonal affective disorder.) The exact cause of this phenomenon is far from certain; one theory is that sufferers have excess melatonin, a hormone that is related to wake cycles and light. Whatever the cause or causes, this disorder usually responds to "light therapy" that is much brighter than ordinary indoor lights. However, many people with apparent SAD will also respond to standard medications for regular depression (see below).

Treatment Options

Because of the potentially dire consequences, getting prompt treatment for depression is important, especially since it can become more firmly entrenched and more difficult to treat the longer it remains unaddressed. With treatment, you may start feeling better as quickly as two to three weeks after starting treatment. Some people need to try several different forms of treatment before they find the one that works the best for them. Following are the most often prescribed treatments for depression:

Antidepressants. Most experts believe these drugs work by influencing the levels of certain neurotransmitters, or chemicals, in the brain, including serotonin (a "feel-good" chemical) and norepinephrine, a hormone that's closely related to epinephrine, or adrenaline. Older antidepressant medications include tricyclic antidepressants (TCAs) and monoamine oxidase inhibitors (MAOIs), and they affect both of these neurotransmitters simultaneously.

Selective serotonin reuptake inhibitors (SSRIs), a newer class of antidepressants, include drugs like Prozac, Zoloft, and Paxil. Most scientists believe that SSRIs work by increasing the amount of serotonin in the brain. It's worth noting, however, that scientists still aren't sure exactly how antidepressants work or why they alleviate the symptoms of depression. Moreover, antidepressants aren't without problems. They can diminish sex drive, and some experts believe that long-term use may be linked to other physical problems such as facial tics. In general, however, SSRIs tend to have fewer side effects than the older antidepressants, which is one reason they have become so popular.

Psychotherapy. Although traditionally thought of as a viable stand-alone treatment only for mild to moderate depression, psychotherapy has recently been gaining adherents as a treatment for all forms of depression. Two types of psychotherapy in particular have gained new respect:

- Cognitive behavioral therapy teaches people to identify negative or distorted thoughts that contribute to their feelings of hopelessness and helplessness—and then attempts to help people control or even eliminate such thoughts.
- Interpersonal therapy helps people pinpoint and cope with the life problems that contribute to the depression.

A 1999 study published in the American Journal of Psychiatry reviewed the previous evidence showing that antidepressants are more effective than psychotherapy in treating major depression and came up with a different conclusion. When the researchers combined the results of four studies, they found that cognitive behavioral therapy is as effective as medication in treating severely depressed people.

St. John's Wort

The jury is still out on this herbal supplement, because studies conducted thus far have yielded conflicting results. Proponents speculate that it works by preventing certain enzymes from destroying mood-boosting brain chemicals like serotonin and dopamine. If you'd like to try the herb, make sure you check with your doctor first, because St. John's wort (also called hypericum) has been shown to interfere with the effectiveness of a number of other drugs, including indinavir, a protease inhibitor used to treat HIV, and cyclosporine, a drug used to reduce the risk of organ transplant rejection.

However, such studies are very difficult to do and many experts still feel that medications are more predictably effective, even though they often take several weeks to produce results.

A combination approach. Typically, a mental health professional will suggest that you try both antidepressants and therapy at the same time, a tactic that has been shown to often yield superior results. A combination treatment is beneficial because, while the medication typically relieves the symptoms of depression in the short term, the therapy can help change your underlying beliefs, attitudes and orientation toward the world. Then, when and if you go off the drugs, you may be better able to cope on your own—and prevent a recurrence down the line.

In about 20 percent of people, depression doesn't respond to standard treatments, according to statistics from the National Institute of Mental Health. Two options are available for this resistant type of illness:

Electroconvulsive treatment (ECT). This treatment, in which an electrical current is passed through the brain, has been shown to be 80 to 90 percent effective in treating severe depression in the short term, perhaps because the electricity alters the sensitivity of the brain's norepinephrine and serotonin receptors. Although it is still regarded as primitive in the public mind, ECT actually has grown in popularity in recent years, because studies have shown that newer methods are usually effective and much less traumatic than with previous techniques. Repeated treatments often are necessary to achieve the desired response, and memory loss is a common side effect, but it is usually short lived. Although it's usually very helpful in relieving depression, there is a high rate of relapse after ECT, so most doctors use it in conjunction with psychotherapy and continual medication.

Vagus nerve stimulation (VNS). VNS is used to treat severe epileptic seizures and may hold promise for treatment-resistant depression. In a study at Baylor College of Medicine in Houston, nearly half of 60 subjects who received the treatment, which requires people to have a pacemaker-like generator implanted in the chest and connected via electrodes to the vagus nerve in the neck, were significantly better after one year. Experts believe VNS may work because the electrical stimulation increases the activity of some neurotransmitters, like serotonin, while decreasing the activity of others. More trials of the approach are under way. Some researchers are also experimenting with implanted electrodes in the brain.

Enhancing Your Recovery

The following activities should also be done in conjunction with any therapy to enhance the recovery process. The most surefire mood-lifting strategies include:

Exercise regularly. A number of studies over the past 20 years have shown that exercise can boost the effectiveness of psychotherapy. It not only provides a sense of accomplishment and fulfillment but also combats the feelings of lethargy and listlessness that usually accompany depression. Likewise, people who exercise regularly are less likely to get depressed, perhaps because physical activity causes the brain to release chemicals called endorphins, the body's natural "uppers." I personally have found that my general mood improves when I exercise regularly.

Maintain a support system. Whether they're family members or close friends, having a few people on tap who you can talk to when you're feeling down or struggling with an issue can often help enormously. And, if you're in treatment for depression, such support can help you meet your goals. For instance, a friend can remind you to practice the coping techniques or problem-solving skills you've learned in therapy or to take your medicine.

Keep caffeine and alcohol to a minimum. Artificial stimulants like caffeine may boost your mood temporarily, but when the feeling wears off, your mood can plummet. Alcohol is even more deceptive. While it gives you an initial warm glow, it is actually a nervous system depressant—the last thing you need when you're feeling low. Unfortunately, it's a common coping tool, especially for men who are struggling with depression. Numerous studies have found that depression is a main cause of problem drinking and that drinking, in turn, fuels the feelings of hopelessness and sadness.

Eat fish. Tuna, sardines, and salmon are chock-full of a type of fat called omega-3 fatty acids. Research has shown that omega-3s may help keep the neurotransmitters in your brain at optimal levels. And such fish can also help prevent heart disease. *(For information on fish and heart disease, see page 14.)*

Find time to do things you enjoy. Although one of the main symptoms of depression is loss of interest in pleasurable activities, it's even more important to push yourself to participate in things you enjoy when you're going through a rough patch emotionally. Having a variety of interests can help prevent the social withdrawal that often characterizes extreme depression.

Maintain a consistent sleep/wake schedule. Going to bed and getting up at the same time each morning may help keep your brain chemicals on an even keel.

It is important to note that none of these activities will "cure" a serious case of depression. However, they can help elevate your mood and will certainly contribute to your overall wellness.

Anxiety Disorders

You feel constantly worried about finances, your health, or your children. You live in dread of the day when you'll have to make a major presentation at work. You're plagued by ugly thoughts that you can't seem to control.

All of these scenarios (and many more) are typical of people suffering from anxiety disorders, now thought to be the most common form of emotional illness in the U.S. Every year, more than 19 million Americans between the ages of 18 and 54 struggle with the frustration and fear that often accompanies this broad category of problems. Although most people experience some feelings of anxiety before an athletic event, a business presentation, or an important exam, people with anxiety disorders are often so consumed by feelings of worry and fear that they avoid any situation in which they're likely to have to face an elevated degree of stress. In a small percentage of people, the illness becomes so severe that they're actually housebound, a condition known as agoraphobia, or "fear of the market place."

Anxiety disorders are complex and probably stem from a number of different causes, including genetic, behavioral, and developmental, but they seem to center on a small structure tucked deep inside the brain, the amygdala. The amygdala is the primitive part of the brain that causes your body to react—to fight or flee—from dangerous situations even before your mind has a chance to process what's happening: That car is coming toward me fast! Those kinds of responses became ingrained in the amygdala. It remembers that you felt fear in a particular setting or situation, and even one or two severe amygdala-stimulating experiences are sometimes enough to make the most benign situations—going to the supermarket, say, or to a party—fraught with anxiety.

There are several main types of anxiety disorders, each with distinctive symptoms and characteristics. Although as with most emotional disorders, statistics suggest that they're more likely to strike women than men, it's worth noting that men may simply be less likely to seek help for these types of problems. Here's a summary of the most common kinds of anxiety disorders:

Generalized anxiety disorder

People with generalized anxiety disorder (GAD) have recurring fears or exaggerated worries about everything from their health and relationships to their financial well-being and professional responsibilities. Although the feeling can wax and wane, it's usually exacerbated by stress. In order to receive a formal diagnosis of GAD, you need to be stuck in worry mode for six months or more. In most people, the feeling of anxiety is accompanied by an unshakable sense of dread, as well as a variety of physical symptoms, such as muscle tension, poor concentration, insomnia, irritability, and fatigue. The cause of the intense feelings of anxiety is often hard to identify (hence the term "generalized"), but the feelings are real and can prevent you from functioning in a normal way. The condition eventually strikes about 3 percent of people in the U.S., half of whom start experiencing symptoms in childhood.

Panic disorder

People with panic disorder are prone to panic attacks—episodes of sudden, intense fear or discomfort, accompanied by physical symptoms like heart palpitations, sweating, trembling, shortness of breath, sensations of choking or smothering, chest pain, nausea, dizziness, light-headedness, chills, blushing, or a full-body flush. The attacks typically build in intensity for about 10 or 15 minutes, tapering off after about a half hour, and people who suffer from them say that they're often afraid of dying or losing control. Although the attacks are usually triggered by a specific event or situation, some people have them at random, in a variety of settings. Panic disorder is diagnosed if you've had at least two panic attacks, and you have begun to worry about having further attacks so much that you've actually altered your normal routine or changed your behavior in some way to prevent a recurrence. In fact, about half of people with panic disorder develop such a pattern of avoidance that they actually become agoraphobic, meaning they stay at home to avoid the embarrassment of having panic attacks in public.

Phobias

A close relative of panic disorder, phobias are intense fears of certain objects or situations—such as dogs, snakes, rodents, spiders, flying, riding in elevators, heights, water, blood, or injections. When phobic people are exposed to the dreaded object, even via video, they suffer intense anxiety and, sometimes, a panic attack. About 8 percent of all adults suffer from one or more phobias, most of which persist for years. Social phobia, a subset of this category, occurs in people who become fearful in social settings or public places. If you're afraid of public speaking, to the point where you avoid it or approach it with unreasonable dread, chances are you have a form of social phobia often known as performance anxiety. Although it's more common in shy people, some public figures have confessed to possessing an excessive fear of public speaking.

Obsessive-compulsive disorder (OCD)

Obsessive-compulsive disorder is a sort of push-pull syndrome. People who have the disorder are plagued by recurrent, uncontrollable, and unwanted feelings, thoughts, or images—actual obsessions—that they perceive as inappropriate or forbidden. These obsessive thoughts cause tremendous anxiety, which in turn elicits the second part of the disorder, the compulsions. A compulsion is a repetitive routine or ritual (hand washing, house cleaning, checking the stove to make sure it's off, counting, or praying) that is designed to prevent the dreaded event envisioned in the obsession from happening. These rituals can take hours to complete. OCD, as it's known, is one of the few disorders that have been found to be equally common in men and women, and it runs in families. It typically starts in adolescence, and the severity fluctuates throughout life, with symptoms becoming worse during times of stress or emotional upset. People with OCD are also more likely to have a history of tics and Tourette's disorder, an illness characterized by severe, multiple tics, including involuntary obscene speech.

Post-traumatic stress disorder

About 9 percent of people who've been through a natural disaster, serious accident, or combat or who've been the victim of a violent crime will develop an anxiety disorder known as post-traumatic stress disorder. Symptoms such as anxiety and a feeling of dreamlike unreality (called dissociation) usually begin within a month of the trauma. Sufferers also typically avoid situations that elicit memories of the trauma and have recurrent flashbacks or sudden, unbidden recollections of the event. As a result, they often feel hopeless and experience a sense of decreased self-esteem and of being permanently damaged—changes that in many cases lead to substance abuse. Mental health professionals are reporting an increase in the numbers of people afflicted with this problem as a result of the World Trade Center tragedy.

Treatment Options

Anxiety disorders are typically treated with a two-pronged approach that includes medication (usually antidepressants or benzodiazepines) and specific types of psychotherapy.

- Behavioral therapy, which has been shown to be effective in treating anxiety disorders, employs techniques like deep, diaphragmatic breathing to subvert the automatic stress response.
- Cognitive behavioral therapy teaches you to understand and change your thinking about stressful events as well changing your body's automatic reactions.

I also want to mention an interesting "treatment" for the phobias described above as "performance anxieties." These can be best understood as moments of predictable anxiety—such as public speaking or a musical recital—when you know you are going to be on display and be nervous. Obviously a certain amount of anxiety in such situations is perfectly normal and even helpful. But for some people, the anxiety becomes overwhelming to the point of interfering with the ability to perform or speak. It has now been demonstrated that the use of beta blockers may be very helpful in such situations. These drugs, as the name suggests, act by blocking so-called beta receptors in various body cells. These receptors can have many different physiologic effects, including many of the physical symptoms of anxiety—such as increased heart rate, elevated blood pressure, and sweaty palms. A beta-blocking drug taken about an hour before the anticipated time of anxiety—giving a speech, for example—can usually reduce these physical signs of anxiety without reducing mental acuity; that is a big advantage over tranquilizers, which usually affect both.

In fact, I have had good experience using a beta blocker about an hour before flying. I have a specific and significant fear of flying, a phobia I developed in the early eighties after almost thirty years of flying without any fear. While the beta blocker does not totally remove my anxiety, it does help reduce the symptoms and therefore helps me tolerate flying better than I would otherwise. (I take 20 milligrams of Inderal, one of the oldest beta blockers.) I have recommended this "treatment" to many friends who have a terrible fear of public speaking and most of them have found it very helpful. (Given what I do for a living, it is good I don't have this phobia!) Before you consider trying this approach to "performance anxiety" I would recommend trying the drug in an ordinary life setting just to make sure it does not affect you in unwanted ways. Using a beta blocker in this way—a single dose—is very safe for most people; suddenly stopping beta blockers that have been taken for long periods can be very dangerous. And since these drugs are available only by prescription, you will have to talk with your doctor about this possibility; by now, most doctors have heard of this interesting use of beta blockers.

Attention Deficit Disorder

If you still think attention deficit disorder (also known as ADD or ADHD, for attention deficit hyperactivity disorder, which is essentially the same illness but with more physical activity) is an ailment that afflicts only children, you're not alone. Until recently, even health professionals believed the illness typically cleared up once children hit their teens. But research has shown that as many as half to two-thirds of children with this frustrating disorder continue to struggle with the symptoms into adulthood. There is also growing evidence that many adults who weren't diagnosed as children (or who were diagnosed with some other learning disability) actually have this problem.

The number of adults with ADD is tricky to estimate and is based largely on estimates in children. According to the Surgeon General, ADD affects 3 to 5 percent of school-age children, and statistics show it is the most commonly diagnosed mental health condition in children in the U.S. It's probable that more adult men have ADD than women, because two to three times more boys than girls are affected by the disorder, according to the National Institute of Mental Health. So far, there are no good explanations for the gender difference.

Common Characteristics

Adults as well as children can undergo neuropsychological testing to determine whether or not you have ADD.

The most common characteristics of the illness are:

Easy distractibility. Men with ADD often have trouble paying attention to details and keeping on task. They make careless mistakes because they're not focused on what they're doing or are in too much of a rush to get on to something else.

Difficulty sustaining attention. They have a hard time sticking with one thing and/or following through on tasks. They may also have trouble listening and following directions when people are speaking to them.

Disorganization. They have tremendous trouble organizing themselves and will typically lose things necessary for tasks and activities.

Forgetfulness. People with ADD often forget about daily activities and appointments.

Symptoms can vary from person to person and between children and adults, but the key feature—severe attention problems—typically remains.

In order to receive a diagnosis of ADD, the behaviors must have appeared before age seven and they must create a real hardship in at least two areas of your life—professionally, personally, or socially. In other words, ADD goes beyond the normal stress and chaos of everyday life.

Scientists have yet to identify the cause of ADD, but the disorder appears to be at least partly genetic. Thanks to new brain imaging techniques, we now know that certain areas of the brain, including the frontal lobe and basal ganglia (parts of the brain that you use to inhibit impulses and control attention) are smaller by about 10 percent in children who have the disorder, and experts believe that certain biological and genetic factors may influence the activity of dopamine, a brain chemical that transmits nerve impulses, in people with ADD.

Treatment Options

ADD is typically treated with a combination of medication and therapy. Ironically, the medications that seem to work the best are stimulants—such as methylphenidate (Ritalin), dextroamphetamine (Dexedrine), and other amphetamines (Adderall)—which may work by modulating certain brain neurotransmitters, including dopamine. Although there has been less work in adults with ADD, studies show that between 70 and 80 percent of children with the disorder respond to medication.

Behavior therapy and cognitive therapy can help sufferers modify problem behaviors, cope with the emotional fallout of the disorder, and learn new organizational skills, including how to prioritize tasks and minimize clutter.

Commonly Used Psychoactive Drugs

The following is a partial list of some of the most commonly used psychoactive drugs today. All of them can have significant side effects and possible interactions with other drugs, so you need to talk carefully with your doctor and pharmacist about any dangers associated with their use.

SELECTIVE SEROTONIN REUPTAKE INHIBITORS (SSRIs)

Examples: fluoxetine (Prozac), sertraline (Zoloft), paroxetine (Paxil), citalopram (Celexa), fluvoxamine (Luvox).

What They're Best For: Depression—most psychiatrists try an SSRI before any other type of antidepressant, because they have more manageable side effects than the other types and they present a lower risk of overdose. They are also used for obsessive-compulsive disorder, post-traumatic stress disorder, and other anxiety disorders. Paroxetine, in particular, has been approved by the Food and Drug Administration for the treatment of social phobia.

TRICYCLIC ANTIDEPRESSANTS (ALSO KNOWN AS HETEROCYCLIC ANTIDEPRESSANTS)

Examples: amitriptyline (Elavil), amoxapine (Aseridin), desipramine (Norpramin), doxepin (Sinequan), imipramine (Tofranil), maprotiline (Ludiomil), nortriptyline (Pamelor), protriptyline (Vivactil), clomipramine (Anafranil), trimipramine (Surmontil).

What They're Best For: Depression—there's some evidence that men with chronic depression sometimes respond better to tricyclics than to SSRIs. These may also be used for obsessive-compulsive disorder if SSRIs fail.

MONOAMINE OXIDASE INHIBITORS (MAOIs)

Examples: isocarboxiazid, phenelzine (Nardil), tranylcypromine (Parnate).

What They're Best For: Depression, and depression with anxiety and phobias; bipolar disorder.

BUPROPION (WELLBUTRIN)

What It's Best For: Depression—it's less likely to decrease sexual desire than the SSRIs, tricyclics, or MAOIs; bipolar disorder.

VENLAFAXINE (EFFEXOR)

What It's Best For: Depression—it has shown promise in treating severe cases of depression. It is also used for anxiety and panic attacks.

NEFAZODONE (SERZONE)

What It's Best For: Severe depression and depression with sleep problems, since it often improves sleep efficiency.

MIRTAZAPINE (REMERON)

What It's Best For: Depression. It blocks two types of serotonin receptors in the brain, thereby increasing the level of serotonin.

LITHIUM (LITHONATE, CIBALITH-S, ESKALITH, LITHOBID, LITHOTABS)

What It's Used For: The manic episodes of manic depression.

DIVALPROEX (DEPAKOTE)

What It's Used For: The manic episodes in manic depression.

BENZODIAZEPINES

Examples: diazepam (Valium), lorazepam (Ativan), clonazepam (Klonopin), alprazolam (Xanax).
What They're Used For: Anxiety disorders (but not for obsessive-compulsive disorder or post-traumatic stress disorder).

BUSPIRONE (BUSPAR)

What It's Used For: Generalized anxiety disorder and nicotine addiction.

CHLORDIAZEPOXIDE (LIBRIUM)

What It's Used For: Anxiety disorders.

STIMULANTS

Examples: methylphenidate (Ritalin), dextroamphetamine (Dexedrine), amphetamine combinations (Adderall), methamphetamine (Desoxyn), pemoline (Cylert).
What They're Used For: Attention deficit disorder.

CHAPTER 9

Stress, Anger, and Coping

Unless you're a monk, and today even that is no guarantee, you probably face stressful situations every day—on the freeway, in your office, at home. Even positive, happy events can be a source of stress. Planning a wedding, traveling to and from a vacation, having a baby, getting a promotion, and moving to a bigger home all can cause tension, because they throw our lives into disarray and place demands on our time and energy, both of which are typically in short supply in our 24-hour culture.

Stress is so prevalent, it has become the plague of modern society. Ask a friend how he's doing, and, chances are, you'll hear the word "stress" in his reply. But calls to eliminate this emotional bugaboo from our lives are not only unrealistic, they're often unnecessary, because the fact is, some stress is good. Without it, it would be more difficult to get motivated to make a sales presentation, write a difficult report, or study for an exam. Stress can sometimes give you an emotional kick in the pants when you need it most. That said, it can do some pretty serious damage, too, not just to your personal relationships but to your physical health.

Reaping the benefits of stress without becoming its victim usually boils down to one key strategy: coping. Unfortunately, for many people, stress leads instead to anger, which leads to aggression or hostility, a chain reaction that is common in men. That's why I have put those issues together in this chapter, along with some concrete advice for breaking this negative cycle.

In short, the issue is not whether you have stress in your life. You do and you will. It's how you respond to stress that will determine in large part whether you use it for your own good or whether it makes you ill.

Stress

Eighty percent of all visits to the doctors' offices in the U.S. are for problems that have a stress component, according to the Centers for Disease Control and Prevention. In other words, many of the problems that make us feel unwell, including chronic backaches, headaches, insomnia, digestive disorders, and emotional problems, can often be traced at least in part back to the dynamic we call "stress." The toll stress takes on our lives is tremendous. It can make you more susceptible to colds, contribute to your risk of heart disease, keep you up at night, and decrease your ability to think clearly, making everything from office mishaps to auto accidents more likely.

Why does stress wreak such havoc on your body? Over the last several decades, researchers have traced a complex cascade of physiological reactions that occur within your body when you're under stress, most of which are triggered by the release of hormones called cortisol and adrenaline. You've probably heard this stress reaction called the "fight-or-flight" response. That's because the reaction was built into our bodies centuries ago, when men out hunting wild animals needed to be able to fight or flee at a moment's notice.

Although most of us are no longer called upon to do battle with fierce animals, we can get that same physiological jolt when we're under pressure in our daily lives. The effects in your body are typical: Your heart rate increases so your body gets more blood-carrying oxygen more quickly. Your pupils dilate so you can see better. Your digestion slows, because your blood is diverted from your abdomen and chest to the big muscles in your legs and arms. In short, your body is in overdrive, ready for quick bursts of physical activity.

In the short term, the condition can be helpful—it can give you the energy to jump out of the way of an oncoming bus, for instance. But when you're sitting at a desk stewing over a deadline, the near-constant emotional stress will easily throw you into physical distress. By putting your body in a state of disequilibrium and, among other things, suppressing elements of your immune system, stress makes minor illnesses and infections more likely and sets the stage for more major problems to possibly develop.

Stress can damage your personal relationships, too. Store up those daily hassles and pressures long enough, and you'll take it out on those you're closest to—your wife, your partner, your colleagues, your kids. Your professional life can suffer as well, because when you're under chronic stress at your job, it can lead to burnout, a state that is characterized by a persistent loss of interest in work-related issues you used to feel passionately about, decreased productivity, and, sometimes, depression. Conversely, it also can lead to workaholism, an issue I'll explore in greater detail later in this chapter.

Just because you're busy, doesn't mean you're "under stress." Many of you have heard about the so-called "Type A personality" (first described in the mid-1950s) as a person who is very competitive and time conscious, always looking at his (usually a he, at least in those days) watch and needing to win even against his own kid when playing a game at home. We haven't heard as much about this concept in recent years because when researchers started to examine it more closely, they found that it was difficult to correlate the external appearances of life (rushing around, long hours, etc.) with harmful stress. And other research has suggested that internal physiological reactions are much more important than external appearances and circumstances. In fact, research into inner physiological reactions to outward circumstances has shown a wide variety of responses among individual men.

I mention this because we sometimes make the mistake of assuming that the person who is very busy is automatically "under stress" while the person who seems placid and passive must be in a much more healthy state. But those assumptions could be very misleading. For example, some research has shown that a person who is very busy but who is his own boss and has control over his own destiny may be much better off than the less busy person who is seething inside because he is at the mercy of many bosses above him. In other words, the "frustration factor" may be more harmful than the "hard work factor." And more recent research on the Type A concept has isolated inner hostility/anger as the most significant among many qualities traditionally attributed to so-called Type A people. In short, I am not minimizing the potential importance of external circumstances in our lives, but I am saying that it is ultimately the way in which we handle such circumstances that really counts.

Fortunately, there are dozens of ways to help keep stress in check. Most aren't time consuming or complicated. As you'll see in the upcoming section, some of them are as simple as, well, breathing.

Learning how to relax

It's impossible to be both physically tensed and relaxed at the same time, so the physical antidote to stress is relatively simple. That is because your body knows how to relax. It wants to relax. All you have to do is give it a little time and space and help, and you'll suddenly find yourself feeling, if not exactly mellow, then at least calmer and more in control. Here are some strategies that will usually help:

Exercise. Working up a sweat every day can help you slough off stress by using up muscle tension and ridding your body of excess adrenaline, the main chemical that causes your body to feel amped up. At the same time, even moderate regular exercise can promote the release of endorphins, chemicals that relieve pain and infuse your body with a sense of well-being. Have a tough morning at work? Take a 20-minute walk at lunchtime and see how much better you feel in the afternoon. Numerous studies have proven that exercise is one of the most potent stress-busters around.

Stretch. As we mentioned in Part One, exercise is the component of a healthy lifestyle that men skip most often, but, along with its myriad other benefits—helping to prevent injuries, maintaining range of motion—it can keep your body feeling looser and less tense. For example, when you're sitting at your desk, gently roll your head in a circle. It'll help ease tension in your neck, a key area where emotional strain takes a toll, and help you stay relaxed. Every hour or two, get up from your desk and gently stretch your arms and legs. Don't push it, however. When you're sitting all day, your muscles can become quite tight, making them more pull-prone. Just stretch to the point where you feel a gentle pulling and hold (don't bounce) for 20 to 30 seconds. As "stressed" in Chapter 2, it is also very helpful to stretch in systematic fashion for 5 to 10 minutes before and after exercise. *(See page 48 for 10 great stretches.)*

Practice deep breathing. The phrase, "Take a deep breath" is more than just a cliché. When you're under stress, your breathing becomes shallow and quick. It's what breath experts call "chest breathing," and it actually exacerbates your body's physiological response to stress. "Belly breathing," on the other hand, in which you breathe deeply, filling out your abdomen to lower your diaphragm and maximally expand your chest, defuses the stress reaction by slowing your heart rate and lowering your blood pressure. (If you don't believe me, try taking your pulse while taking a deep breath and notice how it slows down rather dramatically.) When you're in the middle of a stressful situation, try placing a hand on your abdomen so you can feel it filling out as you deeply inhale. Inhale and exhale through your nostrils. Even three or four deep breaths can help you get control of your body and feel calmer. Get in the habit of breathing deeply at regular intervals throughout the day, and you'll be more likely to think of it when you're ambushed by unexpected stress. The fact is that it is virtually impossible to feel tense at the same time you are taking slow, deep breaths.

Meditate. This Eastern practice has taken the West by storm for good reason: It really works for most people. Study after study has found beneficial effects when you quiet your mind. Although the image of a new-age guru chanting in the lotus position turns some people off, there's really nothing kooky about simple meditation. All you have to do is sit up straight and try to clear your mind of any thoughts—a task that can be both more difficult and more rewarding than it sounds. It can be easier if you try to focus your mind on one thing—your breath going in and out of your body, the flickering of a candle flame, or a repeated sound, like "om" or even a favorite prayer. Breathe deeply, and if your mind wanders (which it will) gently remind yourself to refocus. I still think Dr. Herbert Benson's classic, *The Relaxation Response,* is an excellent guide to simple meditation.

Get a massage. Having a professional massage can relieve stress by relaxing your muscles, almost all of which can become more tense—sometimes painfully so—when you're stressed. When your muscles relax, your mind normally follows suit. I personally find professional massage one of the best ways to unwind.

Take a bath. Warm water can loosen tensed-up muscles. If you're like most men and you've never actually used your bathtub, a warm bath with a few drops of lavender or chamomile oil can be a great antidote to a stressful day.

Go out with a friend. Sharing your concerns with someone you trust can often lessen the burden of stress. Even if you don't feel like talking about your problems, the simple act of being in someone else's company can help you feel better. In my own life, I regard the wise counsel of good friends as so valuable that I consciously nurture such friendships with regular phone calls and e-mail exchanges.

Watch what you eat and drink. Make an effort to eat fruits, vegetables, and whole grains, which may promote the production of serotonin, a calming brain chemical. Meanwhile, keep alcohol consumption to a minimum. Although a drink might make you feel good after a hard day at the office, too much alcohol can have a depressant effect and can make you less able to cope in the long run.

Keep tabs on your caffeine consumption, too. Chronic stress can make you feel tired and run-down, but a caffeine boost will only promote restlessness and anxiety, emotions that fuel your body's stress response. Having said that I should also point out that there is an enormous variation in the response to caffeine from one person to another. Some people can consume large amounts without any effect on the nervous system while in others, even a small amount can put them on edge all day long and well into the night.

Make realistic plans. One of the reasons most of us feel so much stress is that we take on too many projects and make too many promises. As a result, we're chronically overbooked and running late. The simple act of managing your time can go a long way toward keeping your stress level under control.

Develop a hobby. One way to set aside time is to develop a deeper interest in some hobby or pastime. I believe that any of us, if we take the time, can identify something we truly enjoy doing—whether it be woodworking or bird watching (which happens to be my thing). And by taking the time to identify your true interests, you'll be more likely to make the time to indulge them.

Consider professional help. If you're chronically tense and feeling unable to cope with the daily pressures in your life, or if you're suffering from physical ailments that you believe are stress related, it can be extremely helpful to seek the guidance of a mental health professional. A trained professional can help you see new ways of looking at your situation and offer you a variety of coping mechanisms that may be helpful. They might also be able to evaluate whether you're a good candidate for antidepressant or anti-anxiety medication, both of which can help in certain cases.

The importance of sleep

Dozens of recent reports have pointed to an alarming trend in our culture: Americans are chronically sleep deprived. As we push ourselves to squeeze more activities into our busy lives, the thing that gets crunched is sleep, often with devastating results. For instance, the National Highway Traffic Safety Administration found that sleepy people have almost as many automobile accidents as drunk drivers. In addition, there is suggestive evidence that immune function slows in people who are chronically sleep deprived, possibly putting them at increased risk of all sorts of illnesses.

Stress and sleep are intricately linked. On the one hand, stress can cause poor sleep. In fact, about half of all cases of insomnia are related to psychological factors, like anxiety, depression, and stress. On the other hand, sleep deprivation makes it more difficult to cope with stress, both physically and emotionally. It becomes a vicious circle. We all know that a tired child is a cranky child, but we often forget that the same rule applies to adults, too. A number of studies have found that one of the first signs of sleep deprivation is a deterioration of your mood.

The good news: A good night's rest can be a powerful weapon in your daily battles with stress. Here are some tips for getting more restful sleep during stressful times. *(For a more comprehensive look at sleep problems, see page 252.)*

- Allow some time early in the evening (several hours before you go to bed) to think about your worries and concerns. Write them down, along with possible solutions. Research has shown that setting aside a specific time to worry can prevent you from obsessing about your concerns once you're in bed.
- Do something relaxing before bed, like take a warm bath or do some gentle stretches.
- If you're having trouble going to sleep, get up and watch television or read a book. Lying in bed awake can actually make insomnia worse. That said, for some people, the stimulation of a reading light or TV can interfere with sleep—and they're better off resting in bed. You'll need to figure out which approach works best for you.
- Awaken at the same time every morning, even on weekends. That way, you'll program your body to be tired at night.

If you do miss some sleep for a night or two, try not to worry about it. It is an unfair truism that anxiety over sleep only makes it more difficult to get to sleep.

Anger and Aggression

Women and men often respond to stress differently. While women tend to worry and ruminate, men tend to act—and act out. Sometimes that's a good thing. You can release a good deal of pent-up tension with a few hard blows to a punching bag or a sprint down the block. Other times, it's channeled in a less healthy direction, and it comes out as hostility or fury directed at other people, both strangers and friends.

Angry outbursts are not only potentially dangerous, they're also unhealthy.

Over the past two decades, studies of a personality trait known as hostility, which includes anger, aggression, and cynicism, have yielded startling results. High hostility levels in men have been related to increased risk of coronary atherosclerosis (commonly known as hardening of the arteries, a major contributor to heart attacks), high blood pressure, and early death. And the damage begins at a young age, according to researchers in Oakland, California, who recently found that men younger than 30 who score high on tests of hostility already have early signs of coronary atherosclerosis.

Scientists are just beginning to sort out the physiological reasons that hostility damages your health. One reason is probably lifestyle related. Studies have shown that hostile people are more likely to smoke, drink alcohol, and consume more calories than their mellower counterparts—behaviors that have been shown time and again to contribute to ill health.

But there's more to it than that, and a key piece may lie in your body chemistry. Researchers at Ohio State University in Columbus recently found that hostile people have higher levels of homocysteine than calmer people. That's relevant because homocysteine, a dietary by-product of animal protein, may damage the cells lining the walls of your arteries and contribute to the development of arterial plaque—in other words, atherosclerosis. *(For more information on homocysteine and atherosclerosis, see page 139.)*

Clearly, there are a number of good reasons to reign in your anger.

Managing Anger

Fortunately, humans are thinking beings, capable of logic and reason. Without that ability, it would be difficult to control our emotional reactions. With it, however, we can often stem the tide of anger before it overwhelms us. Here are a few tips:

Take a moment to breathe. When you feel your fury rising, take at least three deep breaths. During this momentary pause, take time to consider whether you have a right to be so angry. Does the situation warrant your reaction? Could you be overreacting? Even a breath or two may be enough time for you to see a better way to handle the situation, and deep breathing will serve to defuse some of your rising ire.

Talk yourself out of your anger. Say you're stuck in traffic and it's clear you're going to be late for a meeting. Then a car darts in front of you. Your immediate reaction will probably be anger. But, after a moment's reflection, you'll probably realize that you wouldn't get to your meeting any more quickly even if you were ahead of the rude motorist. If, after reflecting on the situation, you realize your anger is unwarranted, coach yourself through it by coming up with rational reasons why your anger is inappropriate, or simply distract yourself for a while by reading a magazine or doing some simple work, which may give you enough time to leave your initial exasperation behind.

Get some exercise. If you have time before you have to deal with the situation that is making you angry, go out for a walk or run or work out at your health club. Sometimes what you really need is physical, not emotional, release. Exercise has the added benefit of calming you down, which will help you think more clearly about the situation.

Talk it out with a friend. By explaining your situation to someone who's not involved, you may gain insights that you hadn't had before. And simply spending time with a good friend can take the edge off your frustrations.

Think before you speak. If you still feel your anger is justified, think about how to express yourself to best accomplish your goal. Emotional outbursts are rarely effective, because they serve to alienate the people you're communicating with. Instead, speak calmly and express your concerns clearly. If you're being critical of another person, use "I" statements—"I feel angry when you use my good razor to shave your legs, because it makes it dull," rather than "you" statements, like, "How could you be so inconsiderate about my things?"

Workaholism

Balancing your career and personal relationships is tricky in the best of times. But men who are under a significant amount of stress often turn to work for comfort or, if it's increased work demands that are causing the pressure, out of necessity. Men may also escape to work as a place where they can feel powerful or in control of their life. Either way, it creates an imbalance in your life that can lead to unhealthy consequences. Because the social relationships of workaholics usually suffer, they often miss the health benefits of friendship, a key factor in reducing stress and coping with life's difficulties. And, because workaholics are often also perfectionistic, they may not derive much happiness from their main activity—work.

Although there are no concrete definitions of workaholism, you can probably determine if you have a problem by thinking about the following: If the time you spend at work is detracting from other important relationships in your life, or if you feel so caught up in work that it's distracting you even during leisure time, it may be time to examine your values and make an attempt to regain some balance.

Overcoming workaholism can take time, so it's best to make gradual changes. Try spending at least 20 to 30 minutes every day reconnecting with your spouse or partner. Even when you're traveling on business trips, make an effort to have a leisurely phone conversation, so you can catch up on what's happening in each other's lives. Once a week, schedule a dinner or social engagement with a friend or loved one. During the day, take breaks from your desk to take a walk outside or eat lunch at a nearby restaurant.

In addition, it can be helpful to spend some time thinking about your priorities. Career success is undoubtedly important, but what other things are important to you? If you're having trouble coming up with things, play this game: Pretend you're on your death bed and looking back at your life. What are the moments you'll remember and cherish?

If you're having trouble reestablishing a sense of balance in your life or getting out of the overworking rut, you may be dealing with issues that are still too complicated to handle on your own. In those instances, it may be helpful to talk to a professional, who can help you untangle the web of emotional interactions that sometimes push men to work too hard.

CHAPTER 10

Men and Relationships

There may be no more important component of personal happiness than your interpersonal relationships. Think about it: When things are going well with your spouse or significant other, your friends, your associates at work, or your family, you feel robust, cheerful, positive, content. Those feelings of well-being, while worthy of recognition in their own right, also are valuable for another reason: They have a direct impact on your physical health, boosting your ability to ward off illnesses and keep your body functioning at its peak.

This so-called mind-body connection has been increasingly borne out in medical research since the early 1970s. In fact, in the past 20 years, a whole new field of research known as psychoneuroimmunology (PNI) has sprung up to explore the many ways in which our thoughts and emotions affect our physical well-being. What scientists now believe is that your emotions influence the activity of certain hormones and brain chemicals, called neuropeptides. These chemicals carry on an internal dialogue in your body, transmitting messages about your mental state and affecting everything from your heart rate to your immune response when your body is invaded by a cold virus.

These findings have potentially profound implications on a practical level. For instance, in one particularly telling study, published in the Journal of the American Medical Association, researchers found that the death rate of older Jewish men declines right before Passover, a Jewish holiday that carries particular significance for elderly men, who typically lead the ritual celebration. After the holiday, there is a spike in deaths before things settle back to normal. In other words, the excitement and anticipation of sharing a joyful occasion with their loved ones actually seems to help some men postpone their own deaths!

Friendship also has been shown to decrease the incidence of depression in recent heart attack survivors, encourage AIDS patients to stick to complicated medication schedules, increase functioning in people with schizophrenia, help college students maintain a regular exercise regimen, and decrease the risk of heart disease. In our never-ending search for medical magic bullets—supplements that will prevent cancer, herbs that will ward off illness—it appears we could do a lot worse than to simply make a new friend.

What does all this mean for men today? The findings about the impact of personal relationships on health are both good and bad news for most of us. The bad news is this: Troubled relationships can wreak havoc on your emotional well-being and take a toll on your health. And, thanks to a complex interplay of upbringing, socialization, individual temperament, and hormones, men traditionally have had greater difficulty than women in navigating the often-dicey territory of interpersonal relationships.

In her interviews with hundreds of men in the early 1980s, Shere Hite found that many men have never had a best friend and that the friendships most men do have tend to be superficial—they discuss things like business, sports, and politics rather than deeply emotional or personal issues. Although these more shallow relationships undoubtedly provide a certain level of emotional comfort, they skim the surface of the potential benefits that exist within the context of friendship, among them the remarkable health benefits friendship can provide.

Times are changing, however, and men today are becoming more open to the idea of sharing their deeper thoughts and feelings with other people. Meanwhile, a whole new generation of men is being raised by fathers who are more emotionally honest and available than their predecessors. Interpersonal relationships—between men and women, men and men, men and coworkers, and fathers and children—will undoubtedly benefit from this new era of openness, and so will our health.

Until then, why not do what you can to get the most out of your relationships? Here are some of the health-related implications of the everyday interactions most of us take for granted.

The Working Man

Men and work. The two seem almost inextricably linked. It's likely that from the earliest days of humankind, the males of our species have been genetically groomed to toil. The first men spent days in the wild, stalking animals to provide food for their clan or tribe. Today we work for money, which in turn pays for everything we need in terms of food, shelter, clothing, and beyond.

Although the days of hunting wild beasts are largely relegated to prehistoric times, the hunter instinct is alive and well in most contemporary places of business. It's civilized, to be sure, by ties and business suits, executive suites and cell phones, but it's in evidence, nonetheless. Consider the intense competition for attractive jobs, the cutthroat vying for coveted promotions, and the widespread fear of layoffs when profit margins disappear.

Work is a critical element to our health and well-being for a simple reason: We spend so much time there. Despite advances in technology, employees are working longer hours today than 25 years ago. The total time men spend at work has increased 2.8 hours a week—from 47.1 to 49.9—since 1977, according to research conducted by the Families and Work Institute, a nonprofit organization that explores the changing nature of work and family life. Those extra hours, coupled with the increasing demands of a global economy, often translate into decreased well-being. The Institute found that one-quarter of people felt nervous or stressed out very often and 13 percent had a tough time coping with the demands of everyday life. That's not good news, considering the fact that job strain has been shown to increase your risk of high blood pressure, cardiovascular disease, back pain, psychological disorders, and workplace injuries.

Making Room for Wellness

How can you stay healthy in this demanding, fast-paced atmosphere? First, the way you feel about your work is key. Research has shown that stress doesn't take such a deadly toll on people whose job satisfaction is high—in other words, if you enjoy what you're doing, your body actually handles stress more effectively. Fortunately, slightly more than half of men say they're "very satisfied" with their jobs, according to a Louis Harris poll conducted in the year 2000. Another 37 percent are "somewhat satisfied," and 9 percent aren't at all satisfied.

Research has shown that three factors contribute to increased job satisfaction: 1) control over your work, 2) the opportunity to use your talents and skills, and 3) being in an environment in which your work is recognized and appreciated. According to a recent study conducted at the Family Studies Center at Brigham Young University, people with more job flexibility—who can work at home, for instance, or have some control over the hours they work—are actually much more productive and less stressed out than those with more rigid schedules. Everyone has moments of frustration and dissatisfaction at work, but if you feel stuck in an unsatisfying, dead-end job that offers little in the way of personal gratification, you have yet another reason to start looking for greener pastures: your health.

Another factor that will help you cope with increasing job demands is supportive coworkers and bosses. Although the Families and Work Institute found that employees in smaller companies say their workplaces are more supportive than those within larger corporations, the group also found that a majority of workers feel their immediate supervisors are quite supportive and most employees have positive relationships with their colleagues. Developing good working relationships with the people around you can help you cope with the daily demands and hassles of any job.

Finally, you can usually handle work stress more effectively if you have a physical outlet for your frustrations. Although our leisure time is feeling the squeeze of increasing work demands—a Louis Harris poll found that Americans' leisure time has decreased by 37 percent in the past 30 years!—it's important to take at least a half hour every day to do something overtly physical. Start a company softball team. Join a nearby gym that you can visit during your lunch hour. Meet a colleague several times a week for a pre-work jog. Try a number of tactics to squeeze in physical activity to find the one that works for you and that you can stick with for the long haul.

Relationships

The American public has been bombarded of late by books that point out the stark differences between men and women. We've been told that the two genders are from different planets, we don't speak the same language, we have different skills, even our brains are different! It doesn't exactly foster confidence in men who are trying to start a relationship, much less in those who are engaged in the hard work of keeping a long-term relationship alive.

The Benefits and Stresses of Spouses, Partners, and Significant Others

And long-term commitment is hard work. Although most studies have found a 40 to 50 percent divorce rate, researchers at the University of Michigan found that first marriages today stand a 67 percent chance of failing over a 40-year period! Ironically, marriage is particularly dicey in the beginning, perhaps because people are still adjusting to their new circumstances. In any case, studies show that fully half of all divorces occur in the first seven years of marriage. Daunting statistics, to be sure.

Even so, there are lots of good reasons to stay married, some of which are truly surprising. Researchers at the University of Michigan predict that people who stay married live on average four years longer than those who don't. Experts speculate that marriage (or a committed partnership) protects your health on both a macro level—by offering lifelong support and companionship—and on a micro level, by providing an ally who will pester you into being conscientious about everyday health practices, like exercising regularly, eating right, seeing a doctor for routine checkups, and taking your medicine when you're supposed to.

There also appears to be something going on in the bodies of happily married people that keeps them healthier. After analyzing 100,000 cancer deaths from 1960 to 1991, researchers in Norway found that men who had never married and divorced men are 15 percent more likely to die of cancer than married men. Although no one knows the exact mechanisms at work behind this phenomenon, researchers are amassing more and more clues.

John Gottman, Ph.D., cofounder and codirector of the Seattle Marital and Family Institute, has conducted years of research on married couples and has found preliminary evidence showing that people in good marriages actually have stronger immune system responses to foreign invaders than their less happy counterparts. Divorce, on the other hand, depresses the immune system, making you more susceptible to everyday bugs and perhaps even serious diseases like cancer.

Even the short-term stress of a nasty argument can leave your immune system sluggish. When researchers at Ohio State University College of Medicine analyzed the physiological responses of 90 happily married couples during and after a discussion of marital problems, they found that the spouses who exhibited more negative or hostile behavior had greater increases in blood pressure and decreases in their immune system functioning over the subsequent 24 hours than those who remained more positive or supportive.

Psychological well-being also is affected by marriage. Austrian researchers recently analyzed the admission rates at the University of Vienna Department of Psychiatry and found that unmarried people are twice as likely to suffer from depression as married people. Perhaps not surprisingly, the lowest rates of depression in the study were found in employed married men. Likewise, researchers at the University of California at Riverside recently found that divorced men are twice as likely to commit suicide as married men, even though marriage doesn't confer any such protective benefits on women.

So how do you keep your relationship on an even keel? Carrying on a successful relationship requires a fairly high level of diligence and hard work, not just on special occasions, like birthdays and anniversaries, but every day, during ordinary interactions. Although there's no clear roadmap to harmony in couplehood, experts in the field have found indications of what separates a good relationship from a rocky one:

Be emotionally attuned to your partner. Dr. Gottman, one of the foremost researchers in the field, has found that one of the secrets of a successful relationship is paying attention to your partner's minor bids for attention and affection, like an affectionate caress on the arm, a significant look, a smile, or a question or comment. If your partner is reading the newspaper, for example, and says, "I can't believe it! The local YMCA is closing," it may seem like a throwaway comment. You could ignore it or respond to it depending on your mood and other distractions. But Dr. Gottman's research has shown that people in good marriages are more likely to follow up on these everyday observations from their partners. In fact, his studies have shown that husbands who eventually were divorced ignored such bids from their wives 82 percent of the time, compared to 19 percent for men in stable marriages. In other words, paying attention to the little things and cueing into your partner's emotional needs—*on a practical, everyday level*—is one way to give your relationships staying power.

Argue the right way. Research has shown that couples who resolve marital conflict by using a collaborative style—expressing their opinions, then coming to some sort of a mutually acceptable conclusion—have much higher marital satisfaction than those who are competitive, trying to "win" an argument rather than come up with a solution.

Maintain a friendship with your partner. Studies of long-term couples have shown that the foundation of the relationship is friendship. Genuinely liking and enjoying your partner's company helps you ride out the tough times, when your relationship is tested. To keep that basic connection strong, it can help to be diligent about making time for each other, whether it's a half-hour walk together at the end of each day or a special dinner alone once a week.

Accept the fact that there will be hard times. Successful, long-term couples don't have a utopian view of relationships. They know that there will be difficulties, so they don't panic when they enter a tough phase. Instead, they tackle the issues and look for positive solutions. In a study of 50 happily married couples, Judith Wallerstein, Ph.D., found that the couples who recognized the need to adapt and negotiate the relationship were better able to handle difficult times.

Keep your sex life fresh and lively. Studies have found that one of the main reasons men in committed relationships stray is boredom (women, on the other hand, are more likely to commit adultery for emotional reasons), and infidelity is a difficult obstacle for even the best marriages to surmount. With a little extra work and innovation in the bedroom, you can maintain a sense of excitement with your partner, without violating the trust the two of you share. To create an environment in which your sex life can grow and change, it helps to be open and responsive to your partner's ideas and needs. In addition, being affectionate throughout the day—not just in the bedroom—can enhance the sensuality of your relationship.

The Family Man

Depending on your age, you may have very different memories of your father than the ones you want to create for your child. As recently as a generation ago, most men were fairly detached from their children, especially when they were infants, because the care and feeding of babies was considered women's work. Many fathers left for work early in the morning and came home late at night, and when they were home, they were distracted and emotionally distant. Although today more men are likely to be absent entirely—a problem that has reached epidemic proportions in our country—the reverse is true, too. There's a growing movement toward active fatherhood that may signal a sea change in the way American families function.

There is widespread evidence that more and more men are taking a hands-on child-rearing role from the moment their children enter the world. Fathers today are more likely to be involved in and present for their children's births, and studies have shown that in families in which both parents work, fathers are stepping up to the plate, taking responsibility for more child care than they did in previous generations. In a growing number of households, men are the primary caregivers.

Likewise, paternity leave, which was virtually unheard of several decades ago, is slowly gaining momentum as more and more businesses recognize the changing structure of the American family. A U.S. Census Bureau report on 1993 trends in paternal child care found that in families in which the mother worked, 1.9 million fathers were the primary caregiver, providing more hours of child care than any other single provider while the mother was at work.

Such changes, while slow in occurring, have the potential to offer manifold benefits to the family as a whole. Not only is a committed, involved father good for children, it's good for your relationship with your significant other and, in the long term, it may even be good for your health.

Taking Care of Your Children, Taking Care of Yourself

Research on children with involved fathers is compelling. Studies have shown that participatory fathers enhance nonverbal communications in infants as young as one month old, help children develop empathy and a sense of self-control, and instill in children a sense of equality of the sexes. University of Maryland researchers found that when fathers enjoy parenting and play with their children in a nurturing way, the children seem to develop stronger cognitive and language skills.

In addition, men are more likely than women to engage in rough and tumble play with children, a type of play that has surprising benefits. Research has shown, for instance, that children whose fathers roughhouse with them are more popular and have better coping skills than kids with less active fathers. Experts speculate that the type of active play fathers prefer may help children develop self-regulation skills by getting excited and thrilled, then calming down when the game is over. Remember—you can participate and make a huge difference in a child's life as a stepfather, grandfather, uncle, or godfather as well.

Perhaps the biggest impact happens once children reach school age. According to the National Center for Education Statistics, school-age children from two-parent households are more likely to do well academically, participate in extracurricular activities, and enjoy school if their fathers are actively involved in their education (by attending parent-teacher conferences and class events, say, or volunteering at the school.) Meanwhile, father involvement decreases the likelihood that a child will repeat a grade or be suspended or expelled from school.

Research has shown that if you're involved with your child's life early on, you're more likely to remain involved throughout his or her life. In fact, some researchers speculate that the birth of a baby is a sort of window of opportunity for father involvement, and those who choose to get involved at the time of a baby's birth usually remain involved and attached throughout the child's life.

That's good news for your marriage as well as your child. Having children is a notorious marital stressor. In the first year after having a child, 70 percent of wives say they're much less satisfied with their marriages than they were before they had a baby. Men's sense of marital satisfaction tends to plummet shortly thereafter.

Researchers blame this phenomenon on stress, lack of sleep, and increased responsibility. But they have found that there are things you can do to buffer the stress of having an infant in the house, most notably *getting involved*. Helping out with the baby, taking on traditional "women's" responsibilities, like diapering, feeding, and dressing the baby, and being supportive of your partner's child-rearing efforts can ease the strain a newborn places on your relationship—and may actually enhance your relationship. (Conversely, research has shown that being happily married can encourage men to become more involved with their children.)

As children get older, most men find they're able to get more sleep, develop a manageable routine, and adjust to the demands of fatherhood. Once that happens, you'll begin to accrue health benefits from parenting, particularly in the emotional realm. Watching children grow can be deeply rewarding, and the sense of satisfaction some men glean from the experience can permeate the rest of their lives. In fact, research has shown that men who are actively involved in parenting throughout their children's lives develop a nurturing, mentoring attitude that often carries on into their old age. Meanwhile, a survey of more than 500 men found that 84 percent said that being a good father played an important role in their definition of success—proof that many men see their parental duties as an integral part of who they are.

Finally, children often give men an added incentive to take better care of themselves—to stop smoking, to wear a seatbelt, to eat better and get more exercise—probably because the truth of parenthood is hard to deny: While you may very well be replaceable at work, you're utterly irreplaceable in your child's eyes. Your value as a human being literally skyrockets the minute you have a child. This sense of added responsibility and "having something to live for" is sometimes just what a man needs to keep himself healthy, not just for his immediate family but for the generations to come as well.

PART FOUR

Fit for Life

CHAPTER 11

A Final Word

As you may have noticed after reading some or all of the preceding chapters of this book, your risk of many illnesses and ailments increases as you age. The notion of becoming old and infirm isn't a pleasant one for any of us. But more and more medical research points to an optimistic fact: Health problems aren't an inevitable by-product of the aging process. In fact, the more we know about our bodies and how they function, the more optimistic we're becoming about the possibility of most men (and women, thank God) living to old age in robust good health. Considering the fact that the average life span has tripled since the 18th century, from 25 years to 76 years, it's not inconceivable that people born today could routinely live to be more than 100.

Of course, you can't expect to attain such a lofty goal without being committed to certain good health practices—and the sooner, the better. Although genes play a major role in how you age, the contribution of genetics is often less important compared to the influence of lifestyle habits. Our bodies too often become diseased not as a result of chronological age, but as a result of years of abuse. The longer you mistreat your body, whether it's by smoking, eating poorly, drinking too much alcohol, or being sedentary, the more elusive the fountain of youth (or at least youthful good health) will be.

The good news is that it's never too late to make healthful lifestyle changes. Therefore I am closing this book with a couple of checklists for helping you make good health choices as you ponder "the rest of your story."

A "Top 12" List of Men's Good Health Choices

I am now going to engage in the popular game of constructing a list—in this case, of the most important choices for staying sound in body and mind for years to come. In this case, however, we are dealing with the game of life so I am taking this game very seriously. Obviously, there is no scientific way to prove that these are the 12 most important health practices for all men—or that I have ranked them in the right order. But I think I can make a pretty good case for both the list and the order. At the very least, it will be a good way of summarizing what I feel are some of the most important health messages to come out of this book; you can refer back to the pages noted in parentheses for more detail on each one. As you will see, I have cheated a little by combining two items in some cases. And I have chosen both screening tests and preventive practices for the list. But every item shares this one dynamic: They are all under your control. So here goes. (Since I can't reveal them one by one with a drum roll in the background, I will put them in the actual 1 to 12 order.)

1 **Don't smoke.** After reading this book, you will not be surprised by this first choice. Smoking is estimated to kill 400,000 Americans *every single year.* That's the equivalent death toll of three jumbo jet crashes every day! Choosing not to smoke is, without a doubt, the single most important health decision you can make. *(See page 96 for details on the dangers of smoking.)*

2 **Control your weight.** This is not as easy a number two choice for me as was number one. That's because the connection between obesity and actual illnesses or death is often more indirect than is the case with smoking. But I have come to accept the estimates of the Surgeon General's office that obesity is respon-

sible for approximately 350,000 deaths every year and that if American men continue to stop smoking in larger numbers, it might even replace smoking as the number one cause of death for men. *(For information on weight loss, see page 28.)*

3 Drink alcohol in moderation. This message can be taken in both positive and negative terms. As pointed out, truly moderate drinking (one to two standard size drinks a day) does reduce the risk of coronary artery disease, the number one cause of death in our country. However, *excessive* drinking is a major cause of both physical disease and social tragedy. Approximately 10 percent of people who start drinking socially will become alcoholics. The decision to drink even socially should not be taken lightly. *(To determine if you have a drinking problem, see page 170.)*

4 Exercise regularly. This health practice has enormous physical and emotional benefits. Besides reducing the risk for high blood pressure, high blood cholesterol, diabetes, obesity, and osteoporosis, regular exercise can be very helpful in raising our general mood and reducing the risk for depression. *(For specific exercise advice, see Chapter 2, page 36.)*

5 Arrange for regular cholesterol and blood pressure screening. Both high cholesterol and high blood pressure can be described as "silent killers" since they can cause extensive damage to our heart and arteries without producing any telltale symptoms until it is often too late. Therefore, the only way to find out if you have a potential problem is to get tested. *(See page 361 for information on when you should be screened.)*

6 Arrange for regular colonoscopy and PSA testing. As you already know, I strongly believe in the value of both of these tests in detecting two common and potentially lethal diseases—colon and prostate cancer—when they are still curable. There are not many cancers that we can either prevent or detect early enough to make a difference, but these are two where regular screening can make a difference. *(See page 363 for information on when you should ideally have these screenings.)*

7 Take a baby aspirin every day (most of you). Unless you are truly allergic to aspirin (very rare) or at high risk for gastrointestinal bleeding (not very common), this daily dose of aspirin is one of the most beneficial and simple things you can do. It acts to reduce the risk of clot formation in the arteries leading to your heart and brain, thereby reducing the risk of both heart attacks and strokes. And it probably acts in many other beneficial ways we don't yet fully understand.

8 Practice safe sex. In this age of AIDS, you could make a good case for putting this higher on the list. But even less lethal sexually transmitted diseases (STDs) can cause a wide range of disability such as infertility problems and pelvic pain in women. And unless you are in a truly monogamous relationship, there is no good way to tell if a partner is safe, so prevention using condoms is key. *(For more on STDs, see page 296.)*

9 Arrange for regular glaucoma screening. I will probably get some argument on this one versus some other possible choices, but I put it on the list because glaucoma is a major cause of blindness and it usually doesn't produce visual symptoms until it has caused significant damage to the optic nerve. That's why eye doctors call it a "thief in the night." The other benefit of glaucoma screening is that your ophthalmologist will have the opportunity to check for other eye problems such as early macular degeneration. *(For more information on glaucoma, see page 207; on macular degeneration, see page 239.)*

10 Use a sunscreen of at least 15 SPF when in the sun. As you know, skin cancers are the most common of all cancers by far. Fortunately, most of them (basal cell and squamous cell carcinomas) are rarely lethal, though they can certainly cause local disfigurement if not diagnosed early. Melanoma is both disfiguring and lethal so it must be diagnosed as early as possible. But since it is so inconvenient to do a truly thorough check of the skin, at least by yourself, prevention is a very helpful tool. And that means the use of sunscreen and protective clothing and the avoidance of direct sun exposure during the "high hours" (between 10 A.M. and 2 P.M.) when the sun is highest in the sky. *(See page 115 for more information on skin cancer.)*

11 Increase good fats and good carbs in your diet. As I stressed throughout Chapter 1, some of the standard nutritional advice of the past is undergoing change. And this is particularly true in the growing emphasis on making a distinction between good fats and carbs—which should actually be increased in our diet—and bad fats and carbs, which, of course, should be decreased. In other words, just "cutting down" on fats and carbs is not precise enough advice anymore. *(For detailed nutritional information, see Chapter 1.)*

12 Find time for some kind of meditation/relaxation practice. As I pointed out in Chapter 9, it is more important to set aside some time for relaxation than it is to worry about a specific technique for relaxation. Even physical *activity* that is "relaxing" in the sense that it gets your mind away from stressful thoughts can be helpful. All of us should take the time to "get away" mentally and emotionally at least once a day, wherever we are or whatever we are doing.

The prescription I've just outlined for increasing your chances of lifelong health isn't difficult to follow. Seeing your doctor regularly and screening for common diseases can give you the peace of mind that you're healthy (or worst case scenario, that you will have the best odds of beating whatever you do have). Eating right and exercising will actually make you feel better—as will finding appropriate outlets for your stress. By following these 12 bits of very important advice you'll not only be more likely to live to a ripe, old age, you'll also increase your chances of being healthy enough to enjoy those extra years.

Schedule for Tests and Checkups

I will now list the tests that I would recommend for consideration in men under and over age 50. I use age 50 as a dividing line because that is the age when the risk for many diseases starts to increase in both men and women—and therefore the age when it becomes important to undergo certain screening tests on a regular basis. However, age 50 as a dividing line is obviously somewhat arbitrary given that people with existing problems or a strong family history for a certain condition may need specific tests long before age 50.

You may also wonder about the following recommendations in light of my earlier discussion about how often to see your primary care doctor. In chapter 3, I recommended a scheduled visit at least every three years between ages 20 and 40, every two years between 40 and 50, and yearly thereafter. However, I also pointed out that most individuals will end up seeing their doctor more often because of actual symptoms or past problems that need regular checking.

Sometimes these tests can be performed by someone other than a doctor—such as a nurse or physician's assistant in your doctor's office or at work. Therefore I offer the following as a kind of checklist that you should consult to make sure you are covering some important bases. In both age groups, I have arranged the tests in order of importance (more or less)—though obviously that order might vary greatly from one person to another depending on that individual's particular personal and family medical history.

Tests Men Under Age 50 Should Consider

Weighing In. In light of my "top 12" list above, you should not be surprised to see this one. As we all know, it is very easy for our weight to "creep up" (or in the case of our waistline, out) on us without our realizing how quickly we have put on a significant amount of extra weight. Therefore, I personally recommend a monthly weigh-in at home—obviously under the same conditions (no clothes first thing in the morning is easiest) and using the same scale. You might consider investing in a better grade scale available in health stores and checking it against one at your doctor's office sometime. But what really counts is the change on your scale over time. I know some experts will disagree with the monthly recommendation as too frequent and more likely to breed a neurosis about weight. But I would argue for knowing early on when the weight starts to increase because it is much easier to correct the trend before it becomes an established problem.

Checking blood pressure. The recommended frequency for blood pressure checks will vary from one person to another depending on past readings and family history. Obviously someone who has had a blood pressure problem in the past (treated or untreated) will need regular checks, maybe as often as daily or weekly. Someone who has had normal blood pressure readings but who has a strong family history of high blood pressure should have checks every six months or so in my judgment, especially as the individual enters middle age—meaning after 40. For the person with no past problems or family history, at least once a year makes sense. Most of the time, blood pressure readings done by a nurse at work or using a home monitor should be fine. But if your blood pressure is unusually high or when you are just starting treatment or changing drugs, more frequent checking at your doctor's office may be necessary.

Cholesterol testing. As mentioned in the discussion of cholesterol *(page 129),* the latest statement from the National Cholesterol Education Program recommends a complete blood lipid profile every five years in the absence of any reasons to check more frequently. I agree with this recommendation but would stress that many people with a strong family history of high cholesterol will need more frequent testing as will those who are actually being treated for cholesterol problems.

Testicular Exams. As mentioned in the discussion of testicular cancer *(on page 283),* this is the most common cancer in men between the ages of 15 and 35. Therefore I recommend regular self-examination of the testicles every two to three months *(as described on page 285)* and an immediate follow-up exam by your physician whenever anything suspicious is felt. Obviously, if you have any symptoms (swelling or pain) you should have a physician examine you.

Skin exams. As mentioned in the section on skin cancers *(page 115),* regular self exams of the skin make sense, especially for light-skinned persons and those who spend a lot of unprotected time in the sun. The frequency of such exams will vary depending on any past problems and/or family history. And by the age of 50, I believe such exams by a physician make sense on a yearly basis.

Tests for sexually transmitted diseases (STDs). Again, the specifics as to frequency and kinds of testing depend on the specific sexual practices of a given individual. However, anyone who does engage in unprotected sex with a partner who has any chance of being infected should talk to his physician about regular testing. Also, anyone who has received any blood transfusion, no matter how long ago, should talk with his doctor about whether any testing for HIV or hepatitis is indicated. *(See page 299 for info on HIV and page 226 for info on hepatitis.)*

Rectal exams. While this exam makes most sense after age 50 as part of a yearly checkup (see below), I believe it is appropriate as part of any physical exam after age 40. Besides checking for the size and shape of the posterior part of the prostate gland, a rectal exam can detect abnormal growths in the rectum itself and can obtain a stool sample to check for hidden blood as a warning sign of colon cancer.

Vision and hearing tests. It is very difficult to generalize about who should have regular checks of vision and/or hearing. Usually such tests are conducted in response to specific changes or symptoms but some experts are suggesting periodic hearing checks in people regularly exposed to loud noises. Persons with diabetes will require regular eye exams to look for any changes in the retina, the light sensitive back layer of the eye that is so important to vision.

Dental and mouth exams. I assume this will happen when you go to the dentist. Fortunately, dentists today are much more alert to problems in the mouth other than tooth decay. A check for oral cancers is especially important in cigar, pipe, and smokeless tobacco users.

Blood and urine tests. Again, it is very difficult to recommend any regular schedule for blood and urine testing in general. Most people will have many different blood or urine tests by age 50 in response to specific problems or as a part of any comprehensive checkup.

Chest X-rays. I put this on the list simply to stress that there is no good evidence that periodic chest X-rays make any real difference in detecting serious lung disease such as lung cancer early enough to make a difference in survival. However, some physicians will recommend periodic chest X-rays (or some newer scanning procedures such as spiral CT scans) in heavy smokers on the outside chance of detecting lung cancer early enough to cure it.

Tests Men Over Age 50 Should Consider

In addition to the checklist above, certain other tests become more sensible starting at age 50. (Testicular self-exams do not make sense after age 40 since testicular cancer is extremely rare after that age.)

Colonoscopy. As discussed in the section on colon cancer *(see page 89)*, I strongly believe in the value of this endoscopic exam for the early detection of polyps and the prevention of actual colon cancer. Current wisdom suggests that if nothing is found on an initial screening exam at age 50, another screening exam is not needed for 10 years. However, if a polyp is found—or if you are at higher risk for colon cancer because of family history or a long history of ulcerative colitis—you should have colonoscopies more often.

PSA blood tests and rectal exams. As I pointed out in the discussion of screening for prostate cancer *(see page 107)*, this simple blood test is controversial because of many false positives and the absence of definitive scientific evidence that it leads to longer life in men. However, as I pointed out in that discussion, I personally believe that on balance the test is worth doing on a yearly basis starting at age 50 (or earlier in African American men and in men with a family history of prostate cancer) and continuing until age 75. A rectal exam *in addition to PSA testing* is better than either one alone.

Glaucoma testing. This relatively simple test for pressure in the eye can be done in an eye doctor's office and should be a part of any eye exam after age 50—or every few years in the absence of any other reason to see an eye doctor.

Heart stress test. As discussed in the section on diagnosing coronary artery disease *(see page 142)* this test basically involves a continuing electrocardiogram during exercise on a treadmill to stress the heart. (Again I would point out that a resting electrocardiogram is of very little value unless actual symptoms are occurring.) I will tell you that there is also a lot of debate about the value of stress tests in men without any family history or other risk factors for coronary artery disease. However, many physicians, including me, would recommend a screening stress test even for men without any apparent risk factors if they are going to begin a vigorous exercise program for the first time. And as mentioned in my discussion of testing for aerobic fitness *(see page 53)*, the stress test is a very good way to determine overall fitness (as measured during a stress test in so-called METS), and is an excellent predictor of overall survival. Therefore, some experts are recommending stress tests as "exercise tests" that can provide valuable information about fitness status—and possible motivation for increasing regular aerobic exercise.

Again, the value of the above tests in a given individual should be a matter of joint discussion between the person and his primary care physician. These lists are intended to be a starting point for discussion between you and your doctor.

RESOURCES

Continuing Education on Medical Matters

Now that we have reached the end of this guide, I want to offer a final word about keeping up with new information – and finding more in-depth information on a given topic or on topics not treated in this guide. As you might notice, the only book I have recommended within the pages of this guide is Dr. Willett's *Eat, Drink, and Be Healthy* *(see page 19)*. That is because books on medical matters are quickly out of date, at least in parts. And that will be true of this book also even though I have tried to minimize details about treatments which seem to change at the most rapid pace.

I am going to recommend one resource specifically devoted to men's health issues. It is a monthly health letter called *The Harvard Men's Health Watch* and is available by subscription. You can find out more about this—and other Harvard Medical School publications—by going to **www.health.harvard.edu/** and clicking on the appropriate place on the menu. (*Full disclosure:* I am the founding co-editor of the *Harvard Health Letter*, the original publication from Harvard Medical School; while I no longer play an active role in this office, I know the people who run it and can verify their excellence.)

In addition, I reluctantly recommend the internet as a good way to keep up with new health information. My recommendation is "reluctant" because I recognize the difficulty of finding reliable information—and I recognize that not all of you will have easy access to the internet. However, it is ultimately the most timely source of new information.

In addition to the Harvard site, there are many excellent web sites operated by major medical institutions. Two of the best are those of the Mayo Clinic and The Johns Hopkins Medical Center.

www.mayoclinic.com
www.hopkinsmedicine.org/

In addition, the following sites operated by the U.S. government can often be helpful:

The Centers for Disease Control and Prevention: **www.cdc.gov**
800-311-3435

The National Institutes of Health: **www.nih.gov**
301-396-4000

The Food and Drug Administration: **http://www.fda.gov**
888-INFO-FDA ((463-6332)

And, of course, I would encourage you to visit our own ABC News health site, which is updated daily:

www.abcnews.go.com/sections/living/

In addition to medical center and government web sites, there are many sites maintained by disease advocacy organizations. Here are a few examples of such sites:

Alcoholics Anonymous: **www.alcoholics-anonymous.org/**
U.S./Canada AA General Service Office 212-870-3400

Alzheimer's Association: **http://www.alz.org/**
800-272-3900

The Arthritis Foundation: **www.arthritis.org**
800-283-7800

The American Cancer Society: **www.cancer.org**

The American Heart Association: **www.americanheart.org**
800 AHA-USA-1 (242-8721)

The American Diabetes Association:
www.diabetes.org/
800-DIABETES (342-2383)

Index

A

B

D

O

P

T

U

V

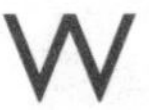

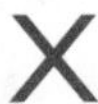

Z